Surgery During Natural Disasters, Combat, Terrorist Attacks, and Crisis Situations

COL Robert B. Lim

Editor

Surgery During Natural Disasters, Combat, Terrorist Attacks, and Crisis Situations

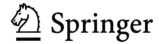 Springer

Editor
COL Robert B. Lim
Department of Surgery
Advanced Laparoscopy and Metabolic Surgery
Tripler Army Medical Center
Honolulu, HI, USA

ISBN 978-3-319-23717-6   ISBN 978-3-319-23718-3   (eBook)
DOI 10.1007/978-3-319-23718-3

Library of Congress Control Number: 2015956334

Springer Cham Heidelberg New York Dordrecht London

Printed on acid-free paper

Springer International Publishing AG Switzerland is part of Springer Science+Business Media (www.springer.com)

Foreword

Colonel Robert Lim's textbook of war and disaster surgery will serve as a guide for all surgeons who are called upon to operate effectively well beyond their current practice and training. A surgeon's professional skill, to be effective and up-to-date, is predicated upon a premise of lifelong learning. The surgeon's usual practice can be disrupted instantly by an accident or disaster, natural or man-made. This book will help all surgeons and physicians interested in war and disaster medicine become better informed about not only the nuances of care and the care continuum, but also reflect on the emotional, spiritual, and moral injuries which providers, physicians, nurses, corpsmen, and other first responders must endure and recognize in order to be resilient and effective. As witnesses and participants to disaster, we must also be able to continue our lives (personal and professional) in a meaningful way after the battle has ended.

This book is comprehensive in its scope of looking at battlefield injuries, resuscitation, and treatment, as well as expanding to cover other natural disasters such as the Haitian earthquake. It also emphasizes the need for preparation, training, rehearsal, and planning in order to have an effective response to these fast moving and deadly scenarios.

The newest information and best practices are given in this textbook. With the rapidity of information relay and technological inventions and innovations, this text serves as a comprehensive update on topics including blast injuries, airway management (awake tracheostomy), operating in austere environments, combat burn injuries, difficult triage decisions, and providing operative care under fire, as well as an interesting chapter on hostage rescue surgery. There are also thoughtful and compelling chapters on some past and recent mass casualty events including the Oklahoma City bombing and the most recent Boston Marathon bombing. Undergirding the entire text is the need for a systematic approach to disaster preparedness including training, preparation, and treatment through well-rehearsed scenarios and team training.

This textbook written by practicing surgeons who have firsthand experience in the topics they present is another important addition to the collection of battlefield and disaster surgery. From the Spanish Siege of Malaga where ambulances were introduced, to Ambroise Pare who introduced surgical dressings and ligatures, to Larrey who introduced the concepts of triage in war surgery, this textbook takes a twenty-first century look at the injuries, science, physiology, and technology all combined to help inform the trauma surgeon how best to care for those injured.

This book does not presume to be the definitive text on wartime and disaster care, but it serves as both an important and an impressive missive on the continuing need to improve and perfect our treatment of the trauma patient with the ever present ideal to preserve life and function and reverse the ravages that nature and man inflict upon humankind. We may never reach that "perfect care" ideal, but we must always strive to keep this as our guiding principle in the care of our brothers and sisters who have been harmed by our hand or nature's.

Adam M. Robinson Jr., MD, MBA, FACS, FASCRS, CPE

Preface

When I first thought about this book, I thought about all the great stories I had heard from my fellow surgeons in the military during their time on the battle-field. Though we were not always clinically busy in Iraq and Afghanistan, it seemed like everyone had a story to tell. Truthfully I would say that most surgeons have one or two experiences that stuck with them because of the amazing story that led to the surgery. Many civilian surgeons, for instance, provided care in events like the Oklahoma City bombing and the Asiatic Airline crash. The power from these stories did not always come from a rare, fantastic surgical case but rather the uniqueness of the injury or the personal story behind the reason for the surgery.

One of my surgical mentors from my fellowship in Minimally Invasive Surgery at Beth Israel Deaconess Medical Center in Boston, Massachusetts, is Dan Jones, MD. In April of 2013, he and I, from separate locations, were headed to Baltimore for a surgical conference. We were both scheduled to arrive on Monday April 2013, which was the day of the Boston Marathon bombing. Dr. Jones told me later that he was in Logan Airport, almost ready to board his plane, when he heard the news. He immediately called back to his hospital and asked if he needed to come back. Boston area hospitals had a good Massive Casualty (MASSCAL) plan, there were plenty of surgeons on hand, and he was told that he was not needed. He later confessed to me that it was a good thing he wasn't needed because he wasn't sure he would know what to do.

Now, Dan Jones is a brilliant man and a great surgeon, and I have no doubt that he would have performed admirably and would have known exactly what to do if thrust into that situation. But his admission got me to thinking. Is there a way to prepare medical providers for natural disasters, terrorist attacks, surgery in austere environments, or even combat itself? Now there are many programs designed to prepare for MASSCAL events and even for combat, but I think all who have been in these events would agree that, even with all of that training, there is still chaos during these events. Moreover that nothing truly prepares you emotionally or psychologically for what you might face or what decisions you may have to make.

The stories in the book cover the surgical aspects of several of the significant natural disasters, terrorist attacks, and battlefield experiences from the past 20 or so years. They also cover unique experiences like caring for hostage victims or providing care for highly wanted criminals. The personal side of the stories allows the readers to put themselves in the author's position. It is my hope that readers will have a better understanding of what to expect in these unusual events should they ever have to experience it themselves. Additionally I hope that these stories will allow readers to feel more comfortable when participating in these events.

Finally I would like to say that these stories are not just for physicians and other health care providers. In addition to being highly entertaining, they demonstrate the strength of the human spirit. When faced with unusual surgical emergencies, highly political cases, limited equipment, or the lack of a safe and intact surrounding infrastructure, these surgeons made difficult but correct decisions. Surgery is often thought of as an exact science but any physician knows there is a lot of art in medicine; and that a successful outcome sometimes requires innovative and progressive thinking. This book demonstrates this creative mind, which led to successful outcomes in some simply amazing cases. I hope you enjoy it.

Honolulu, HI, USA   COL Robert B. Lim

Author Biography

COL Robert B. Lim, M.D., is currently on Active Duty in the United States Army and he has been deployed five times to the combat zone. He was amongst the first surgeons to arrive in Baghdad during the initial invasion in Iraq. He has earned the Combat Medic Badge, the Combat Action Badge, and a Bronze Star.

Disclaimer
The views expressed in this work are those of the authors alone and do not represent the views of the Department of Defense or of the Department of the Army.

Contents

Contributors

Julie E. Adams, MD Department of Surgery, University of Vermont Medical Center, Burlington, VT, USA

Alec C. Beekley, MD Divisions of Trauma/Acute Care Surgery and Bariatric Surgery, Department of Surgery, Thomas Jefferson University Hospitals, Philadelphia, PA, USA

George E. Black IV, MD Department of Surgery, Madigan Army Medical Center, Fort Lewis, WA, USA

Susan M. Briggs, MD, MPH Department of Surgery, International Trauma and Disaster Institute, Massachusetts General Hospital, Boston, MA, USA

Sean M. Bryant, MD Emergency Medicine/Medical Toxicology, Cook County Hospital (Stroger), Chicago, IL, USA

Eileen M. Bulger, MD Department of Surgery, Harborview Medical Center, University of Washington, Seattle, WA, USA

Yong U. Choi, MD, FACS Department of Surgery, Dwight D. Eisenhower Army Medical Center, DDEAMC, General Surgery Clinic, Fort Gordon, GA, USA

Rochelle A. Dicker, MD Department of Surgery, UCSF at San Francisco General Hospital, San Francisco, CA, USA

Matthew J. Eckert, MD, FACS Department of Surgery, Madigan Army Medical Center, Tacoma, WA, USA

Trauma and Acute Care Surgery Service, Legacy Emanuel Medical Center, Portland, Oregon

Joseph M. Galante, MD Division of Trauma, Acute Care Surgery and Surgical Critical Care, Department of Surgery, Davis Medical Center, University of California, Sacramento, CA, USA

Jennifer M. Gurney, MD, FACS Department of Surgery, San Francisco General Hospital, San Francisco, CA, USA

LCDR Jami L. Hickey, MD, MC, USN Emergency Department, Naval Medical Center Portsmouth, Portsmouth, VA, USA

Seon Jones, MD, FACS Department of General Surgery, Naval Medical Center San Diego, San Diego, CA, USA

David R. King, MD, FACS Division of Trauma Emergency Surgery, and Surgical Critical Care, Department of Surgery, Harvard Medical School, Massachusetts General Hospital, Boston, MA, USA

Booker T. King, MD US Army Burn Center, San Antonio Military Medical Center, San Antonio, TX, USA

US Army Insititue of Surgical Research, Cibolo, TX, USA

M. Margaret Knudson, MD, FACS Professor of Surgery, Univeristy of California San Francisco, San Francisco General Hospital, San Francisco, CA, USA

COL Robert B. Lim, MD, FACS Department of Surgery, Advanced Laparoscopy and Metabolic Surgery, Tripler Army Medical Center, Honolulu, HI, USA

Henry Lin, MD General Surgery and Urology, Naval Hospital Camp LeJeune, Uniformed Services University of the Health Sciences, Camp LeJeune, NC, USA

Matthew J. Martin, MD Department of Surgery, Madigan Army Medical Center, Tacoma, WA, USA

Trauma and Acute Care Surgery Service, Legacy Emanuel Medical Center, Portland, Oregon

Tomaz Mesar, MD Division of Trauma, Emergency Surgery, and Surgical Critical Care, Department of Surgery, Harvard Medical School, Massachusetts General Hospital, Boston, MA, USA

John S. Oh, MD, FACS Department of Surgery, Walter Reed National Military Medical Center, Bethesda, MD, USA

Carlos J. Rodriguez, DO, MB Department of General Surgery, Walter Reed National Military Medical Center, Bethesda, MD, USA

Michael R. St. Jean, MD, FACS Eastern Maine Medical Center, Northeast Surgery of Maine, Bangor, ME, USA

Scott R. Steele, MD, FACS, FASCRS Department of Surgery, Division of Colorectal Surgery, University Hospitals Case Medical Center, Case Western Reserve University, OH, USA

David W. Tuggle, MD Department of Trauma, Dell Children's Medical Center of Central Texas, Austin, TX, USA

Gordon Wisbach, MD, FACS Department of General Surgery, Naval Medical Center San Diego, San Diego, CA, USA

Zaradhe M.S. Yach, BS, MS Mercy Medical Group, Roseville, CA, USA

Disaster Medicine: Lessons Learned from the Crash of Asiana Airlines Flight 214

M. Margaret Knudson

On July 6, 2013, Flight OZ214 took off from Incheon International Airport in South Korea carrying 291 passengers and 16 crewmembers bound for San Francisco International Airport (SFO). The majority of the passengers were from China, including 70 students and teachers traveling to the USA for a summer camp in Southern California. The flight was cleared for a visual approach to runway 28 L at SFO. At 11:28 A.M., *the plane crashed short of the runway, with the landing gear and the tail striking the seawall that projects into the San Francisco Bay*. Both engines and the tail section separated from the aircraft. The remainder of the fuselage and wings rotated counterclockwise approximately 330° finally coming to rest 2400 ft from the initial point of impact on the seawall. It was later determined that the plane was flying too low and too slow on its approach. The cause of the crash was recently attributed to pilot error by the National Traffic Safety Board [1]. Shortly after impact, a ruptured oil tank above the right engine began to leak and the hot engine ignited (Fig. 1.1). Two evacuation slides were deployed on the left side of the airliner allowing many passengers to walk away on their own. On the right side, evacuation slides deployed inside the airplane, pinning some flight attendants in their seats. Three of the four flight attendants seated at the rear were ejected from the aircraft in their seats; remarkably all three survived. The majority of injuries occurred to the passengers in the rear of the plane as seats collapsed on them and many had to be physically cut out of their seatbelts. Two Chinese students traveling to the summer camp who were ejected died on the runway. Sadly, one was killed by an emergency vehicle that ran over her in the ensuing aftermath. Despite the potential for chaos, however, the emergency crews from both the airport and from several surrounding communities responded promptly and conducted a remarkably efficient triage operation, assuring that the most critical were identified quickly and immediately transported to the most appropriate treatment facilities [2]. In all, 181 patients were injured, 12 critically. Nine different hospitals received patients, with ten in critical condition being transported immediately to San Francisco General Hospital and Trauma Center. Stanford University Medical Center received the other two critical patients. The crash of Asiana Flight 214 was the first commercial airline crash to result in fatalities in over 4.5 years in the USA.

M.M. Knudson, M.D., F.A.C.S. (✉)
Professor of Surgery, Univeristy of California
San Francisco, San Francisco General Hospital, 1001
Potrero Avenue, San Francisco,
CA 94110, USA
e-mail: pknudson@sfghsurg.ucsf.edu

© Springer International Publishing Switzerland 2016
C.R.B. Lim (ed.), *Surgery During Natural Disasters, Combat,
Terrorist Attacks, and Crisis Situations*, DOI 10.1007/978-3-319-23718-3_1

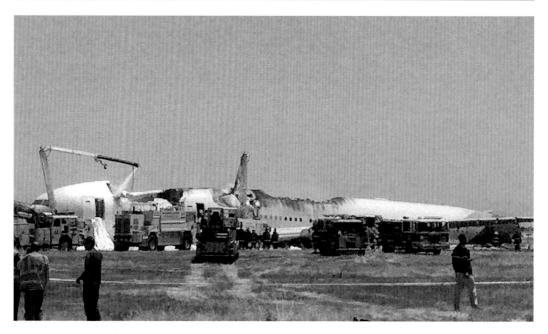

Fig. 1.1 The plane shortly after the crash

1.1 San Francisco General Hospital and Trauma Center

San Francisco General Hospital and Trauma Center (SFGH) is the only major trauma center for the City and County of San Francisco and also serves half of the population of the adjoining county to the south (San Mateo County). It is also the closest trauma center to SFO just 11 miles away. The hospital has a long history of responding to crises, including resistant tuberculosis, the AIDS epidemic, and the violent crimes associated with the 1960s drug culture in San Francisco [3]. It also has an illustrious history of pioneering trauma care, and was one of the first hospitals in the nation to have a dedicated trauma surgical team. However, the challenges presented by this international disaster were unprecedented.

Communication is always challenging in the initial phase of disaster response and this occurrence was no exception. We were first told that a small cargo plane with few victims had crashed; however it soon became clear that this was a much larger event. Our hospital Incident Command Center was quickly activated, including the four core functions of planning, operations, logistics, and finance, allowing our facility to organize the response to the disaster in an orderly fashion [4]. Even while the Command Center was being organized however, the first six critical patients arrived simultaneously. Each member of the in-house trauma team was assigned to evaluate one patient, with the trauma surgery attending performing triage until the formally assigned triage officer (an emergency room physician) took over that role. This allowed the trauma team to concentrate on the three patients who required immediate operative therapy.

The response from outside the hospital was immediate. Staff responded promptly when they heard about the crash on the radio and TV, or via social media. As has been noted by others, social media has an increasingly recognized important role in disaster response [5, 6]. Residents, fellows, attending physicians from all disciplines, and members of the hospital administration responded in person and conducted their duties. Beds were cleared in the emergency department and ICU, and some non-acute patients were sent to awaiting rehabilitation centers. The pediatric clinic was used as a staging center for the involved children.

Five attending anesthesiologists expanded operating room capacity and four attending radiologists gathered to speed up diagnostic imaging. Additional responders including nurses, social workers, interpreters, environmental service personnel and kitchen staff. In all, during the first few hours after the crash, 67 patients were evaluated at SFGH, with 36 admitted to the hospital.

1.2 Nature of the Injuries

According to the National Traffic Safety Board, just over 400 transportation-related deaths each year in the USA can be attributed to general aviation accidents [1]. Each month, there are approximately 90 aircraft crashes in the USA, with a mortality rate of 20 %. The great majority of these crashes involve small private airplanes. In contrast, few physicians have had experience caring for victims of major commercial airline disasters.

Data on injuries sustained by survivors of airline crashes is almost nonexistent. Baker and others searched the Nationwide Inpatient Sample for aviation-related injuries and found that 27 % had lower extremity fractures, 11 % head injuries, and only 9 % had an internal injury [7]. This data is somewhat misleading however, as 1/3 of these injuries occurred in parachutists. The in-house mortality in that report was 2 %. In contrast, in a review of recent UK and Netherlands crash data, head injuries and spine fractures were common, with in-hospital mortality rates between 7 and 34 % [8]. Johnson and others reviewed injuries sustained by aircraft accident survivors admitted to their burn unit and reported that almost 40 % had fractures, and 8 % sustained TBI (Traumatic Brain Injury), but less than 1 % had internal injuries [9]. Table 1.1 summarizes the types of injuries that we treated after the crash. As can be seen, sternal fractures and spine injuries were found in many patients. The relatively rare spine fracture that occurs with violent forward flexion over a fixed point (termed a Chance fracture) and that is associated with internal organ injuries was seen in some of our patients (Fig. 1.2). Damage control surgery, usually reserved for patients who

Table 1.1 Summary of patient data

Hospital service	Number of patients
Initially evaluated	67
Admitted to the hospital	36
Required ICU admission	6
Required ventilatory support	4
Operations performed within 48 h	10
Injuries/body region[a]:	
Head	6
Spine	13
Chest (chest well, sternum, lung)	8
Abdominal	2
Extremity fractures	7
Burn wounds	4
In-hospital deaths	1

[a]Note: Many patients sustained injuries to more than one body region

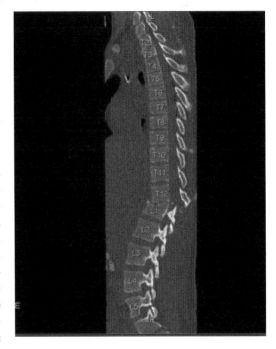

Fig. 1.2 Spine films demonstrating a Chance fracture from one of the patients

have physiologic derangements making definitive surgery unsafe, is performed for a different reason during a disaster; that is, the least amount is done during the first surgery in order to move the surgical team on to the next patient.

During the 48 h after the crash, our surgical teams utilized 100 units of packed blood cells, even with judicious use of blood and blood products guided by point-of-care viscioelastrography. The need for coordinating, compiling and constantly updating patient data and the importance of the tertiary survey for potentially delayed diagnosis of injuries during a disaster such as this cannot be overemphasized. Although none of our patients sustained burns induced by the fire, some had severe "road burns" that were deep second and third degree and required excision and grafting over the ensuing weeks. The ICU care in these patients was particularly challenging, with many developing complications that required repeated abdominal procedures, care of intestinal fistulas, hemodialysis, advanced rescue techniques for respiratory failure including prone positioning, and treatment of sepsis. Only one patient who reached the hospital died, primarily from CNS injury. Prolonged hospitalization was necessary for others, with the last patient leaving the hospital after more than 30 operations and 4 months of hospitalization.

1.3 Other Unique Challenges

1.3.1 Toxicology

In some patients we observed a strange metabolic/physiologic pattern consisting of extremely low ionized serum calcium levels, cardiac arrhythmias, acidosis out of proportion to the trauma wounds incurred, and hypotension. A nearly continuous infusion of calcium was required to rescue these patients. We eventually postulated (but never proved) that given the numerous hazardous materials found at the crash scene (smoke, jet fuel, fire retardant) a toxic exposure might have occurred, especially in the patients with open wounds. There is a huge body of literature on aviation combustion toxicology which is beyond the scope of this review [10]. However, the pattern we observed has also been reported from exposure to hydrogen fluoride in fire suppression systems in military vehicles [11]. In the future, decontamination of exposed skin and early treatment with nebulized calcium should be considered for victims of similar crashes.

1.3.2 International Considerations

There were initial concerns regarding the potential that this was a terrorist attack (that fortunately were later proven to be unfounded) which required increased security presence at the hospital. The manifest from the plane could not be shared with the hospitals (only the Red Cross has access to this list), so many patients who departed the plane without belongings were initially unidentified. Parents and their children were sent to different hospitals depending upon the severity of their injuries and many children were traveling alone. While we waited for families to arrive from South Korea and China, some patients remained unidentified for days. Because so few spoke English, the demand on Korean and Chinese interpreters was heavy. Obviously, none of our patients had cleared customs, so Homeland Security and Customs Agents set up stations in our hospital cafeteria. The cultural differences surfaced with the need to release information to the media (see below) which, while within HIPAA guidelines, sometimes fell outside of the cultural norms for these Asian families.

1.3.3 Media

The media play an important role in any disaster; this is how the rest of the world finds out what has happened. Thus, it is important to acknowledge that role and use it to full advantage. Through our director of media relations, we established several rules of engagement. First, we provided hourly briefings and updates using a website combined with regularly scheduled press conferences. We insisted that each member of the media was given the same message fairly and without prejudice. All of our patients and their families declined interviews with the media so we protected them from unwanted advances by reporters. It is important to identify physician speakers to provide credible medical information but these conferences should be carefully scripted for accuracy and patient protection. As mentioned earlier, social media can be incredibly helpful during a disaster especially if the source is the treating facility [5, 6, 12].

1.3.4 Psychological Support

The aftermath of this disaster impacted our trauma center for months. During the acute event, the rush of adrenaline keeps the teams motivated but eventually physical and emotional fatigue sets in and the horrors associated with this tragedy, including lives lost and others permanently altered, set in. Additionally, the month of July marks the beginning of surgical residency and many of those who worked with us were just a few days out from completion of medical school. Several decompression sessions open to all hospital staff and employees were provided by mental health specialists and spiritual advisers throughout the ensuing months. Also important is taking the time to praise all that went well and to identify areas for improvement for when the next disaster strikes.

1.4 The Way Forward

Fort Hood, Aurora, Sandy Hook, the Boston Marathon, Asiana Flight 214: All of these recent disasters required a different response but also share a common theme: the need to be prepared. Each of these mass casualty events resulted in *physical* injuries, despite the public's broader concerns about the potential for chemical or nuclear attacks. Formal training in disaster medicine should be required of every licensed physician [13]. For surgeons, the American College of Surgeons Committee on Trauma's Disaster Management Course (www.facs.org/trauma/disaster/dmep_course.html) is an excellent starting point. Publications such as these of the lessons learned after mass casualty events need to be widely disseminated [14, 15]. Importantly, the advances made by our military colleagues over the past 10 years of war in response to multiple casualty incidents and their developments in combat casualty care need to be incorporated into the civilian medical disaster arena. Military-civilian collaboration in the response to the earthquake in Haiti has previously been highlighted in the New England Journal of Medicine *Journal* [16]. More dramatic, however, was the rapid transfer of hemorrhage control techniques from the battlefields of Iraq and Afghanistan to the streets of Boston, clearly salvaging patients who might otherwise have been lost [17]. Propper, Rasmussen, and others recently summarized the surgical response to multiple casualty incidents following explosive events in a US Military Combat Hospital in Iraq [18]. Of the 50 patients contained in that report 75 operations were required (average 3.8 procedures per casualty), 25 (50 %) required mechanical ventilation, and a total of 74 units of blood were transfused in the first 72-h period. These data, along with the numbers we present in Table 1.1, provide receiving centers with at least some reasonable numbers of what to expect in mass casualty events of similar magnitude. Continuing to translate the lessons from modern wartime trauma care, which has resulted in the lowest case fatality rate ever recorded, will undoubtedly save many civilian lives and preserve the knowledge gained from the sacrifices of a generation of military service personnel [19, 20].

Editor's note: Dr. Knudson continues to practice Trauma Surgery in the San Francisco area. She was tasked to lead the collaboration between the American College of Surgeons and the Department of Health Affairs to combine the experiences of military surgeons and those of civilian surgeons in an effort to improve surgical care in trauma and in disaster situations like the one described here.

References

1. http://www.ntsb.gov/aviation. Accessed 24 Jun 2014.
2. Lerner EB, Schwartz RB, Coule PL, et al. Mass casualty triage: an evaluation of the data and development of a proposed national guideline. Disaster Med Public Health Prep. 2008;2 Suppl 1:S25–34.
3. Schecter W, Lim R, Sheldon G, et al. The history of the surgical service at San Francisco General Hospital. Wilmington, NC: Broadfoot; 2008.
4. Frykberg E, Weireter L, Flint L. 10 Questions and answers about disasters and disaster response. Bull Am Coll Surg. 2010;95:6–13.
5. Huang CM, Chan E, Hyder AA. Web 2.0 and internet social networking: a new tool for disaster management? –lessons from Taiwan. BMC Med Inform Decis Mak. 2010;10:57.
6. Merchant RM, Elmer S, Lurie N. Integrating social media into emergency-preparedness efforts. N Engl J Med. 2011;365:289–91.

7. Baker SP, Brady JE, Shanahan DF, Li G. Aviation-related injury morbidity and mortality: data from U.S. Health Information Systems. Aviat Space Environ Med. 2009;80:1001–5.

8. Postma ILE, Winkelhagen J, Bijisma TS, et al. Injury. 2012;43:2012–7.

9. Johnson M, Kerr L, Harris M et al. Mortality associated with injuries sustained by aircraft accident burn survivors. Internet J Rescue Disaster Med. 2008;8(2). http://ispub.com/IJRDM/8/2/11492.

10. Chaturvedi AK. Aviation combustion toxicology: an overview. J Analyt Toxicol. 2010;14:1–16.

11. Zierold D, Chauviere M. Hydrogen fluoride inhalation injury because of a fire suppression system. Mil Med. 2012;177:108–12.

12. Gribble KD. Media messages and the needs of infants and young children after Cyclone Nargis and the WenChuan Earthquake. Disasters. 2013;37:80–100.

13. Merchant RM, Leigh JE, Lurie N. Health care volunteers and disaster response-first, be prepared. N Engl J Med. 2010;362:872–3.

14. Wild J, Maher J, Frazee RC, et al. The Fort Hood Massacre: lessons learned from a high profile mass casualty. J Trauma Acute Care Surg. 2012;72:1709–13.

15. Jacobs LM, Wde D, McSwain NE, et al. Hartford consensus: a call to action for THREAT, a medical disaster preparedness concept. J Am Chem Soc. 2014;218:467–78.

16. Auerbach PS, Norris RL, Menon AS, et al. Civil-military collaboration in the initial medical response to the earthquake in Haiti. NEJM. 2010;363:e32.

17. Schneidman D. Surgeons put planning, preparation, past experience to work in efforts to save Boston marathon bombing victims. Bull Am Coll Surg. 2013;98:9–17.

18. Propper BW, Rasmussen TE, Davidson SB, et al. Surgical response to multiple casualty incidents following single explosive events. Ann Surg. 2009;250:311–5.

19. Elster EA, Butler FK, Rasmussen T. Implications of combat casualty care for mass casualty events. JAMA. 2013;310:475–6.

20. Rasmussen TD, Gross KR, Baer DG. Where do we go from here? J Trauma Acute Care Surg. 2013;S:S105–6.

Disaster Preparedness and Response

2

Susan M. Briggs

2.1 Introduction

No one can predict the time, location, or complexity of the next disaster. The management of the medical and public health effects of contemporary disasters, whether natural or man-made, is one of the most significant challenges facing surgeons today. Disaster medical care, including surgery, is NOT the same as conventional medical care. Disaster medical care requires a fundamental change ("crisis management care") in the care of disaster victims in order to achieve the objective of providing the "greatest good for the greatest number of victims" [1, 2]. Demand for resources always exceeds the supply of resources in a Mass Casualty Incident (MCI) (see Fig. 2.1).

The demands of surgical disaster care have changed over the past decade, in the scope of care, the spectrum of threats, and the field of operations. Increasingly, surgeons are being asked to respond to complex disasters, the spectrum of threats ranging from natural disasters to man-made disasters such as terrorism [2, 3].

S.M. Briggs, M.D., M.P.H. (✉)
Department of Surgery, International Trauma and Disaster Institute, Massachusetts General Hospital, 8 Hawthorne Place, Suite 114, Boston, MA 02114, USA
e-mail: briggs.susan@mgh.harvard.edu

Disasters involving weapons of mass destruction (WMD) are a significant challenge for all disaster responders. Many of today's disasters occur or result in "austere" environments. Access, transport, resources, or other aspects of the physical, social, economic, and political environments may impose severe constraints on the adequacy of immediate care to the population in need (see Fig. 2.2).

Most surgeons will not be involved in a MCI during their career; but in reality, MCIs can happen anywhere. The Boston Marathon bombing and the Oklahoma City bombing showed that big cities are susceptible to these events. Multi-casualty events, such as auto accidents with multiple casualties, can overwhelm smaller communities in a similar manner, especially if transportation of these critically injured patients to trauma centers is delayed or impossible due to weather. The concepts discussed in this chapter highlight the principles healthcare providers should follow in MCI events.

2.2 Epidemiology of Disasters

Natural disasters may be classified as sudden-impact (acute) disasters or chronic-onset (slow) disasters. Sudden-impact natural disasters generally cause significant mortality and morbidity immediately as a direct result of the primary event (e.g., traumatic injuries, crush

© Springer International Publishing Switzerland 2016
C.R.B. Lim (ed.), *Surgery During Natural Disasters, Combat, Terrorist Attacks, and Crisis Situations*, DOI 10.1007/978-3-319-23718-3_2

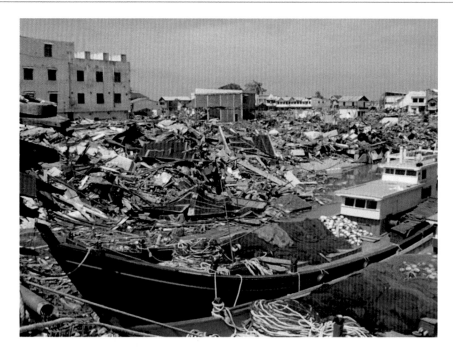

Fig. 2.1 Banda Aceh tsunami

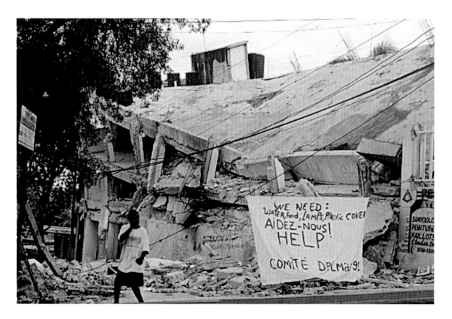

Fig. 2.2 Haiti earthquake (2010)

injuries, drowning). Chronic-onset disasters cause mortality and morbidity through prolonged secondary effects (e.g., infectious disease outbreaks, dehydration, and malnutrition) [4].

Sudden-impact disasters include:

- Earthquakes.
- Tsunamis.
- Tornados.

- Floods.
- Tropical cyclones, hurricanes, or typhoons.
- Volcanic eruptions.
- Landslides and avalanches.
- Wildfires.

Chronic-onset disasters include:
- Famine.
- Drought.
- Pest infestation.
- Deforestation.

Man-made disasters may be unintentional or intentional (terrorism) and range from technological disasters to MCI involving WMD (radioactive, biological, and chemical agents). Disasters involving WMD, whether accidental or man-made, are a significant challenge for medical providers for several reasons [1, 2].

- WMD have the potential to produce casualties in numbers large enough to overwhelm healthcare systems, including surgical capacities.
- WMD may produce large numbers of "expectant" victims. This denotes a category of disaster victims not expected to survive due to severity of injuries or underlying diseases and/or limited resources. This term was first used in conjunction with chemical warfare.
- WMD may produce a "contaminated" environment. Surgeons must be able to perform triage, initial stabilization, and possible definitive surgical care outside traditional healthcare facilities.
- WMD produce significant numbers of "psychogenic" casualties, greatly complicating rescue and triage efforts. Terrorists do not have to kill people to achieve their goals.

Creating a climate of fear and panic to overwhelm the medical infrastructure achieves their goals. During the Sarin attack in Tokyo (1995), 5000 casualties were referred to local hospitals. Fewer than 1000 individuals were suffering from the effects of the gas. The remainder of the individuals were experiencing psychological symptoms.

The spectrum of agents used by terrorists is limitless and includes conventional weapons, explosives, and biological, chemical, and radioactive agents. Over 70 % of terrorist attacks involve the use of explosive weapons and are a significant challenge for surgeons due to the complexity of injuries (primary, secondary, tertiary, and quaternary blast injuries) (see Fig. 2.3). Responders must also be aware of the potential for secondary strikes directed at harming emergency response personnel.

2.3 Principles of Disaster Response

2.3.1 Principle #1

Surgeons cannot utilize traditional command structures when participating in disaster response. The Incident Command System (ICS) is a modular/adaptable system for all incidents and facilities, including hospitals, and is the accepted standard for all disaster response. Functional requirements, not titles, determine the ICS hierarchy. The organizational structure of the ICS is built around five major management activities (Incident Command, Operations, Planning, Logistics, and Finance/Administration). Operations directs all disaster medical personnel.

The structure of the ICS is the same regardless of the nature of the disaster. The difference is in the particular expertise of key personnel. Surgeons, often used to working independently, must adhere to the structure of an ICS in order to integrate successfully into the disaster response team and avoid many negative consequences including:

- Death of medical personnel due to lack of safety and training.
- Lack of adequate medical supplies to provide care.
- Staff working beyond their training or certification.

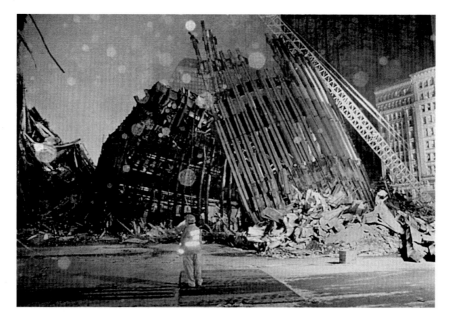

Fig. 2.3 Terrorist attack, World Trade Center, New York (2001)

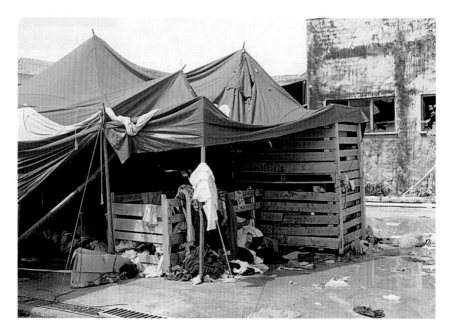

Fig. 2.4 Temporary shelter, Turkey earthquake (1999)

2.3.2 Principle #2

Similar to the ABCs of trauma care, disaster response includes basic concerns that are similar in all disasters [1, 2]. The ABCs of disaster care include the following:

2.3.3 Public Health Concerns (See Fig. 2.4)

- Water.
- Food.
- Shelter.

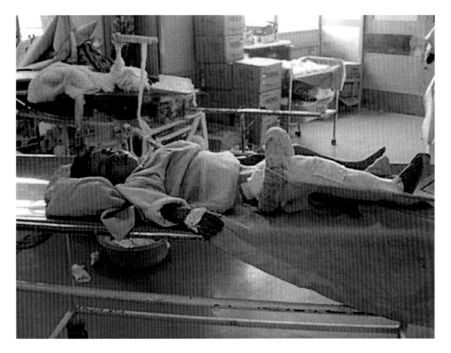

Fig. 2.5   Pakistan earthquake (2005)

- Sanitation.
- Security/safety.
- Transportation.
- Communication.
- Endemic/epidemic diseases.

2.3.4   Medical Concerns (See Fig. 2.5)

- Search and rescue.
- Triage.
- Definitive care.
- Evacuation.

The difference in disasters is the degree to which certain capacities are needed in a specific disaster and the amount of outside assistance (regional, national, and international) required to meet disaster needs. Rapid assessment by experienced personnel will determine which surgical assets are needed in the acute phase of the disaster to augment local capacity. Surgeons are uniquely qualified to participate in all four aspects of disaster medical response given their expertise in triage, emergency surgery, care of critical patients, and rapid decision making.

2.3.5   Principle #3

Effective "surge capacity" is not based on well-intentioned and readily available volunteers. Surgeons must understand the basic principles of disaster response (ICS, disaster triage, gross decontamination) to be effective members of the disaster team. Surgeons must be willing to care for non-disaster-related diseases/emergencies as well as disaster-related injuries. Pre-disaster training is an essential part of disaster preparedness.

2.3.6   Principle #4

Disaster surgical care requires a fundamental change in the approach to the care of victims. The objective of disaster care is the "greatest good for the greatest number of victims." This is in contrast to the objective of conventional care which is the "greatest good for the individual patient." It is important to apply the principles of crisis management care to all phases of disaster management:

Phase 1: Preparedness; planning/training.
Phase 2: Mitigation; hazard vulnerability.
Phase 3: Response; emergency phase.
Phase 4: Recovery; restoration.

2.4 Role of Surgeons in Disaster Response

2.4.1 Search and Rescue

The local population near any disaster site is the immediate search and rescue asset, but the technical equipment and expertise to facilitate extrication of victims trapped in the rubble are usually lacking. Many countries have developed specialized search and rescue teams, and surgeons are frequently part of these teams. Search and rescue teams respond to a broad range of disasters, including earthquakes, mine collapses, bomb-

ings, and hurricanes and are involved both in the extrication and initial stabilization of victims, including field amputations and fasciotomy as necessary (see Fig. 2.6) [1, 5]. Search and rescue teams are generally composed of specialists in the following areas:

- Acute care specialties (surgery, emergency medicine, anesthesia).
- Technical search.
- Hazardous materials.
- Communications and logistics.
- Trained canines and their handlers.

2.4.2 Disaster Triage

Triage is the process of prioritizing casualties according to the level of care they require. It is the most important, and psychologically most difficult, mission of disaster medical response, both in the pre-hospital and hospital phases of the disaster. Disaster triage requires a fundamental change in the approach to the surgical care of patients. The objective of conventional civilian triage is to do the greatest good for the individual

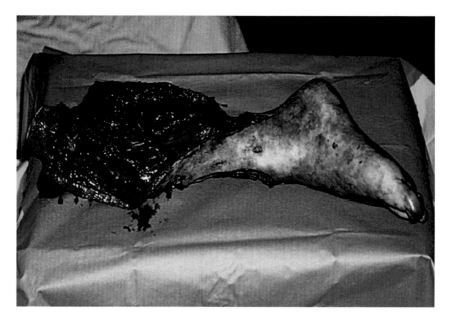

Fig. 2.6 Field amputation

patient. Severity of injury/disease is the major determinant for medical care. The objective of disaster triage is to do the greatest good for the greatest number of patients. The determinants of triage in disasters are, however, based on three parameters:

- Severity of injury.
- Likelihood of survival.
- Available resources (logistics, personnel, evacuation assets).

The major objective and challenge of triage is to rapidly identify the small minority of critically injured patients who require urgent life-saving interventions, including operative interventions, from the larger majority of non-critical casualties that characterize most disasters. In a mass casualty event, the critical surgical patients with the greatest chance of survival with the least expenditure of time and resources are prioritized to be treated first.

Triage is a dynamic decision-making process of matching victims' needs with available resources. Many MCI will have multiple different levels of triage as patients move from the disaster scene to definitive medical care. Disaster medical triage maybe conducted at three different levels depending on the level of casualties (injuries) to capabilities (resources).

Field Triage

Field triage, often the initial triage system utilized at the disaster scene or casualty collection centers, is the rapid categorization of victims potentially needing immediate medical care "where they are laying" or at triage sites. Victims are designated as "acute" or "non-acute." Simplified color coding may be used. Once the victims are transported to casualty collection centers (fixed or mobile medical facilities), medical triage according to severity of injury may be performed (see Fig. 2.7).

Medical Triage

Medical triage is the rapid categorization of victims, at a casualty collection site or fixed or mobile medical facilities, by the most experienced

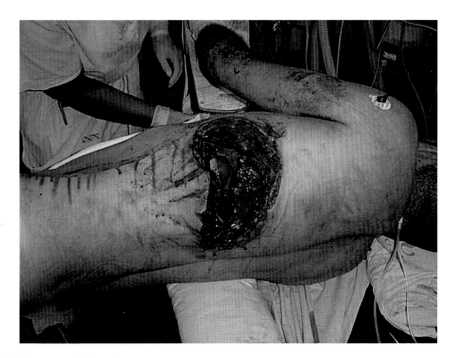

Fig. 2.7 Red category of triage (urgent)

Fig. 2.8 Medical triage categories

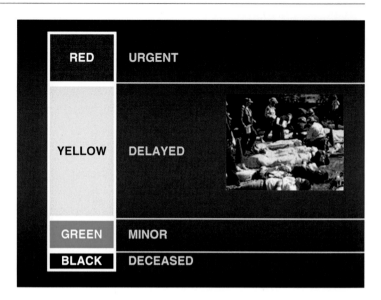

medical personnel available to identify the level of medical care needed based on severity of injury. Triage personnel must have knowledge of the medical consequences of various injuries (e.g., burn, blast, or crush injuries or exposure to chemical, biological, or radioactive agents). Color coding may be used (see Fig. 2.8):

Evacuation Triage

Evacuation triage assigns priorities to disaster victims for transfer to definitive care facilities. Burns, crush injuries, and pediatric trauma are among key priorities for early transfer due to the complexity of injuries and frequent need for multidisciplinary surgical teams.

2.4.3   Definitive Care

Definitive surgical care refers to care that will improve, rather than simply stabilize, a casualty's condition. Both small- and large-scale disasters may require the mobilization of disaster surgical teams to participate in the field medical response or supplement surgical capacities at facilities in the disaster region. Alternatively, the evacuation of disaster victims to regional surgi-

cal facilities outside the disaster region may be required to provide definitive care (fixed or mobile facilities). The care that surgeons deliver in mass casualty incidents is significantly more austere than the care medical providers deliver on a day-to-day basis.

In mass casualty incidents, it is usually possible only to deliver "minimally acceptable care" in the initial phases of the disaster due to the large number of casualties in contrast to the "maximally acceptable care" that is delivered in non-disaster situations [5, 6].

2.5   Disaster Management Teams

Current disaster preparedness and response emphasizes the need for an all-hazards approach. The need for multidisciplinary, mobile surgical teams that can provide a graded, flexible response to the need for definitive care is the key to an effective disaster response, especially if hospitals are destroyed or contaminated. Clinical competencies, not titles, determine the roles of surgical providers in disaster response. Disaster management teams are designed and trained to provide specific "functional" areas of disaster

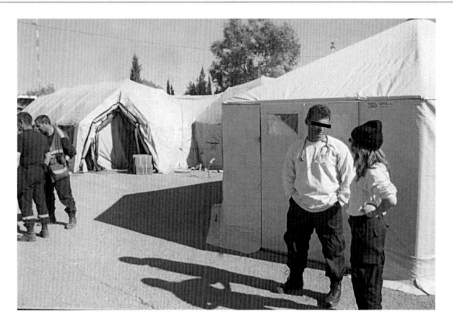

Fig. 2.9   US Field Hospital, Bam Iran earthquake (2004)

care such as critical care, pediatrics, obstetrics, and acute and trauma surgery, especially when the casualty load is unknown. The complexity of today's disasters demands civilian and military partnerships as key to effective disaster response [3, 6, 7].

2.6   Mobile Medical Facilities

Deployable, rapid-assembly medical facilities with the capacity for initial stabilization, operative interventions, and critical care are frequently used by both civilian and military medical teams and significantly increase the flexibility of disaster response (see Fig. 2.9). In recent disasters such as the Indonesian tsunami and the Haiti earthquake, hospital ships have proven valuable definitive care assets [8–10]. Sterilization of surgical instruments is a significant problem in mobile field hospitals. An accepted method of sterilizing instruments in austere environments is the use of Glutaraldehyde Solution 2 %, a method utilized by many civilian and military field hospitals when conventional sterilization is not possible due to limited water and/or electricity (see Fig. 2.10).

2.7   Damage Control Surgery

Damage control surgery is frequently employed in disaster settings and is an important component of crisis management care. In many disasters, local hospitals are destroyed, transportation to outside medical facilities may not be immediately feasible, or the environment may be contaminated. Damage control surgery limits surgical interventions to control of hemorrhage and contamination. This provides the opportunity to stabilize patients hemodynamically and correct hypothermia, acidosis, and coagulopathy. Surgical patients can then undergo definitive repair of injuries at a later date. Damage control surgery was initially developed for abdominal trauma with uncontrolled hemorrhage, but has expanded to most other surgical specialties, such as orthopedic and vascular surgery (see Fig. 2.11).

Spinal and regional anesthesia as well as conscious sedation for minor procedures and debridements are important adjuvants to surgical therapy. Intraosseous infusion is used frequently in field hospitals in the initial resuscitation of surgical patients.

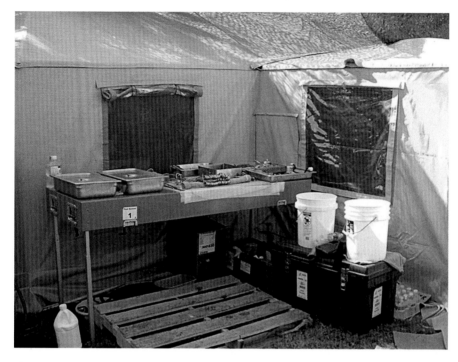

Fig. 2.10 Sterilization area, Haiti earthquake (2010)

Fig. 2.11 Damage control surgery, Haiti earthquake (2010)

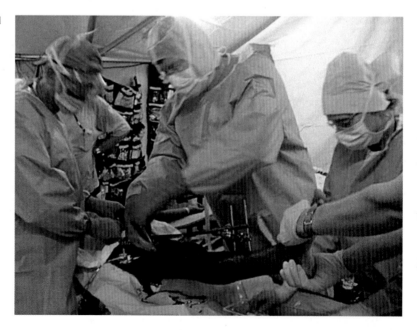

2.8 Disaster Drills

Disaster preparedness must include practical drills to ascertain the true magnitude of system problems, not just tabletop exercises. Mass-casualty drills must include three phases:

- Preparation phase.
- Exercise management phase.
- Patient treatment phase.

The preparation phase must include clear definition of functional areas of responsibility that can be evaluated objectively, not subjectively, during the disaster drill. The exercise management phase includes objective evaluation of all key functional roles in the ICS. The patient treatment phase includes objective evaluation of well-defined functional capacities such as:

- Triage.
- Initial resuscitation.
- Definitive care.
- Evacuation.
- Care of dead victims.

2.9 Summary

The goal of disaster medical response is to reduce the critical mortality associated with a disaster. Critical mortality rate is defined as the percentage of critically injured survivors who subsequently die. Numerous factors influence the critical mortality rate, including [7, 8, 11–13]:

- Triage accuracy, particularly the incidence of over-triage of victims.
- Rapid movement of patients to definitive care.
- Implementation of damage control procedures.
- Coordinated regional disaster preparedness.

Those who volunteer to help in these disaster responses should utilize these guidelines to help coordinate care and maximally utilize their personnel and resources. While most surgeons in their careers will not have to the opportunity to participate in these events, they may experience an MCI for their hospitals' level of care. Again the principles here should be employed to help providers and surgeons direct their efforts to caring for the most patients that their resources can support.

Editor's note: Dr. Briggs has been deployed to six other natural disasters around the world aside from Haiti to include Armenia, China, El Salvador, Iran, Russia, and the Virgin Islands. In the USA, she led surgical teams during Hurricanes Andrew and Katrina and during the terrorist attacks of 9/11 in New York and marathon bombing in Boston. Dr. Briggs also spent 6 years in the US Army Reserves and was deployed as a surgeon in Desert Storm I.

References

1. Briggs SM. Advanced disaster medical response manual for providers. 2nd ed. Woodbury, CT: Cine-Med; 2014.
2. Born CT, Cullison TR, Dean JA, et al. Partnered disaster preparedness: Lessons learned from international events. J Am Acad Orthop Surg. 2011;19 Suppl 1:S44–48.
3. Briggs SM. Role of civilian surgical teams in response to international disasters. Bull Am Coll Surg. 2010;95(1):14–7.
4. Briggs SM. Natural disasters: an overview. In: Partridge RA, editor. Oxford handbook of disaster medicine. New York, NY: Oxford University Press; 2012.
5. Raines A, Lees J, et al. Field amputation: response planning and legal considerations inspired by three separate amputations. Am J Disaster Med. 2014;9(1):53–7.
6. Briggs SM, Guy Lin. Disasters. In: John Meara et al. (eds), Textbook of global surgery. CRP Press, 2014; 443–453.
7. Lin G, Lavon H, Gelfond R, et al. Hard times call for creative solutions: medical Improvisations at the Israel Defense Forces Field Hospital in Haiti. Am J Disaster Med. 2010;5(3):188–92.
8. Ahmed H, Ahmed M, et al. Syrian revolution: a field hospital under attack. Am J Disaster Med. 2013;8(4): 259–65.
9. Kearns R, Skarote MB, Peterson J, et al. Deployable, portable and temporary hospitals; one state's experiences through the years. Am J Disaster Med. 2014;9(3):195–207.
10. Sechriest VF, Wing V, et al. Healthcare delivery aboard US Navy hospital ships following earthquake disasters: implications for future disaster relief missions. Am J Disaster Med. 2012;7(4):281–94.

11. Weiner DL, Manzi SF, Briggs SM, Fleisher GR. Response to challenges and lessons learned from hurricanes Katrina and Rita: a national perspective. Pediatrics. 2011;128:S31.

12. Bartal C, Zeller L, Miskin I, et al. Crush syndrome: saving more lives in disasters, lessons learned from the early-response phase in Haiti. Arch Intern Med. 2011;171(7):694–6.

13. Latifi R, Tiley E. Telemedicine for disaster management: can it transform chaos into an organized, structure care from the distance. Am J Disaster Med. 2014;9(1):25–37.

Trauma Surgery in an Austere Environment: Trauma and Emergency Surgery in Unusual Situations

3

Seon Jones and Gordon Wisbach

3.1 Introduction

Using the rich history and vast experiences that led to the establishment of a mature trauma surgical facility during Operation Enduring Freedom (2012–2014), we hope to provide ideas from experiences in deployed settings that may work well for the prospective trauma teams in similar situations. Trauma care can involve numerous fields of expertise including trauma system development, primary injury prevention programs, trauma epidemiology, prehospital care, trauma resuscitation, trauma operative management, trauma critical care, and rehabilitation. In-depth discussions of these subjects are beyond the scope of this chapter. We will focus only on the topic of trauma and acute care surgery at forward-deployed casualty-receiving facilities with surgical capabilities (Fig. 3.1). This chapter should serve as a conceptual tool kit to organize a trauma and surgical treatment facility that includes pre-planning, preparation, supplies and equipment, personnel, team organization, team training, and effective turnovers to replacement teams. The intent of the following material is to offer an advanced starting point with emphasis on the process not the end product of a trauma/acute care surgery (ACS) facility in unusual circumstances that are variable and evolving. The material is a synthesis of our experiences and lessons learned at a combat receiving hospital that had more surgical capability than the local host nation medical centers. The terminology used for this type of hospital varies depending on the military service branch involved and can include Level II, Role II, Role IIe, or Forward Resuscitative Surgical System [4]. The interested reader is encouraged to review how these mobile hospitals have evolved over the past wars and conflicts [5–7]. For the purposes of this document, it is sufficient to know only that our facility and team were designed to perform operations focused on providing immediate life, sight, and limb-preserving procedures adequate enough to be definitively managed at higher echelons of care [4]. In addition, deployed surgical teams may be asked to provide resuscitative care and definitive care for the local population, particularly if deemed the highest level of care in the area. When confronted with this particular humanitarian responsibility, an emphasis on ensuring the highest standards of trauma and acute care surgery care in resource limited settings is warranted.

S. Jones, M.D., F.A.C.S.
G. Wisbach, M.D., F.A.C.S. (✉)
Department of General Surgery, Naval Medical Center San Diego, BLDG 3, 4th Floor, 34800 Bob Wilson Drive, San Diego, CA 92134, USA
e-mail: Gordon.g.wisbach.mil@mail.mil

© Springer International Publishing Switzerland 2016
C.R.B. Lim (ed.), *Surgery During Natural Disasters, Combat, Terrorist Attacks, and Crisis Situations*, DOI 10.1007/978-3-319-23718-3_3

Fig. 3.1 Entryway to the trauma center

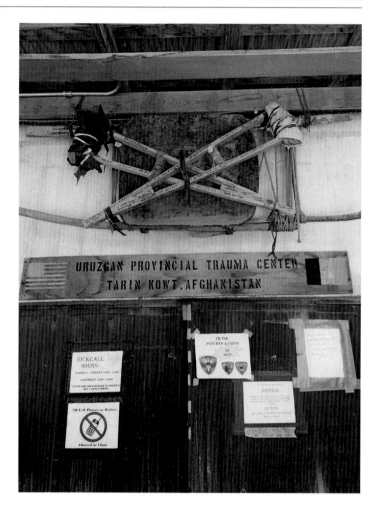

Good resources are available for guidance on ensuring the essential components of establishing and maintaining high-quality trauma or casualty-receiving facilities [1, 4, 8]. Some of these resources are listed later. To complement those general guidelines, we illustrate how those concepts can be put into real-world situations at casualty-receiving facilities in austere, hostile settings. To reiterate, the concepts emphasized in this chapter with the most leverage in providing quality trauma surgical care in these settings are briefly listed:

• Careful planning and training of personnel.
• Consideration of the social, cultural, and political milieu.

• Development and implementation of essential checklists.
• Ongoing team training, development, and welfare considerations.
• Continuous process assessment and improvement.
• Thoughtful and thorough turnover of lessons learned to the replacement team.

Through the use of publicly available guidelines with an emphasis on the above listed concepts, we hope to supplement these resources to provide guidance for setting up and providing quality trauma surgical care in unusual situations.

3.2   Preparation

3.2.1   Medical Rules of Engagement: Policies and Politics

Well-organized regional and local trauma systems have been shown to reduce morbidity and mortality [9–14]. The recent Boston bombing event is a stellar example of a successful trauma system where the mortality and morbidity of a terrorist attack was minimized largely due to the well-organized and rehearsed trauma system and disaster response plans [15]. Unfortunately, such a robust, well-prepared, and organized trauma system is outside the reach of those countries hosting US and coalition military presence [2, 3]. Yet, the US military has been able to set up an effective trauma system within a short time by duplicating the necessary elements of a first world trauma system in any setting (as demonstrated by the Joint Trauma System, JTS) [13, 16]. Ideally, a trauma team would be located in a region where a functioning trauma system existed and would serve a parallel or complimentary role. Due to the evolving missions in areas of conflict or disaster relief, the deployed trauma team may also have the privilege of caring for the local population. This would involve the integration of the host nation's local and regional medical resources into a unified triage and disposition decision tree (Fig. 3.2). For the majority of patients in these settings, air assets may be available to transfer them out using medical evacuation helicopters (Fig. 3.3). When the number of casualties or the severity of their injuries overwhelms the local hospital, the deployed trauma team may receive civilian patients. Survivability and long-term prognosis in the resource-constrained host nation will likely influence the transfer decision from the trauma team's facility and demand a continual awareness of alternative resources. On one hand, patients initially deemed expectant by the local population may receive basic lifesaving treatments that are both feasible and sustainable in the austere environment. For example, a local population may presume a traumatic limb amputation or chest trauma is fatal but simple control of hemostasis and uncomplicated chest tube management can be life-saving interventions. After the initial resuscitation, these patients can return back to the local hospital without undue burden on their resources. Also for most of these patients, when further treatment of the patient cannot be provided by the military facilities, nongovernmental organizations and other charitable organizations can be queried for further assistance.

Due to the variability in the patient population, forethought on the anticipated care that certain patients would receive plays a major role in whether a patient will receive temporarily stabilizing or definitive surgical management at the initial surgically capable facility. In addition to the usual reasons why patients cannot be sent to a higher level of care due, such as weather restrictions and the patients' stability for transport, the trauma team should also consider the continued care eligibility of the patient within the deployed trauma system. Occasionally, the forward deployed facility may be deemed the highest level of care the patient will receive. Unfortunately, being able to provide this assistance may not always be possible or practical. For example, a critically injured patient with severe traumatic brain injury may continue to require resource intensive, life-sustaining therapy upon transfer to the host nation's local or regional hospital where such resources are nonexistent or scarce. The disposition for such patients will vary on a case-by-case basis, and exploring all resources available for these difficult situations should be a priority upon arrival to the area.

In addition to orienting the team to the social and political environment and how this information affects the trauma team, adequate predeployment training tailored to the expected needs of the team is essential. The level of training of each team member is a quantifiable commodity that can optimize or limit his or her utility for the team. Various commercial courses are available that may help prepare for trauma care. Some of the curriculum is designed to meet the needs of the surgical team in austere environments. For additional information and resources, the American College of Surgeons website under "Trauma Education" lists additional course that

Fig. 3.2 Patient disposition algorithm

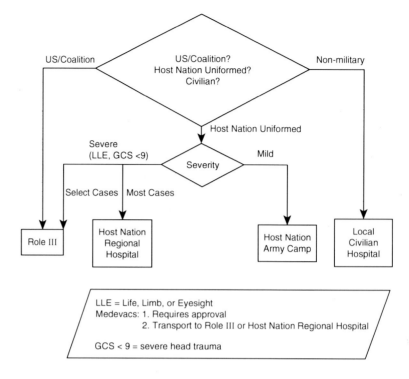

Fig. 3.3 Blackhawk helicopter as Army Medevac UH-60Q

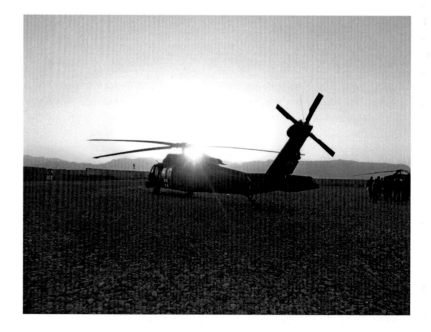

may be helpful. The following is a short list of such courses that should be considered prerequisite to deployment:

- Advanced Trauma Life Support (ATLS): This course is taught around the world and has improved the survivability of trauma patients [17, 18]. Prior to the existence of this systematic approach to trauma care, a majority of the care received by trauma patients was disorganized, haphazard, and incomplete and led to many patients dying of wounds that would otherwise be survivable with minimal intervention. Realizing the benefit of having this training, topics from ATLS can be incorporated into ongoing training curriculum during the deployment period.
- Advanced Surgical Skills for Exposure in Trauma (ASSET): This is an advanced course highly recommended for the surgeon who may need to control traumatic hemorrhage rapidly. The most common cause of death in trauma remains exsanguination.
- Emergency War Surgery (EWS): This course addresses the military perspective of the care for casualties of war. More insight is provided for those unique mechanisms of injury resulting from war such as high-velocity ballistic injuries, blast injuries, unique burn injuries, and casualties of chemical, biological, and nuclear warfare.
- Naval Expeditionary Medical Training Institute (NEMTI): As part of the medical unit deploying to war, the principles of ATLS and EWS are reinforced and practiced in a simulated setting with familiarization to the principles of triage, resuscitation, preoperative preparation, field operating rooms, postoperative management, transfer of patients including aeromedical en route care, and team dynamics.

Since 2001, a joint civilian and military venture with three major, US civilian, academic trauma centers has evolved and trained members of the US Army, Navy, and Air Force in the management of trauma casualties. The Army program is located at the University of Miami, Ryder Trauma Center. The Navy has a similar program at the University of Southern California, Los Angeles County Medical Center. The Air Force has programs at R. Adams Cowley Shock Trauma Center at the University of Maryland in Baltimore, Saint Louis University in St. Louis, and the University Hospital at the University of Cincinnati in Cincinnati. The training is state of the art involving didactics, simulations, expeditionary medicine, and clinical exposure to trauma care [19, 20].

In addition to the above high-yield courses, consideration should be given to attending some additional supplemental courses listed:

- Tactical Combat Casual Care Course (TCCC) is a short course designed to train the hospital corpsmen and medics in the prehospital care of the injured combatant, including unique training for care under dangerous situation.
- The Joint En route Care Course (JECC) provides training for medical personnel in trauma transport care during aeromedical operations in rotary wing platforms.
- The Trauma Evaluation and Management (TEAM): This course serves as a basic introduction to trauma management. The program is appropriate for medical students but lecture presentations and course manual can be adapted into the staff training schedule (discussed below).

Books and other informative resources for reference that are beneficial in preparing for trauma care in austere environments are available as well (see Table 3.1).

3.3 Supplies and Equipment

Communications: Access to communication equipment should be one of the first priorities of the trauma team. Fortunately, the military will provide a system for essential communication. This system may include the use of secure telephones and electronic mail. However, other commercial forms of communication may be available to the trauma team and can provide the

Table 3.1 List of high-yield references

• The World Health Organization: Guidelines for essential trauma care [1] is an excellent reference that outlines feasible standards in the treatment of injured patients in resource-limited countries (http://www.who.int/violence_injury_prevention/en/)
• Surgery and Healing in the Developing World [47]
• Joint Theater Trauma System (JTTS) command clinical practice guidelines [48]
• Tactical Combat Casualty Care course manual [49]
• PHTLS: Prehospital Trauma Life Support [50]
• ATLS manual [51]
• ASSET manual
• EWS manual [5]
• Combat casualty care: lessons learned from OEF and OIF [52]
• Manual of definitive surgical trauma care [53]
• Pediatric advanced life support: provider manual [54]
• Pediatric surgery and medicine for hostile environments [55]

needed transfer of vital information with local health care providers. Although not as secure, mobile phones can be utilized to call local surgeons, particularly in urgent situations. It is important to establish a reliable form of communication to provide the necessary components of transitions of care to the receiving facility. When using two-way radios, the security of the information relayed cannot be ensured and coded terminology should be implemented.

Use caution when using non-secure mobile phones to take pictures of patients or parts of their documentations to avoid violating their privacy. Illustrations may be used for quality assurance and training; however, personally identifiable information (PII) must be removed from these images.

Proper documentation serves as the hard copy, durable communication of patient care. During a chaotic trauma resuscitation or operative management requiring the total and prolonged attention of the multiple providers caring for the patient(s), documentation of care tends to be an afterthought and important details of the injuries and treatments rendered can be lost. In this regard, the trauma team members designated as medical recorders, or scribes, is an important component of this form of written communication. In addition, the team should consider keeping a logbook of the care provided through all phases of care in the facility including the clinic, resuscitation bays, critical care unit, inpatient wards, and operating room. These logs will require periodic review and can be used for reference when patients returned for follow up or required further care. The patients' medical records are on paper forms, but can be scanned and sent to other care providers as long as those lines of communication are secure. The first page of the JTS resuscitation form is displayed in Fig. 3.4. Keeping copies of the records allowed the peer review officer (described below in the peer review process) to refer back to these records for process improvement. As supplemental means of communication for process improvement, the After Action Report (AAR) summaries (explained below) can serve as a continued repository of what processes go well and which could be improved.

The list of consumable medical and surgical supplies, surgical instruments, their quantities, and wait times for replenishment is vital information. Equally important, is determining how supplies are reordered or how resupply is obtained. Visualization of what supplies are actually available should be compared with the items listed on the supply list. An additional benefit of this process is that the team can become familiar with the location of the supplies and can check the veracity of the supply lists.

RESUSCITATION RECORD
Part I, Nursing Flow Sheet

1. PATIENT INFORMATION

1.1 TRAUMA TEAM DATA

Service	Time Called	Time Arrived	Name
ED Physician			
Trauma Surgeon			
Respiratory Therapy			
Anesthesiology			
Lab/Blood Bank			
Radiology			
Pharmacy			
Consult (i.e., Ortho)			

1.2 ARRIVAL
Date _____
Time of Arrival _____
Time of Injury _____
Date of Injury _____
Transit Time _____ minutes

1.3 EVAC FROM
☐ 1st Responder
☐ Forward Resuscitative Care
☐ Theater Hospital
Location _____

1.4 MODE OF ARRIVAL
☐ Walked/Carried
☐ CASEVAC - Air
☐ CASEVAC - Ground
☐ MEDEVAC - Air
　Mission # _____
☐ MEDEVAC - Ground
　Mission # _____
☐ CCAT
☐ Ship EVAC
☐ AE
☐ Other

1.5 INJURY TYPE
☐ Blunt
☐ Burn
☐ Penetrating

1.6 INJURY CLASSIFICATION
☐ Battle
☐ Non-Battle
☐ Unknown

1.7 TRIAGE CATEGORY
☐ Immediate
☐ Delayed
☐ Minimal
☐ Expectant

1.8 VALUABLES FOUND
☐ None
☐ Given to Patient
☐ Secured by PAD
Time _____

1.9 PATIENT CATEGORY
☐ USA
☐ USAF
☐ USMC
☐ USN
☐ USCG
☐ USPHS
☐ Civilian - Local
☐ Civilian - Other
☐ Contractor
☐ EPW
☐ NATO - Coalition
☐ Non-NATO - Coalition
☐ Other

1.10 INJURY CAUSE
☐ Building Collapse
☐ Bullet/GSW/Firearm
☐ Burn
☐ EFP
☐ Fall
☐ Fire/Flame
☐ IED
☐ Inhalation Injury
☐ Mine
☐ Mortar/Rocket/Artillery Shell
☐ Multi-Frag
☐ MVC
☐ Sports
☐ UXO
☐ Other

2. CARE DONE PRIOR TO ARRIVAL

2.1 PREHOSPITAL TOURNIQUET

Upper Extremities:
Type:
☐ CAT ☐ SOFTT
☐ Other _____
Time On _____ Off _____
☐ R How many? ☐1 ☐3 ☐2 ☐4
Effective? ☐ Y ☐ N
☐ L How many? ☐1 ☐3 ☐2 ☐4
Effective? ☐ Y ☐ N

Lower Extremities:
Type:
☐ CAT ☐ SOFTT
☐ Other _____
Time On _____ Off _____
☐ R How many? ☐1 ☐3 ☐2 ☐4
Effective? ☐ Y ☐ N
☐ L How many? ☐1 ☐3 ☐2 ☐4
Effective? ☐ Y ☐ N

2.2 PREHOSPITAL VITALS
GCS
Eye _____ /4
Verbal _____ /5
Motor _____ /6
Total _____ /15
T _____
P _____
RR _____
BP _____ / _____
O$_2$Sat _____

2.3 PREHOSPITAL HEMORRHAGE CONTROL MEASURES
☐ Celox
☐ ChitoFlex
☐ Combat Gauze
☐ Direct Pressure
☐ Field Dressing
☐ HemCon
☐ QuikClot
☐ None
☐ Unknown
☐ Other

2.4 PREHOSPITAL WARMING
☐ Blanket
☐ Body Bag
☐ HPMK
☐ Space Blanket
☐ Other _____

2.5 PREHOSPITAL MEDS
_____
_____
_____
_____

2.6 PREHOSPITAL INTERVENTIONS
Prehospital Airway
☐ Y ☐ N
Intubated ☐ Y ☐ N
Cric ☐ Y ☐ N
Trach ☐ Y ☐ N
Needle Decompression ☐ Y ☐ N
C-spine Immobilized ☐ Y ☐ N
Pelvic Binder ☐ Y ☐ N
IO Infusions ☐ Y ☐ N
Eye Shield OS ☐ Y ☐ N
　　　　　OD ☐ Y ☐ N
CPR prior to arrival ☐ Y ☐ N

3. PRIMARY SURVEY

3.1 VITALS
P _____
RR _____
BP _____ / _____
O$_2$Sat _____
Pain Scale (0 - 10) _____

3.2 AIRWAY
☐ Patent
☐ Stridor
☐ Drooling
☐ Obstructed
☐ Oral/Nasal Airway
☐ BVM
☐ Intubated
☐ Combi Tube
☐ Other _____

3.3 HYPO / HYPERTHERMIA CONTROL MEASURES
Arrival Temp _____ ☐ F ☐ C
Time _____ Date _____
Route ☐ Oral ☐ Axillary ☐ Rectal
Temperature Control Procedure:
☐ Bair Hugger ☐ Warming Blanket
☐ Fluid Warmer ☐ Cooling Blanket
☐ Other _____

3.4 CPR IN ED
☐ Y ☐ N
Start Time _____
End Time _____

3.5 BREATHING
☐ Unlabored
☐ Labored
☐ Flaring
☐ Retraction
☐ Absent

Breath Sounds:
Clear ☐ R ☐ L
Rales ☐ R ☐ L
Wheeze ☐ R ☐ L
Absent ☐ R ☐ L

Chest Symmetry:
☐ Equal ☐ Left > ☐ Right >
Flail ☐ R ☐ L

Trachea:
☐ Midline
☐ Deviated

3.7 DEFICIT / NEURO
☐ Alert - Obeys Commands
☐ Responds to Verbal Stimuli
☐ Responds to Painful Stimuli
☐ Unresponsive to Painful Stimuli

GCS:
Eye _____ /4
Verbal _____ /5
Motor _____ /6
Total _____ /15

3.6 CIRCULATION
Skin:
☐ Warm ☐ Cool ☐ Hot
☐ Pink ☐ Pale ☐ Cyanotic
☐ Dry ☐ Moist ☐ Diaphoretic
Heart Sounds:
☐ Clear ☐ Muffled
Capillary Refill:
☐ < 2 Seconds (normal)
☐ > 2 Seconds (delayed)

Pediatric Broselow Tape Color:
_____

PATIENT IDENTIFICATION

Name: Last _____ First _____ MI _____ Rank _____

Patient ID/SSN _____ BRN _____ Medical Record # _____ DOB _____ Age _____ Gender ☐ M ☐ F

Facility Name _____ Facility Location _____ MOS/AFSC/NEC _____ Deployed/Assigned Unit _____

Nurse Name _____ Nurse Signature _____

DD FORM X601, 20110930 Page 1 of 5

Fig. 3.4 Sample resuscitation record

Fig. 3.5 C-arm fluoroscope in the operating room

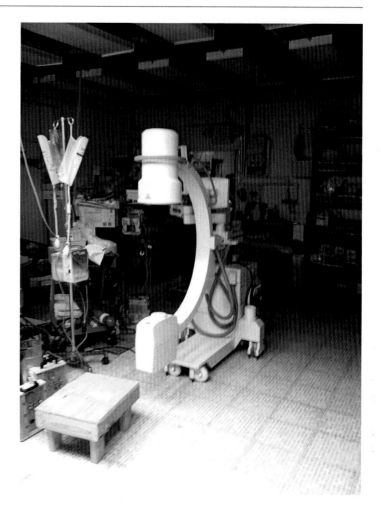

3.3.1 Equipment

Below is a list of equipment that is considered essential for providing trauma care in an austere setting; however, it is neither exhaustive nor authoritative.

Imaging equipment: A portable X-ray unit with a digital imaging system is quite useful for the evaluation of chest trauma, abdominal trauma (for free air, contrast extravasation, foreign bodies, ballistic fragments, etc.), fractures, radiopaque fragments in extremities, and spot angiography. With the aid of contrast material, ureterograms and cystograms among other gastrointestinal and urinary contrast studies are feasible.

The fluoroscopic C-arm is paramount in the operating room for the alignment and reduction of fractures and visualization of foreign bodies (Fig. 3.5).

Of note, the C-arm (and X-rays) may be used frequently in the tight spaces of the resuscitation bays and the operating room; therefore, it is important to ensure that lead aprons are widely available.

Portable ultrasound units are crucial for rapid diagnosis of pericardia tamponade, hemoperitoneum, hemothorax, and pneumothorax. The ultrasound can also aid in the evaluation of the gallbladder, appendix, uterus, adnexa or in the placement of peripheral intravenous, central venous, and arterial catheters.

Power supply: Having a steady, reliable electrical source is important especially for running a functioning operating room with the anesthesia equipment demanding priority. When needed, battery-operated headlights to operate and illuminate the surgical field with additional handheld flashlights is adequate.

Additional vital equipment to consider:

- Warmers: for fluids, blood products, ultrasound gel, and blankets.
  - Coolers for blood products.
  - Anesthesia machines.
  - Oxygen tanks.
  - Oxygen concentrators.
  - Oxygen generators.
  - Oxygen tank fillers.
  - Transport oxygen tanks.
  - Vitals machines.
  - Portable pulse oximeter.
  - Ventilators.
  - Portable suction machines.
  - Electrocardiogram.
  - Cardiac defibrillator/cardioverter.

Specific supplies for pediatric emergency medical, surgical, and trauma care must also be available. Although the mission of the trauma team may be focused on adult casualties, unfortunately the most vulnerable populations affected by prolonged armed conflict are children [21–23]. Even without violent injuries occurring, children are prone to sustaining injuries from accidents. Some of the more serious injuries could perhaps be curbed with the institution of some safety policies and adoption of a culture of safety among the children themselves. Simple measures such as wearing seatbelts and helmets could spare many lives in third-world countries as in the first-world countries [24–27]. Establishing such primary injury prevention programs is a huge and complicated undertaking involving multiple parties, financial resources, social marketing, and public education to effect lasting improvements [27–31]. However, as healthcare providers, we should still promote primary injury prevention practices whenever possible and appropriate. A brief educational discussion that is culturally sensitive with the child or parent may be adequate enough to impact their future attitude and behavior towards injury prevention [32]. Trauma care provider should keep in mind that in addition to pediatric injuries sustained from armed conflict, non-violent injuries such as falls from height, bicycle accidents, burns, and motor vehicle crashes are still prevalent among children in austere and hostile areas, and these types of injuries, mostly orthopedic, may form the majority of pediatric trauma surgical care.

Emergency pediatric resuscitation systems, such as the Broselow™ (trademark) System, that provide prepackaged and readily accessible pediatric supplies based on the height estimate of the child can be quite useful when quick medication dosing decisions and access to size specific equipment is needed during pediatric trauma resuscitations. One possible limitation of such systems is that the height-to-weight estimated correlation to develop such a system is based on population studies of children of high income countries, and it may not be accurate all the time and for all body habitus. Consider, however, that these systems usually underestimate the weight class based on height [33], but in those countries with limited resources, the children tend to be underweight. Become familiar with the contents of these kits in advance. If commercial kits are unavailable, the general principle can still be applied to gather, create, and package such a kit. Such pre-staging methods to give a quick and easy color-coded estimate of the equipment and medication dosing needs of the child of various sizes and ages can be helpful when time is limited [34].

Ambulance gear bag: The contents of the gear in the basic ambulance should be reviewed and adjusted to anticipate the life preserving equipment that may be needed during the transport of a patient in the ambulance. A sample list essential gear bag inventory is available in Table 3.2: Contents of gear bag to take on ambulance for patient pick up. The list can be used to inventory the contents and ensure that used supplies are

Table 3.2 Contents of gear bag to take on ambulance for patient pickup

1.	Airway/breathing
(a)	Adult bag-valve-mask
(b)	Pediatric bag-valve-mask
(c)	Oral airway (pediatric and adult sizes)
(d)	Nasopharyngeal airway (pediatric and adult sizes)
(e)	Facemask, non-rebreather mask (pediatric and adult sizes)
(f)	Oxygen tank
2.	Circulation
(a)	IV fluid
(b)	IV kit
(c)	IV tubing
(d)	IV flush
(e)	IV tourniquet
3.	Disability
(a)	Penlight
(b)	Headlight
4.	Exposure
(a)	Trauma shears
(b)	Heating blanket
5.	Miscellaneous
(a)	Eye protection
(b)	Latex-free gloves
(c)	Gauze
(d)	Elastic bandages
(e)	SAM® (registered trademark) splint
(f)	QuikClot® (registered trademark) Combat Gauze™ (trademark)
(g)	Tourniquets × 4

replenished in the gear bag. The ambulances can be any basic form of motorized transport with enough room to carry two non-ambulatory patients on litters (Fig. 3.6). Any expensive or sophisticated permanent contents of these vehicles would not be essential because the necessary equipment and supplies can be carried in the ambulance gear bag as described in Table 3.2.

3.4 Personnel

The trauma team members and support staff should be familiar to the recommended guidelines by the American College of Surgeon

Committee on Trauma and the World Health Organization on essential trauma care [1, 35]. In general, the essential member of the trauma team can be one to two general surgeons, an orthopedic surgeon, an emergency physician or physician assistant, two anesthesia providers, two to three registered nurses, a laboratory technician, a radiologic technician, two to three operating room technicians, a medical administrator, and three to four additional hospital corpsmen or medics. In addition to providing basic medical care, the level of training of the team members should allow for capabilities to receive and stabilize multiple blunt, blast, and penetrating wound casualties. The team should have enough expertise to perform life-saving resuscitative surgeries such as resuscitative thoracic, abdominal, vascular, and orthopedic surgeries. Limited neurosurgical procedures such as decompressive craniectomies may be achievable. Other nonsurgical capabilities should be the ability to admit and manage of post-resuscitation and postoperative patients on the inpatient wards or critical care unit settings for about 72 h. The personnel should also be proficient in the preparation and organization of expeditious and safe patient transfer to higher levels of care.

3.5 Organization

Mass casualty plan and rehearsal: Upon arrival to the area of operation, one of the first priorities of the team should be to evaluate the mass casualty plan. The review of this plan can also help to orient everyone on the team and assist in the familiarization of the layout of the facility and surrounding environment. Along with the response plan for mass casualty, the rehearsal of the plan is mandatory. This team familiarization can be as simple as a review of the plan in a brief format or as creative as a game to engage all of personnel, enhancing team building at the same time (see Fig. 3.7). The key component of the mass casualty response plan is full participation in periodic rehearsal of the plan in the form of mass casualty drills.

Fig. 3.6 Basic ambulance

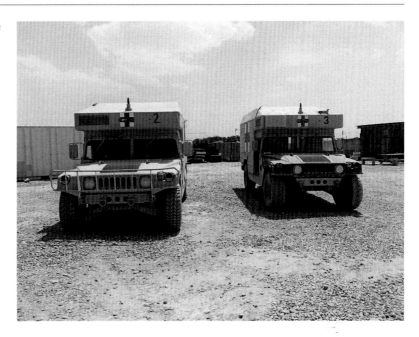

The trauma bay (see Figs. 3.8 and 3.9): The actual details on the setup of a casualty receiving facility and trauma resuscitation bay will vary, but most will follow a general guideline which will ensure that the immediately necessary equipment is available and easily obtainable.

Team positions: In addition to standardized locations of supplies and equipment, defined positions of the team members with respect to the patient according to the team member's role can help organize trauma resuscitations. The Trauma Team Leader (TTL) standing at a position near the foot of the bed may have the best overview of all of the activities around the patient. The physical examiner can start on the right side of the patient performing the primary and secondary trauma assessments. The registered nurse (RN) can be stationed on the left of the patient. The anesthesia provider can be stationed at the head of the patient with easy access to the patient's airway and materials needed to assess and manage the patient's airway and ventilation needs. Additional assistants for patient transfer and clothing removal can be stationed at the far right and/or far left of the patient.

Team roles: Prior to the arrival of casualties, team members should be assigned a defined role and positioned as above to minimize confusion,

missing essential tasks, or performing repetitive tasks needlessly. The roles and names of the team members should be easily visible for quick reference near the TTL. One of the most important roles is identifying a recorder who will keep the medical record and enter all of the salient details. In the event of a mass casualty, this role will be of even higher importance. Every patient should be assigned one recorder.

Role-based checklists: Trauma checklists are essential tools to ensure that critical supplies, equipment, and considerations are not overlooked [36, 37]. Each team member assigned to a role is responsible for verifying their respective checklists posted at their stations and then provide confirmation to the team leader that their respective checklist has been completed (see sample checklists in Table 3.3). The leadership of the trauma team should anticipate some noncompliance and plan to explore and address possible barriers to adherence [38].

Resuscitation team training and rehearsal: The trauma team training curriculum for the deployed units can have a positive impact on the quality of the trauma care delivered by those units [39]. The trauma resuscitation plans using team roles and role-based checklists should be reviewed and rehearsed. Successful implementation of a training

"THE AMAZING RACE"

Teams: 3 - consisting of 3 members
Pit Stops: 6 Casualty Collection Points (CCPs) – Located in _____
Objective: Familiarize the Mass Casualty Response Plan. Complete the course. Do not be in the last place!

1) Each team will start at _____
2) When music starts, each team will proceed to designated Pit Stop
   a. Team 1 -> _____
   b. Team 2 -> _____
   c. Team 3 -> _____
3) At first Pit Stop, team will obtain mass casualty medical supply box, place on stretcher and will need to recruit one non-medical person to assist as stretcher bearer to _____
4) At _____, team will find out next Pit Stop
   a. Team 1 -> _____
   b. Team 2 -> _____
   c. Team 3 -> _____
5) At next Pit Stop (similar to Step 3), team will obtain mass casualty medical supply box, place on stretcher and will need to recruit a different non-medical person to assist as stretcher bearer to _____
6) At _____, team will inventory both mass casualty medical supply boxes and determine missing items
7) When step 6 complete, team will need to complete quiz of 10 questions - correctly
8) 1st two teams finished win
9) Last team will ensure mass casualty medical supply boxes have correct inventory, then all three teams will return items to proper CCP

MASS CASUALTY QUIZ

1) A medical emergency involving multiple casualties which overwhelms existing medical support systems is called?
2) The triage category for "seriously injured casualties requiring urgent treatment".
3) The scene must be _____ before removing casualties to the nearest CCP.
4) Minimal, delayed and expectant patients will be directed to where?
5) Traffic flow for the ambulances will be _____
6) Triage the following patients as delayed, minimal, immediate or expectant.
   a. Young adult with GSW to head with large exit wound
   b. Young adult with GSW to abdomen with faint palpable radial pulse
   c. Senior adult with traumatic right leg amputation and strong radial pulse
   d. Young adult with right arm shrapnel injury, good palpable radial pulse
   e. Senior adult with forehead abrasion that is fully alert

Answers:
1) MASS CASUALTY
2) Immediate
3) Safe
4) Dining Facility
5) Counter-clockwise
6) Triage
   a. Expectant
   b. Immediate
   c. Delayed (First place functional tourniquet!)
   d. Minimal
   e. Delayed (or minimal)

Fig. 3.7 Mass casualty response plan familiarization game

program that incorporates simulation and team enhancement tools such as the TeamSTEPPS program is feasible in an austere, hostile environment [40]. Improving team communication and collaboration using such evidence based approach as the TeamSTEPPS model is critical to achieving optimal outcomes from the initially chaotic presentations of severely injured, multiple casualties.

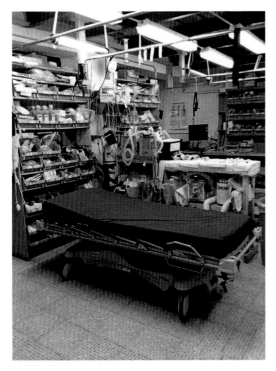

Fig. 3.8 Trauma bay

In addition to the simulations and rehearsals, prior to the arrival of each casualty, the team roles, role-based checklists, and the anticipated resuscitation plan should be verbally reviewed by the TTL.

TTL guide: Although it may seem repetitive, stating the roles and resuscitation plans for each incoming trauma casualty may help focus the trauma team and clarify leadership, and can remind the team members about commonly forgotten steps such as donning personal protective equipment, exercising noise discipline, and using clear-closed-loop communication.

To avoid adding to confusion with various providers giving multiple and sometimes conflicting orders, it is helpful to agree in advance that only the TTL gives specific resuscitation orders to team members. With this simple hierarchy established, information about the patient status and management suggestions will flow up to the TTL to help him or her maintain situational awareness. At certain critical points during a resuscitation (i.e., before intubation, after blood

Fig. 3.9 Trauma bay diagram. *RN* registered nurse

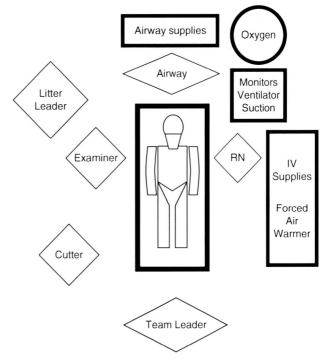

Table 3.3 Trauma resuscitation bay role-based checklists

Airway checklist

(a) Make sure functioning IV access for meds (sedation/paralytics)

(b) TTL or airway person to verbalize drug and doses

(c) Oral airway

(d) Nasal airway

(e) Supplemental oxygen (face mask, nasal cannula, non-rebreather)

(f) Laryngoscopes (present and functioning)

(g) Bag-valve-mask

(h) Oxygen tank check (remember to turn on when using)

(i) Suction

(j) CO_2 detector

(k) Stethoscope

(l) ETT holder or tapes

(m) NG/OG tube

Difficult airway list

(a) LMA

(b) Bougie

(c) GlideScope®

(d) Bronchoscope

(e) Cricothyroidotomy kit

(f) Tracheostomy kit

(g) 6–0 tracheostomy tube, cuffed

(h) 15 blade

(i) Suture/needle driver

Trauma/Tactical Operations Center (TOC) checklist

(a) Prehospital information (time of injury, MOI, injuries, vitals, estimated blood loss)

(b) TOC watch stander sends (mass texts and calls)

(c) Notify force protection

(d) Notify Joint Operations Center

(e) Check generator status

(f) Corpsmen grab ambulance gear bag oxygen tank and pick up patient

(g) Interpreter(s) available and notified

(h) Medevac potential

(i) Weather status for flight

(j) Medevac availability

Registered nurse/vital signs checklist

(a) Resuscitation fluid (warm crystalloid and colloids)

(b) Intravenous line placement kits

(c) Have fluid warmer ready

(d) Tetanus dose ready

(e) Cefazolin dose ready

(f) Thoracotomy set available

(g) Chest tube supplies available

(h) Central line cart ready

(i) Ultrasound available and check battery

(j) Doppler available and check battery

Radiology/lab/blood bank checklist

(a) Notified radiology technician

(b) Plasma warmer on

(c) Number and type of blood products available displayed on central dry-erase board

Litter/whiteboard checklist

(a) Whiteboard(s) ready

(b) Whiteboard holder identified

(c) Heater blanket on bed

(d) Regular blanket available

(e) Forced-air warming system on

(f) Cervical immobilizer-collar open and nearby

(g) Trauma shears available

(h) Paperclips for radio-opaque wound markers available

(i) Combat tourniquets available

Primary and secondary examiner's checklist

(a) Double gloves

(b) Otoscope functioning

(c) Stethoscope

(d) Surgical lubricant packet inside glove

(e) Ensure medical record keeper is assigned

(continued)

Table 3.4 Trauma team activation checklist

Trauma team activation
Planning for team
Prehospital information (time of injury, mechanism of injury, injuries, vital signs, estimated blood loss)
Trauma administrative center hospital corpsman makes calls
Trauma team
Force protection
Joint Operations Center
Medics grab gear bag and pick up patient
Medevac potential
Weather
Air transport availability
Team roles—identify and check status
Primary assessment (ABCDE), secondary assessment
Airway management
Nurse/vital signs
IV placement/blood for laboratory
Radiology technician and assistants
Laboratory technician/blood bank
Clothes cutter/white slider board/litter bearers
Recorder
Checking equipment
Airway equipment (pediatric equipment; cricothyroidotomy set)
Make sure functioning IV access for meds (sedation/paralytics)
Trauma Team Leader (TTL) or airway to verbalize drug and doses
Oral airway
Nasal airway
Supplemental O_2 (FM, NRB, NC)
Laryngoscopes (present and functioning)
Bag valve mask
Oxygen tank check (remember to turn on when using)
Suction on
CO_2 detector
Stethoscope
ETT holder or tapes
NG/OG tube
Difficult airway tools
LMA
Bougie
GlideScope® (registered trademark)
Bronchoscope
Cricothyroidotomy kit
Tracheostomy kit

(continued)

Trauma team activation
6–0 tracheostomy tube, cuffed
15 blade, suture, needle driver
Resuscitation fluid (warm crystalloid and colloid stock)
IV kits
Combat tourniquets
Central venous catheter kit (large bore only)
Chlorhexidine
Monitors and defibrillators
ACLS medications
Thoracotomy set and/or chest tube
White patient slider board ready
Cervical-collar nearby
Turn on plasma warmer
Get heater blanket
Regular blanket
Have fluid warmer ready
Forced-air warming system on
Trauma shears
General sequence
Prior to patient arrival, perform a pre-brief
Upon patient arrival, perform primary survey including a brief neurologic exam and full exposure for trauma evaluation
Get patient off the white slider board (logroll and examine posterior surfaces and rectum)
Monitors placed
Vitals reported to TTL
X-rays ordered
Report from medic received
Secondary survey done
Additional X-rays as needed
To operating room or transfer out
Team leader communication
Noise discipline: limit to one person talking, there should not be a need for shouting
Reminder: closed loop communication (i.e., confirm all orders verbally, report when the order is performed)
Pre-brief is important before patient arrival
Clear, concise communication
Allow patient to enter the room and on to the bed
Threat assessment ongoing
May need decontamination for hazardous materials
If you use a sharp instrument, place it in sharps box
Proper personal protective gear (eye protection and gloves)
Potential difficulties or patient care issues
Encourage team members to voice concerns

pressure stabilization, or after return of pulses), the TTL should update his or her team with a brief summary of the patient status and overall plans to reciprocate situational awareness to the team. To improve noise discipline, the locations of supplies and equipment in and near the resuscitation bay should be familiar to each of the resuscitation team members to minimize calling out for supplies.

The TTL should realize that providing high-quality trauma resuscitation care to injured patients depends less on sophisticated technology or equipment and more on organization, clear communication, and teamwork [36, 40–42]. Even in deployed or remote settings, applying useful, evidence-based concepts in team dynamics and team communication to improve patient safety is feasible without adversely affecting efficiency [40].

The role of the TTL outlined below is a review of the broader role that the TTL must consider with each resuscitation:

- Lead the resuscitation.
- Ensures systematic patient assessment.
- Obtain appropriate consults.
- Obtain appropriate adjuncts (X-ray/FAST/vascular access/labs).
- Efficient transfer from the resuscitation bay (OR, wards/ICU, medevac, or ambulance).
- If multi-trauma, appropriate prioritization of resources and personnel.
- Facilitate treatment in OR.
- Sufficient personnel support (need nurse, circulator, tech, or surgeon).
- Sufficient supplies (equipment, blood products, etc.).
- Arrange for appropriate disposition or postoperative care.
- Determine need for medical evacuation, ambulance, prolonged intubation, ICU, or ward care.
- Assist in ensuring the proper use of personnel and resources.
- Completion of role as TTL.
- If plan changes or complications arise, the medical director will direct patient care.

- Ensure proper documentation and transfer of care.
  - Trauma flow sheet.
  - Operative notes.
  - Progress notes and discharge summaries.
  - Transfer summary and notes.
  - Orders as needed.
  - Surgery database.

For reference before and during resuscitation, the TTL should have easy access to a "Trauma Team Activation" checklist (see Table 3.4).

3.5.1 Additional Notes on Trauma Resuscitation

Depending on the resources available at a particular facility and treatment guidelines available, treatment algorithms may need to be customized for the surgeons specific situation (as an example see Fig. 3.10). Availability of timely transport to a higher level or care for the patient is a key factor in developing these algorithms.

Blood product protocols: There will be a limited store of blood on site at an austere setting. Notably, resuscitation with fresh blood is associated with lower morbidity and mortality. Following evidence-based guidelines, attempts can be made to institute Massive Transfusion Protocols (MTP) when needed [43–45], but anticipate this to be constrained by the lower supply of plasma and platelets. Patients needing the MTP will likely receive greater than the recommended blood product rations of 1:1:1 for red blood cells:fresh frozen plasma (FFP):platelets, respectively.

Walking blood bank is a viable option, but the protocols on setting up a walking blood bank should be carefully reviewed. Ideally, those with prior experience should be recruited to assist. This setup requires a considerable amount of preplanning and prior commitment by the nonmedical personnel who would be providing the blood.

Fluid warmers: Two warmers that could each thaw four units of FFP at a time may be adequate to provide clotting factors to major trauma patients. However, the time required to thaw FFP

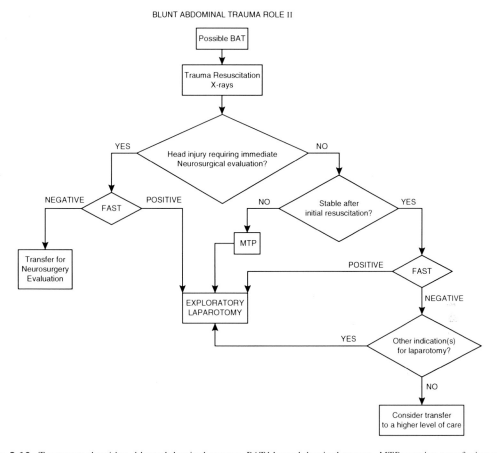

BLUNT ABDOMINAL TRAUMA ROLE II

Fig. 3.10 Treatment algorithm, blunt abdominal trauma. *BAT* blunt abdominal trauma, *MTP* massive transfusion protocol, *FAST* focused assessment with sonography for trauma

can affect the transfusion times and blood product transfusion ratios.

The operating room (Figs. 3.11 and 3.12): Operating team members should inventory this area of care to ensure that the room is clean with enough space for the patient(s), and that the necessary personnel, supplies, and equipment are present. Cleanable floors, a sterilizer, overhead lights, operative lights, headlights, and surgical consumables supplies should be readily available. As in the other areas of the facility, checklists can be valuable in the OR. These preoperative, intraoperative, and postoperative checklists are available and easily modifiable to suit the team's needs [41]. The benefit of checklists cannot be overstated [42]. As an example, see Table 3.5, Anesthesia checklist from JTTS Clinical Practice Guidelines.

Post-anesthesia care unit (PACU): Post-anesthesia care should be provided in an area where patients can be closely monitored until criteria are met for transfer to the inpatient wards and the critical care unit or prepared for en route care and transfer to an outside facility.

Critical care unit (CCU): This area can be in the same large room as the wards if space is limited. But specific beds with additional monitoring and positions closer to the nursing station should be designated as the CCU area (Fig. 3.13).

Inpatient wards should be climate controlled, relatively clean, quiet, and able to provide privacy. Basic medical observations, parenteral fluid therapy, and wound management should be easily performed here.

Clinic: Clinic visitation days are necessary for follow up of patients and new patients that the

Fig. 3.11 Basic operating room after a major trauma resuscitation

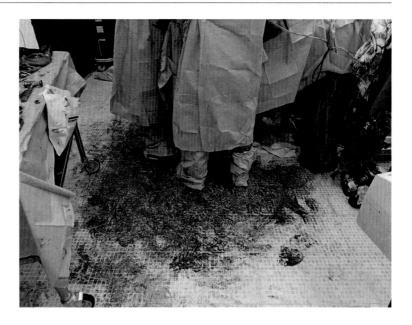

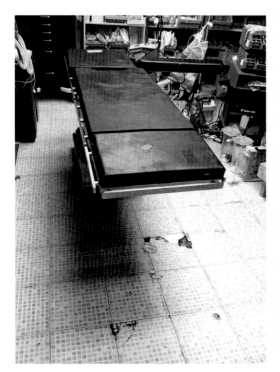

Fig. 3.12 Basic operating room table

acute appendicitis, and complicated anorectal disease.

Labs: Limited lab capabilities may be available using point-of-care devices in austere environments (glucometer, i-STAT® (registered trademark) system, urine test strips, blood typing cards).

Radiology: Basic X-ray machines can be very useful and usually provided adequate images on digital processors. Other imaging modalities that are practical in austere environments are portable ultrasound machines and C-arm fluoroscopy. Patients requiring more advanced imaging studies should be sent to a higher level of care.

Pharmacy: Strictly controlled substances should be managed and secured by the registered nurses and anesthesia providers. Other essential medications such as antibiotics, non-narcotic analgesics, and topical medications can be stored and dispensed from a locked room designated as the pharmacy.

3.6 Team Strengthening

3.6.1 Team Dynamics

local health care providers may send for assistance in management of diagnoses such as nonunion or malunion of fractures, fresh closed or open isolated fractures, non-healing wounds,

The leadership of the trauma team should not ignore the fact that individual team members are

Table 3.5 Anesthesia checklist from JTTS clinical practice guidelines

Before patient arrival
Room temperature ≥25 °C
Warm IV line
Machine check
Airway equipment check
Blood bank notified to have blood available per unit SOP
Patient arrival
Patient identified if possible
Blood bank notified to deliver blood per unit SOP
Ensure large bore IV or CVC access
Monitors (SaO$_2$, BP, ECG)
Pre-oxygenation
Induction
Sedative hypnotic (ketamine vs. propofol vs. etomidate)
Neuromuscular blockade (succinyl choline vs. rocuronium)
Intubation (per Trauma Airway Management CPG)
(+) ETCO$_2$
Place orogastric tube
Anesthetic
Consider TIVA
(Volatile anesthetic and/or benzodiazepine) +narcotic
Insert additional IV access and/or arterial line if needed
Resuscitation (per DCR CPG)
Send baseline labs, type, and cross if not yet done
Follow MAP trends
Goal FFP:PRBC:plt 1:1:1 if massive transfusion
Goal urine output 0.5–1.0 mL/kg/h
Consider TXA if <3 h from injury and indicators for massive transfusion identified
Consider calcium chloride 1 g
Consider hydrocortisone 100 mg
Consider vasopressin 5–10 IU
Administer appropriate antibiotics
Special considerations for TBI as indicated in several head injury CPG
Closing/postoperative
Low-volume ventilation per acute respiratory failure CPG

unique with various temperaments and backgrounds. As professionals, we expect our team members to perform optimally all the times from beginning of the mission to the end. In reality, we should anticipate stress and conflicts to arise so

that we can detect and address them before it adversely affects the quality of the team performance. It would be wise to refer to some models of team formation to use as a framework to anticipate and mitigate such difficulties. One such model is Bruce Tuckman's revised stages of group development consisting of five stages: forming, storming, norming, performing, and adjourning (Fig. 3.14) [46].

Passively allowing "compassion fatigue" to overwhelm our teammates is counterproductive. Providing tools to mediate conflict and ensuring a supportive environment is a duty for all of the team members especially in such a stressful environment where mutual trust and respect can be a valuable asset. Training all the team members on how to detect conflict or psychological stress in others is important to maintain the psychological health of the individual resulting in better functioning and better communicating teams.

3.6.2 Morale

Attention should be given to ensure enough time to decompress and discuss the stress of a particularly difficult case or stressful multiple casualty cases for emotional and psychological support of the adversely affected team members. Facilities for exercise can be important and may ward off illnesses associated with stress. Some form of Morale, Welfare and Recreation (MWR) service is as vital as any of the other components of a deploying unit. As an important service of the MWR programs, providing the ability to communicate with family can aid in reducing stress for both the persons deployed and for the family members at home. Other reminders of home in the form of access to news, entertainment, food, games, etc. should be made available as well.

3.6.3 Role Changing and Cross-Training

Being the TTL is challenging. Intense focus is required to prioritize the attention given to a multitude of verbal, visual, and tactile information

Fig. 3.13 Critical care unit/wards

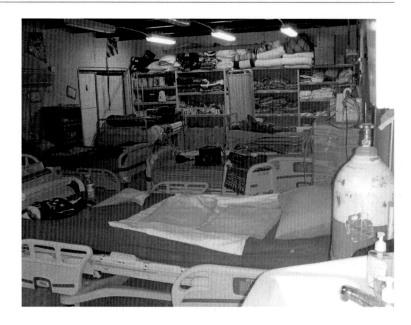

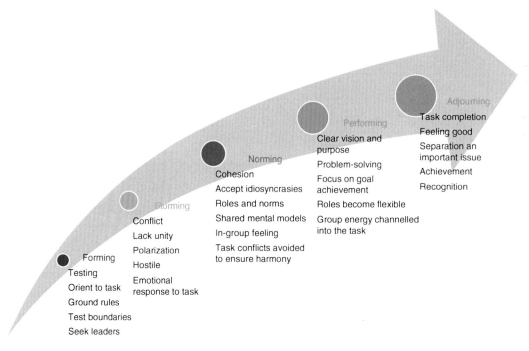

Adjourning
Task completion
Feeling good
Separation an important issue
Achievement
Recognition

Performing
Clear vision and purpose
Problem-solving
Focus on goal achievement
Roles become flexible
Group energy channelled into the task

Norming
Cohesion
Accept idiosyncrasies
Roles and norms
Shared mental models
In-group feeling
Task conflicts avoided to ensure harmony

Storming
Conflict
Lack unity
Polarization
Hostile
Emotional response to task

Forming
Testing
Orient to task
Ground rules
Test boundaries
Seek leaders

Fig. 3.14 Tuckman's model of group development

that are thrown at the TTL simultaneously or in rapid succession. At the same time, the TTLs consider the injuries, give orders in a rational way (in accordance to ATLS concepts), and coordinate the actions of the multiple team members involved. However, being the TTL can be rewarding and many of the team members, including providers from other facilities, will likely volunteer to be mentored and trained to perform this role. Having additional, trained TTLs will allow for efficient and effective resuscitation of multiple trauma patients simultaneously.

With the personnel resources that are limited, the lack of a particular skill set among the team members may limit the capabilities of the team as a whole. Cross-training all the members on various skills is one way to address this potential problem. Cross-training can be used to become proficient on the use of the X-ray machines, portable ultrasound, laboratory equipment, blood product preparation, intravenous catheter placement, intraosseous line placement, central venous catheter placement, external fixator placement, intubation, emergency surgical airway placement, wound care, and operation of the rapid fluid/infuser.

In addition, didactic training should be scheduled regularly. A sample month of the scheduled lectures and training sessions is shown below (Fig. 3.15). The entire contents of the ATLS course and the JTTS Clinical Practice Guidelines can be considered as one way to organize the training curriculum.

3.7 Process Improvement

After action reports (AAR): AARs are essential meetings dedicated to evaluate for areas of improvement for each trauma resuscitation including the review of prehospital transport and treatment, communications issues, trauma bay resuscitation, operating room events, PACU/CCU/ward events, and transfer/disposition issues. All cases warrant review. When fortunate enough to get it, feedback from previously treated patients or their providers from facilities at higher levels of care should be shared to give closure for all the team members involved in the care for those patients. All interested members including other coalition medical personnel in the area can be invited to attend these sessions. To consolidate and reinforce the learning points from the AARs, written summaries of these debriefs were documented and shared with the members of the team for review. Also, these documents were passed on to the next team for learning and process improvement purposes. Examples of the AAR summaries are in Fig. 3.16: Examples of the AAR summa-

ries. These debriefs should be scrubbed of all identifiable information to conform to the privacy guidelines set forth. The discussions and any related documents are needed for quality improvement.

Peer reviews: Peer reviews should be conducted regularly to ensure best medical practices were exercised. It should be mandatory for all providers. Both inpatient and outpatient charts can be reviewed.

In contrast to the AARs, the peer review process involves only the providers more responsible in the clinical decision making thereby emphasizing more on improving the quality of the executive processes of the trauma team. The peer review officer should thoroughly review selected patient documentations and pose questions or address issues with the providers in a systematic way.

The peer review instructions and forms should be included in the turnover file. Records of the peer review sessions should be kept in a secure file to maintain documentation of the peer review process. Periodic peer review may motivate the team members to continuously strive for excellence in providing medical and surgical care even in remote areas with limited resources and avoid complacency.

3.8 Trauma Team Turnover

As the prior team or members of the team rotate out of the area, it is important to ensure that important specific lessons learned are passed onto the next team. The unique knowledge obtained by the prior team and the resultant suggestions can be evaluated and improved or disregarded as the mission and settings change for the unique situation of the oncoming combat surgical team. See Table 3.6 for the details on how turnover can be achieved.

In brief, a description of the capabilities of the individual personnel and the team as a whole should be reviewed with the oncoming team. This discussion should encompass critical items that impact the overall capability such as surrounding

Monday	Tuesday	Wednesday	Thursday	Friday
1 PEER Review for June TCCC topic	2 Splenectomy vaccination	3 ATLS Topic	4 Joint Conference	5 Urologic Trauma Management
8 AAR from 5JUL Frozen Blood	9 Topical hemostatics	10 15:30-M&M	11 Joint Conference	12 Nutrition
15 MRI in mTBI	16 Cold Injuries	17 M&M Sport Supplements	18 Joint Conference	19
22 Heat Injuries	23	24 15:30-M&M	25 Joint Conference	26 Military working dogs
29 Acoustic Trauma and Hearing Loss	30	31 15:30-M&M		

Fig. 3.15 Example of a monthly training calendar

Trauma Resuscitation Debrief for _____(Date)

Here is our debrief. If you have any questions, suggestions, or comments, please let me know.

This information is peer review material designed to improve the quality of patient care and is privileged and confidential.

The cases and images are presented here solely for the educational purposes of the staff. Neither the text nor the images presented in these cases are to be forwarded to persons or organizations outside our facility. Text and images presented here are not to be posted on the internet, copied, published or distributed in any other manner without permission; please contact me with questions regarding this issue.

Here are the cases debriefed:

Case 1 *was a 12 y/o boy who had jumped or fell off a tree and suffered and left femur fracture. He was initially seen at the local hospital around 1AM, and he was brought to us later in the morning. He underwent the standard trauma resuscitation in the trauma bay and was stable except a heart rate in 110's. His only injury turned out to be an open comminuted left femur fracture. He received tetanus prophylaxis in the trauma bay and cefazolin 750mg in the OR.*

Fig. 3.16 Examples of the AAR summaries

Points brought up were:

1. *There was an extra patient who jumped into the ambulance and insisted on being seen at our facility.*

   a. *We DO NOT let local nationals come to our facility on a nonlocal national clinic day.*

2. *The patient and family member was checked for contraband at the gate, but it turned out that the family member had a knife that was not confiscated until a second search was done at the gate.*

3. *There was some confusion about calling out secondary exam findings or just telling the findings later.*

   a. *When asked for by the TTL, the secondary exam findings should be called out to keep the TTL aware of all pertinent positive and negative findings.*

4. *There is an overall impression that some of our equipment such as the pulse oximeters do not work very well so that if there is no reading or if it is a low number we tend to assume the oxygenation is normal and that the machine is failing to pick it up.*

   a. *While most of the time, it may be true that the pulse oximeter is not working well, we should verify such critical data to reassure ourselves.*

Case 2 was a 14 year-old male involved in an MVC. From the constellation of findings, he was likely a pedestrian struck by a vehicle on the right side with injuries in his left leg, left ribs, left clavicle, left face and left head. He was comatose on arrival. We established a definitive airway with,and an ETT wasplaced. He was apneic, hypoxic, and tachycardic, with a GCS <8 (eyes 1, verbal 1, motor 4 = 6). He did have a gag reflex and withdrawing all four extremities on initial presentation. He was hypothermic to 95 degrees F, coagulopathic (INR 3.3), and acidotic (pH 6.8). He had blood coming out of his nose, ears, and mouth.

The points brought up were:

1. *There was some confusion because a lot of the providers were involved in another case at the same time, we were short on people, and the corpsman covering the desk had to leave to pick up the trauma patient.*

   a. *We've decided that the duty corpsman should stay in the operations center and assign someone else to go to pick up the patient if possible.*

   b. *The corpsman at the desk should then proceed to make the required calls.*

      i. *We've identified the need to have a checklist for whom to call when a trauma is en route.*

         1. *This list should include force protection.*

Fig. 3.16 (continued)

2. There were no supplies or equipment in the ambulance and therefore no good way to provide emergency care en route by the HM's if needed.

    a. We should take a pack of all the necessary supplied that may be needed for the ambulance.

        i. This pack should be kept in the armory and everyone on the team should know where it is and what should be in it.

        ii. At the least, it should have a bag-valve-mask with different sized masks, oral and nasal airway, facemask, oxygen tank, c-collar, IV supplies, and tourniquet. A detailed list is pending.

3. We decided that the preferred ambulance to take for trauma pick up should be the #2 ambulance because it is reported to be the most reliable for now.

    a. Please use the other vehicles for nonessential travel.

4. HM2XXXXX did a great job placing a left AC large bore IV, but unfortunately it became dislodged before it could be secured.

    a. It may help to communicate to those nearby that you are trying to secure the IV and that the patient should not be moved.

    b. Securing the IV should be done expeditiously

        i. Some tips given were:

            1. Have tape and securing devices within reach and prepared for one handed use.

            2. Have an assistant

            3. Just cap the IV after saline flush while securing it instead of waiting for a IV fluid line

5. Lab results should be given to the TTL first then it can be handed off to the recorder so that the TTL has overall situational awareness

6. This patient was hypothermic and we did not have a heat blanket on the trauma bay gurney.

    a. We should make placing the heat blanket on the gurney as part of the initial checklist.

Thanks everyone for all your efforts on the above trauma resuscitations and to all who keep this facility going.

Fig. 3.16 (continued)

Table 3.6 Turnover document and turnover plan

Turnover plan
General: location of electronic document: _____
Early tasks—supply liaison, security clearances
A. Leadership
(a) Welcome/orientation
(b) Logistics (room turnover)
(c) Safety (weapons conditions, fire safety, badges)
(d) Multinational base—familiarization/tour
(e) Medical counterinsurgency mission
B. Clinical
(a) Trauma/general (weekly morbidity and mortality conferences)
• Clinical practice guidelines
(b) Orthopedics
(c) Anesthesia
(d) Other hospitals and clinics nearby
(e) Nursing
C. Ancillary support
(a) Pharmacy (monthly narcotic reconciliation)
(b) Laboratory
(c) Radiology
(d) Supply
(e) Equipment/BioMed
(f) Electronic medical records
D. Personnel
(a) Linguists
(b) Custodian
E. Programs (weekly schedule)
(a) Mass casualty plan
(b) Peer review
(c) MWR (propane tank, food ordering/cooking)
(d) Commando clinic
(e) Commando training
(f) Local national clinic
(g) Walking blood bank
(h) Vampire blood program
(i) Motor pool/motor stables
(j) Medevac
F. Other organizations

resources, relations with the host nation, supplies, equipment, and level of expertise of the team members. Also, important information regarding points of contact should be passed on.

Another point to emphasize to the next team is the importance and feasibility of specific trauma team cross-training even in the austere setting.

In addition, the importance of the Trauma Team Activation Checklist and the Role Based Checklists can be stressed with similar emphasis as the use of the checklists in the operating room. The team training schedule can be handed down to use as a modifiable template for the next team.

Finally, the importance of continuing the process of improvement using the peer review processes and AARs after every trauma cases should be emphasized during turnover. If the prior team was diligent, the records of these peer reviews and AARs can serve as a repository of lessons learned for the oncoming team.

3.9 Conclusion

Well-developed and working guidelines do exist as good resources that provide ways to achieve best practices in trauma care that can be applied in many settings with minor adjustments. Above is a brief description of how the actual applications of these guidelines can be implemented in the unique situation of being a part of a surgical team deployed to an austere, hostile environment. To meet this unique challenge, the essential components of a quality trauma casualty receiving facility have been described. A complement of well-prepared and skilled individuals with a common goal as well as gathering and ensuring access to the essential supplies and equipment listed above should be a starting point. With this foundation of human and material resources, the trauma team can provide most effective trauma resuscitative treatments to various population groups in an area of responsibility that may be resource deprived. Careful and detailed attention to the organization, training, team dynamics, vital checklists, and continuous process improvement procedures seem to have the most positive impact on the trauma team's mission of providing a high standard of trauma care in suboptimal conditions.

Future missions and teams will be unique in their own ways and our experience will not likely mirror theirs exactly, but this chapter may add to their compendium of resources available to help prepare and guide their own trauma teams.

Editor's note: CDR Gordon Wisbach, M.D., USN, is currently serving on Active for the US Navy. He has served on two combat tours in support of Operation Enduring Freedom and he helped establish a hospital in Western Afghanistan.

References

1. Mock C, World Health Organization, International Society of Surgery, International Association of Trauma Surgery and Intensive Care. Guidelines for essential trauma care. Geneva: World Health Organization; 2004.
2. Latifi R, Ziemba M, Leppaniemi A, Dasho E, Dogjani A, Shatri Z, et al. Trauma system evaluation in developing countries: applicability of American College of Surgeons/Committee on Trauma (ACS/COT) basic criteria. World J Surg. 2014;38(8):1898–904.
3. Wisborg T, Murad MK, Edvardsen O, Husum H. Prehospital trauma system in a low-income country: system maturation and adaptation during 8 years. J Trauma. 2008;64(5):1342–8.
4. Borden Institute. Emergency war surgery. 3rd U.S. revision. Washington, DC: Dept. of Defense, USA; 2004.
5. Woodard SC. The AMSUS history of military medicine essay award. The story of the mobile army surgical hospital[corrected]. Mil Med. 2003;168(7): 503–13.
6. Beekley AC. United States military surgical response to modern large-scale conflicts: the ongoing evolution of a trauma system. Surg Clin North Am. 2006;86(3):689–709.
7. Grathwohl KW, Venticinque SG. Organizational characteristics of the austere intensive care unit: the evolution of military trauma and critical care medicine; applications for civilian medical care systems. Crit Care Med. 2008;36(7 Suppl):S275–83.
8. Eastman AB. Resources for optimal care of the injured patient – 1993. Bull Am Coll Surg. 1994; 79(5):21–7.
9. Jurkovich GJ, Mock C. Systematic review of trauma system effectiveness based on registry comparisons. J Trauma. 1999;47(3 Suppl):S46–55.
10. Mann NC, Mullins RJ, MacKenzie EJ, Jurkovich GJ, Mock CN. Systematic review of published evidence regarding trauma system effectiveness. J Trauma. 1999;47(3 Suppl):S25–33.
11. Simons R, Eliopoulos V, Laflamme D, Brown DR. Impact on process of trauma care delivery 1 year after the introduction of a trauma program in a provincial trauma center. J Trauma. 1999;46(5):811–5. discussion 5–6.
12. Nathens AB, Jurkovich GJ, Cummings P, Rivara FP, Maier RV. The effect of organized systems of trauma care on motor vehicle crash mortality. JAMA. 2000;283(15):1990–4.
13. Eastridge BJ, Costanzo G, Jenkins D, Spott MA, Wade C, Greydanus D, et al. Impact of joint theater trauma system initiatives on battlefield injury outcomes. Am J Surg. 2009;198(6):852–7.
14. Durham R, Pracht E, Orban B, Lottenburg L, Tepas J, Flint L. Evaluation of a mature trauma system. Ann Surg. 2006;243(6):775–83. discussion 83-5.
15. Gates JD, Arabian S, Biddinger P, Blansfield J, Burke P, Chung S, et al. The initial response to the Boston marathon bombing: lessons learned to prepare for the next disaster. Ann Surg. 2014;260(6):960–6.
16. Bailey, J., Spott, M. A., Costanzo, G. P., Dunne, J.R., Dorlac, W., & Eastridge, B. Joint Trauma System: Development, Conceptual Framework, and Optimal Elements, U.S. Department of Defense, U.S. Army Institute for Surgical Research, 2012. Web. 1 Nov. 2014.
17. Ali J, Adam R, Stedman M, Howard M, Williams JI. Advanced trauma life support program increases emergency room application of trauma resuscitative procedures in a developing country. J Trauma. 1994;36(3):391–4.
18. Ali J, Adam R, Butler AK, Chang H, Howard M, Gonsalves D, et al. Trauma outcome improves following the advanced trauma life support program in a developing country. J Trauma. 1993;34(6):890–8. discussion 8-9.
19. Thorson CM, Dubose JJ, Rhee P, Knuth TE, Dorlac WC, Bailey JA, et al. Military trauma training at civilian centers: a decade of advancements. J Trauma Acute Care Surg. 2012;73(6 Suppl 5):S483–9.
20. Pereira BM, Ryan ML, Ogilvie MP, Gomez-Rodriguez JC, McAndrew P, Garcia GD, et al. Predeployment mass casualty and clinical trauma training for US Army forward surgical teams. J Craniofac Surg. 2010;21(4):982–6.
21. Djeddah C, Shah PM. The impact of armed conflict on children: a threat to public health. Contribution of the World Health Organization to the United Nations Study on the Impact of Armed Conflict on Children. Geneva, Switzerland: World Health Organization (WHO); 1997.
22. Machel G. The impact of war on children : a review of progress since the 1996 United Nations report on the impact of armed conflict on children. New York: Palgrave; 2001.
23. UNICEF. Children UNOotSRotS-Gf, Conflict A. Machel Study 10-year Strategic Review: children and conflict in a changing world. Office of the Special Representative of the Secretary-General for Children and Armed Conflict; 2009.
24. Newman RJ. A prospective evaluation of the protective effect of car seatbelts. J Trauma. 1986;26(6):561–4.
25. Marine WM, Kerwin EM, Moore EE, Lezotte DC, Baron AE, Grosso MA. Mandatory seatbelts: epidemiologic, financial, and medical rationale from the Colorado matched pairs study. J Trauma. 1994;36(1):96–100.
26. American College of Surgeons; Committee on Trauma. Statement on bicycle safety and the promo-

tion of bicycle helmet use. Bull Am Coll Surg. 2014;99(9):45.

27. Lindqvist K, Timpka T, Schelp L, Ahlgren M. The WHO safe community program for injury prevention: evaluation of the impact on injury severity. Public Health. 1998;112(6):385–91.

28. Bablouzian L, Freedman ES, Wolski KE, Fried LE. Evaluation of a community based childhood injury prevention program. Inj Prev. 1997;3(1):14–6.

29. Gofin R, De Leon D, Knishkowy B, Palti H. Injury prevention program in primary care: process evaluation and surveillance. Inj Prev. 1995;1(1):35–9.

30. McClure RJ, Davis E, Yorkston E, Nilsen P, Schluter P, Bugeja L. Special issues in injury prevention research: developing the science of program implementation. Injury. 2010;41 Suppl 1:S16–9.

31. Gittelman MA, Pomerantz WJ, Schubert CJ. Implementing and evaluating an injury prevention curriculum within a pediatric residency program. J Trauma. 2010;69(4 Suppl):S239–44.

32. Sacks JJ, Kresnow M, Houston B, Russell J. Bicycle helmet use among American children, 1994. Inj Prev. 1996;2(4):258–62.

33. DuBois D, Baldwin S, King WD. Accuracy of weight estimation methods for children. Pediatr Emerg Care. 2007;23(4):227–30.

34. Lubitz DS, Seidel JS, Chameides L, Luten RC, Zaritsky AL, Campbell FW. A rapid method for estimating weight and resuscitation drug dosages from length in the pediatric age group. Ann Emerg Med. 1988;17(6):576–81.

35. Trauma ACoSCo. Resources for optimal care of the injured patient. American College of Surgeons, Committee on Trauma; 1990.

36. Kelleher DC, Jagadeesh Chandra Bose RP, Waterhouse LJ, Carter EA, Burd RS. Effect of a checklist on advanced trauma life support workflow deviations during trauma resuscitations without pre-arrival notification. J Am Coll Surg. 2014;218(3):459–66.

37. Parsons SE, Carter EA, Waterhouse LJ, Fritzeen J, Kelleher DC, O'Connell KJ, et al. Improving ATLS performance in simulated pediatric trauma resuscitation using a checklist. Ann Surg. 2014;259(4):807–13.

38. Nolan B, Zakirova R, Bridge J, Nathens AB. Barriers to implementing the World Health Organization's Trauma Care Checklist: a Canadian single-center experience. J Trauma Acute Care Surg. 2014;77(5):679–83.

39. Steinemann S, Berg B, Skinner A, DiTulio A, Anzelon K, Terada K, et al. In situ, multidisciplinary, simulation-based teamwork training improves early trauma care. J Surg Educ. 2011;68(6):472–7.

40. Kellicut DC, Kuncir EJ, Williamson HM, Masella PC, Nielsen PE. Surgical team assessment training: improving surgical teams during deployment. Am J Surg. 2014;208(2):275–83.

41. Tobin JM, Grabinsky A, McCunn M, Pittet JF, Smith CE, Murray MJ, et al. A checklist for trauma and emergency anesthesia. Anesth Analg. 2013;117(5):1178–84.

42. Sewell M, Adebibe M, Jayakumar P, Jowett C, Kong K, Vemulapalli K, et al. Use of the WHO surgical safety checklist in trauma and orthopaedic patients. Int Orthop. 2011;35(6):897–901.

43. Holcomb JB, Wade CE, Michalek JE, Chisholm GB, Zarzabal LA, Schreiber MA, et al. Increased plasma and platelet to red blood cell ratios improves outcome in 466 massively transfused civilian trauma patients. Ann Surg. 2008;248(3):447–58.

44. Stinger HK, Spinella PC, Perkins JG, Grathwohl KW, Salinas J, Martini WZ, et al. The ratio of fibrinogen to red cells transfused affects survival in casualties receiving massive transfusions at an army combat support hospital. J Trauma. 2008;64 Suppl 2:S79–85 discussion S.

45. Shaz BH, Dente CJ, Nicholas J, MacLeod JB, Young AN, Easley K, et al. Increased number of coagulation products in relationship to red blood cell products transfused improves mortality in trauma patients. Transfusion. 2010;50(2):493–500.

46. Tuckman BW, Jensen MAC. Stages of small-group development revisited. Group Organ Manag. 1977;2(4):419–27.

47. Geelhoed GW. Surgery and healing in the developing world. Georgetown, TX: Landes Bioscience; 2001.

48. Joint Trauma System Director. United States Army Institute of Surgical Research. Joint Trauma System Clinical Practice Guidelines. 4 Dec. 2014. Web. 1 Nov. 2014.

49. Baker MS. Tactical combat casualty care. Mil Med. 2008;173(3):iv.

50. Salomone JP, Pons PT, McSwain NE, eds. PHTLS Prehospital Trauma Life Support: Military Version. 6th ed. St. Louis: Mosby, Inc., 2007. Print.

51. American College of Surgeons. Committee on Trauma. ATLS, advanced trauma life support program for doctors. 7th ed. Chicago, IL: American College of Surgeons; 2004.

52. Savitsky E, Eastridge B, United States. Department of the Army. Office of the Surgeon General, Borden Institute (U.S.). Combat casualty care: lessons learned from OEF and OIF. Fort Detrick, MD: Office of the Surgeon General, Department of the Army; 2012.

53. Boffard KD. International Association of Trauma Surgery and Intensive Care. Manual of definitive surgical trauma care. 3rd ed. London: Hodder Arnold; 2011.

54. Chameides L, Ralston M, American Academy of Pediatrics, American Heart Association. Pediatric advanced life support: provider manual. Dallas, TX: American Heart Association; 2011.

55. Fuenfer MM, Creamer KM, Lenhart MK, eds. Pediatric surgery and medicine for hostile environments. Falls Church, Virginia: Office of The Surgeon General, United States Army; Washington DC: Borden Institute, Walter Reed Army Medical Center; Fort Sam Houston, Texas: US Army Medical Department Center and School, 2010. Print.

Difficult Triage Decisions in the Combat or Austere Environment

4

Matthew J. Martin and Matthew J. Eckert

4.1 Setting and Background

The material and cases described in this chapter were derived from the experiences of the authors on multiple combat deployments in support of Operation Enduring Freedom and Operation Iraqi Freedom from 2005 to 2015.

4.2 Mass Casualty Scenarios and Difficult Triage Decisions

4.2.1 Severe Abdominal Injuries and Limited Resources

Case: A severely wounded local national solder arrives by helicopter at a Combat Support Hospital in Iraq. He was hit with several rounds from a .50 caliber machine gun in the abdomen and was unconscious and hypotensive in the field. On arrival you note that half of his lower abdominal wall is missing with exposed viscera and active bleeding (Fig. 4.1). He is the only patient that you

M.J. Martin, M.D. (✉) • M.J. Eckert, M.D.
Department of Surgery, Madigan Army Medical
Center, 9040 Fitzsimmons Avenue, Tacoma, WA
98431, USA

Trauma and Acute Care Surgery Service,
Legacy Emanuel Medical Center, Portland, Oregon
e-mail: matthew.j.martin16.mil@mail.mil

have in the emergency medical treatment tent at this time, and he is triaged in the "Immediate" category for clearly having life-threatening injuries. Within 2 min of arrival he goes into cardiac arrest with no palpable pulses but with some organized cardiac electrical activity on the monitor. You begin resuscitation and perform an emergency department thoracotomy with an aortic cross clamp. He now has clearly organized cardiac activity and a weakly palpable carotid pulse. He is taken immediately for surgical exploration and continued resuscitation with blood products. In the operating room you start on his abdomen while anesthesia continues to resuscitate with blood products. He has so many injuries you don't know where to begin, but you get to work and are finally gaining ground when the pagers go off again. Seven "urgent surgical" patients are inbound, and your anesthesiologist tells you he just hung the tenth unit of blood, which is half of your total blood supply. You will be unable to get any resupply of blood products for at least 12 h due to weather conditions. All eyes in the operating room are now on you—what are you going to do? Do you continue and exhaust your unit's blood supply on this patient with a low probability of survival? Do you stop and re-triage this patient as "expectant" even though he is currently alive on the OR table, allowing him to die so that you can tend to the other injured patients? [1].

Discussion: Although triage is certainly discussed and practiced in the civilian environment,

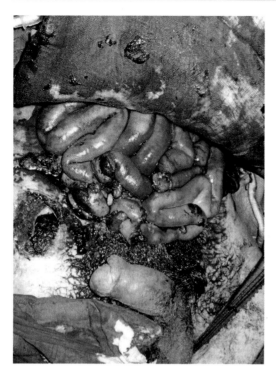

Fig. 4.1 Preoperative photo of the patient showing a massive abdominal wound secondary to a high-powered and high-velocity gunshot wound

these types of very tough life and death decisions about constrained resources and levels of care are very rarely encountered. Even if a particular civilian center has constrained resources, they almost always have the ability to rapidly obtain the needed resources (resupply of blood products for example) or to transfer the patient to a higher level of care. The types of decisions regarding the provision, withholding, and withdrawal of aggressive care are ones rarely faced within the typical civilian practice, but will be frequently encountered in the deployed setting or during natural disasters when the numbers of patients clearly outmatch the available resources.

Triage is a frequently discussed but often misunderstood process that bears little importance in most trauma scenarios involving one or a few patients with ample resources and personnel available to provide whatever care they need. Alternatively, triage in the resource-constrained environment and with overwhelming numbers of patients is the critical foundation to achieving optimal outcomes and maximize salvage of life

with minimal morbidity. For instance, a small community hospital may be the first facility to be able to provide care of a bus accident involving 20 or more passengers. Figure 4.2 outlines some of the key concepts and lessons learned about triage and MASCAL scenarios from the past decade of combat operations, as well as multiple civilian MASCAL events.

There are several common misconceptions that often lead to poor triage decisions that bear mention. First is that triage does not start with a sorting of patients, or "sifting and sorting" as it is often referred. Triage starts with a rapid but detailed assessment of the situation, including your capabilities and resources, followed by as much preparation as possible prior to patient arrival. This should focus on questions like the following: How many open ER beds do I have? How many providers and what specialties do I have available? How many OR beds are open and available for patients that need immediate surgery? How much surge capacity do I have? What options do I have for the transfer of select patients? What are the security concerns and the local tactical situation? All of this information is critical to have before you can effectively decide how to triage incoming patients and what types of injuries you can or cannot care for at that time. In the military, we have now coined the term for this process the "Zero Survey," as it needs to occur before even the primary ATLS survey of an injured patient.

Another common mistake is to base triage primarily on the severity of injury, with the worst injured triaged first and then following in descending order of severity. Triage is not about doing everything for everybody, and doing this in proportion to the nature and severity of injuries. Triage is about maximizing the number of optimal outcomes in any given MASCAL scenario, and requires very high level decision making that considers both sides of the equation regarding resources versus patient needs and chance of survival. Closely linked to this misperception is the idea that anyone can do the triage job, and the outdated concept of making the "least valuable" provider the senior triage officer (STO). The large body of experience in battlefield medicine

MASCAL and Triage Decisions: Top 10 Lessons Learned

1. No one is safe! MASCAL events are only likely to increase in frequency, and can occur ANYWHERE and at ANY TIME (usually the worst place/time), so be prepared.

2. The first phase of triage is preparation, so assess your assets and capabilities as these can significantly change your triage decisions

3. Appropriate scene triage can turn a potential MASCAL event into a much more orderly Mass Casualty event (example: the Boston Marathon bombing)

4. The most important job is the senior Triage Officer; this should be an experienced and trusted provider with trauma expertise and who works well with others

5. An organized security plan is essential to protect personnel, limit entrance of non-essential personnel, and control entry points

6. MASCAL execution is all about patient flow and throughput; establish a one-way flow pattern and disposition patients out of the ER as soon as possible

7. Establish a separate area for the minimally injured (aka "walking wounded"), either in the ER or preferably in a separate area; outpatient clinics are often ideal locations

8. Hemorrhage control is the initial priority, followed by airway and breathing issues

9. Minimize unnecessary imaging! Extremity xrays, spine CTs, etc. are not needed in the initial evaluation

10. The Triangle of Success: Leadership and Expertise are the critical foundation that must be present for successful MASCAL care, but they will not suffice without TRAINING and REHEARSAL.

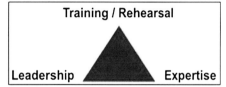

Fig. 4.2 Top ten lessons learned in triage and MASCAL management

has taught the importance of initial triage in setting the stage for success or failure of a MASCAL event. In fact the STO should be one of the more senior, mature, and knowledgeable providers, preferably a trauma surgeon or emergency medicine physician. Outside of the military setting, the importance of active and expert triage has been demonstrated to be a key factor in improving outcomes and minimizing preventable deaths in civilian MASCAL events (Fig. 4.3) [2].

There are several universal aspects to performing good triage. The first is to pick a triage system for your facility or group and ensure that everyone is thoroughly trained in using and understanding the system. The purpose is to put the patients into defined categories to prioritize their care. There are many well-described triage systems available to choose from, with the most common being the SALT system, the START system, and the DIME (delayed, immediate, minimal, and expectant) system used by the US military and most NATO allies (Fig. 4.4) [1, 3–5]. All of these systems follow a similar protocol of sorting patients into simplified categories that determine their priority of care. This typically includes categories for immediate or urgent care (life- or limb-threatening but correctable injuries), delayed (significant injuries present but not immediately life or limb threatening), minimal (minor injuries, frequently called the "walking wounded"), and expectant (non-survivable injuries or requires life-saving resources that are not available). It is critical to the success of any mass casualty event that all of the providers and key team members understand the triage criteria and meanings, and also are intimately familiar with the local MASCAL plan. This should be a detailed document that outlines the plan for triage and initial assessment, patient flow and location of care, priorities for resource utilization,

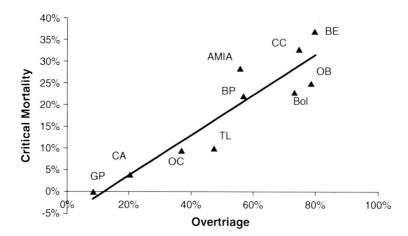

Fig. 4.3 Graph showing critical mortality (*Y*-axis) as a function of the degree of overtriage (*X*-axis) for civilian MASCAL events. The critical mortality increases directly with the degree of overtriage that was identified on review of the initial triage decisions. Reprinted with permission from Frykberg ER. Medical management of disasters and mass casualties from terrorist bombings: how can we cope? J Trauma 2002;53(2):201–12

Triage and Evacuation Categories

- Standard NATO nomenclature is recommended, often called "DIME"
  - **Delayed** (yellow tag) – may be life-threatening, but intervention may be delayed for several hours with frequent reassessment – (fractures, tourniquet-controlled bleeding, head or maxillofacial injuries, burns)
  - **Immediate** (red tag) – immediate attention required to prevent death – usually "AABC" issue – airway, arterial bleed, ventilation, circulatory
  - **Minimal** (green tag) – ambulatory, minor injuries such as lacerations, minor burns or musculoskeletal injuries – can wait for definitive attention
  - **Expectant** (black tag) – survival unlikely, such as extensive burns, severe head injuries

- Triage categories differ from Medical Evacuation categories :
  - **Urgent** – save life or limb, evacuate within 2 hours
  - **Urgent surgical** – same but must go to higher Level surgical capability
  - **Priority** – evacuate within 4 hours, or may deteriorate into urgent
  - **Routine** – evacuate within 24 hours to continue medical treatment
  - **Convenience** – administrative movement

Fig. 4.4 The DIME triage system used by NATO (*top*) and the NATO medical evacuation categories (*bottom*). With kind permission from Springer Science + Business Media: Lammie J, Kotora J, Riesberg J. Combat triage and mass casualty management in front line surgery: a practical approach. Martin MJ, Beekley A, eds. Springer, New York; 2011

mobilization of hospital assets and surge capacity, security and crowd control plan, decontamination activities for suspected or known chemical/biologic/radiologic agent use, transfer and evacuation plans, and all contingency plans in the event of possible complicating factors (power loss, damage to facility, etc.). And most importantly, even the most detailed MASCAL plan is worthless unless the personnel know it and have undergone effective and realistic training drills at regular intervals.

As demonstrated in these scenarios, triage is also not a static or one-time process, and even after a patient has been triaged to a certain category they may require re-triaging to a different category if there is a significant change either to their clinical status or to the available resource pool. A common example of this includes a patient who initially appears stable and minimally injured but then either decompensates or has an unsuspected severe injury identified. This will happen in even the best triage systems, and the triage officer needs to be flexible and immediately re-triage these patients to the appropriate level. Alternatively, there may be patients triaged to the most urgent category, but then have injuries identified that are non-survivable or that are beyond the scope of available care (Fig. 4.5) [6]. These are most commonly severe head/brain injuries and massive thermal injuries (see the next case for an example of a severe burn triage decision). Finally, as demonstrated in this case, the scenario may rapidly change and force you to have to make a very tough decision based on limited or imperfect information. Not infrequently the answer will be that you cannot provide aggressive care or need to cease aggressive care and re-triage the patient as an "expectant" casualty. This is most common when a patient has a low probability of survival or functional recovery and continued efforts at care and resuscitation may exhaust your limited supply. The case initially described illustrates such a scenario, with initial very aggressive management of the patient when he was the only casualty at the facility, but then is subsequently downgraded to "expectant" due to both the nature and severity of injuries as well as the likely continued massive transfusion requirement that would have exhausted the local blood bank and compromised the care of patients with survivable injuries.

These difficult triage scenarios are typically made with imperfect and incomplete information, and also are based on a general estimate or gestalt of the likelihood of survival. Without any exact criteria or evidence-based guidelines on which to base these decisions, the responsible provider is left to rely on their individual judgment and prior experience. In addition, they are often required to be made in a chaotic and rapidly evolving environment that may further confuse the picture. Finally, there are usually multiple providers and ancillary staff involved with the ongoing care of the patient, and the opinion about how to triage the patient might not be universally agreed upon by all team members. We have found that involving all of the key team members in these decisions to be an incredibly useful practice that helps avoid conflicts, misunderstandings, and feelings of guilt after the decision has been made. In the case described above, the operating surgeon stated a summary of the current status ("I don't think these injuries are survivable and we are burning through all of our blood products") and then asked for input from the team members ("Do you see any hope in continuing? Do you have any other ideas before we change to expectant care?"). Consensus was rapidly obtained to halt all aggressive care efforts and conserve resources for the multiple incoming patients, and the patient was transitioned to expectant status with comfort measures provided.

4.2.2 Difficult Triage Decision in a Case of Severe Burns

"Above all, let us remember that our duty to our patients ends only with their death, and that in the preceding hours there is much that we can do for their comfort. At the very least, we can stand by them." Alfred Worcester, 1855–1951

Case: A 48-year-old Afghani male awakens early to start the morning fire outside his family home in southern Afghanistan. Using an accelerant mixture of oil and diesel fuel he dowses the wet debris of the trash pile and lights it, only to be consumed in flames. Quickly smothered in a blanket by his family, the man sustains extensive burn injury to most of his body, sparing his face. Approximately 6 h after injury the patient and his family arrive by foot at a US military forward operating base with a small surgical team. The patient is quickly taken to the treatment area

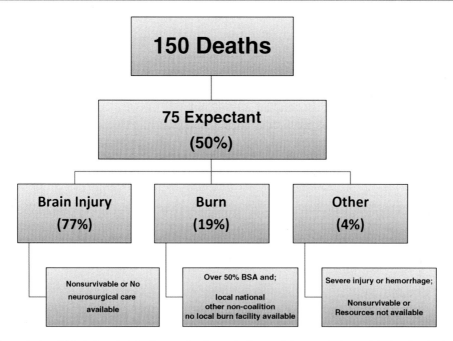

Fig. 4.5 Analysis of 150 in-hospital deaths at a Combat Support Hospital over 1 year [6]. Note that 50 % of these were managed as "expectant" and consisted of primarily head injury and burn patients. With kind permission from Springer Science+Business Media: Rush R, Martin M. Expectant and end of life care in a combat zone in front line surgery: a practical approach. Martin MJ, Beekley A, eds. Springer, New York; 2011

where initial examination and resuscitative measures are begun. Peripheral venous access fails and a subclavian central venous line is placed. Small doses of intravenous ketamine are used for analgesia while he is intubated for airway protection due to oral soot and auditory wheezing. Careful attention to use of warmed irrigation and ambient warming measures is initiated while completely exposing the burns and removing sloughing skin. After complete exposure, his estimated total body surface area burn is 70 %. With no capacity for evacuation to a civilian or military burn center and a lack of resources to adequately care for a severe burn injury at the forward medical facility or in the local civilian hospitals, the providers are now facing the difficult decision of what to do for this patient.

Discussion: The principles of initial burn injury management in both civilian and military casualties are the same. However, extensive burn injury or other catastrophic injury in the setting of austere environments, zones of conflict, and medically underserved/under resourced nations necessitates appropriate and humane triage discussions whenever evacuation to higher levels of care capable of providing for these patients is not available [7–9]. Extensive burn injuries in local national patients encountered by deployed military providers frequently generate a heart-wrenching and labored discussion of appropriate resource allocation. Similar situations are encountered in humanitarian and disaster medical missions.

Medical triage and evacuation categories traditionally recognize separate patient groups based upon time required for intervention to save life, limb or eyesight, as well as the extent of injury severity (Fig. 4.4). These triage categories are typically applied in MASCAL situations to ensure appropriate utilization of medical resources for maximal benefit to salvageable patients. While this framework applies well in the setting of multiple patients, it is difficult to apply to single patients with critical injury. Emotional, ethical, religious, and professional considerations are frequent contributors in the discussion of appropriate care for this unfortunate group of patients. Furthermore, serious but survivable injuries treated in developed and well-resourced settings may be non-survivable in the austere and under-resourced environments. Providers unfamiliar with the constraints and limitations outside their normal practice may find medical decision making in the austere setting very difficult.

Existing data from civilian disaster situations involving the care of burn patients may be used to extrapolate mortality estimates for burn injuries in austere environments, but these data do not account for lack of medical resources, pre-existing disease, or malnutrition that may be encountered among these populations [10]. A burn surface area threshold of > 50 % in civilian casualties in war zones with the aforementioned limitations appears to correlate with near 100 % mortality [1]. Applying the survivability that can be obtained in modern and fully resourced medical centers is inaccurate in the austere environment, and makes decision making all the more difficult when faced with these scenarios. In those cases where deployed forward medical treatment facilities have attempted to provide definitive burn care to patients with more than 50 % body surface area burns, the results have been uniformly dismal with the patients dying either from sepsis or from multi-system organ failure.

While survival may be beyond reasonable expectation in severe burn injury in the austere environment, humane care and attention to comfort measures are typically well within the capacity of medical teams. Once the non-survivable condition is recognized, emphasis upon comfort care should be paramount, for the well-being of the patient, family, and providers. An example of comfort care orders from a deployed military medical team are shown in Fig. 4.6. The decision to extubate an expectant patient, or consciously avoid intubation, frees additional intensive care resources. Appropriate treatment of oral secretions, anxiety and pain management are paramount. With minimal instruction, many of these comfort care measures, aside from medication administration can be provided by nonmedical

personnel or family members, with careful intermittent observation by trained providers. While the intensive care area may provide the easiest location to care for expectant patients, these beds should be prioritized for potentially salvageable patients. A quiet and private area for patient and family is often a more appropriate setting for comfort care [1].

Finally, always remember that these events can take a real toll on the hospital staff and providers. Patients who are brought into the hospital alive and subsequently die will often weigh heavily on providers of all types and experience levels. It is important to know how your people are doing—especially your nursing staff—because they are constantly at the patient's bedside executing the minute-by-minute care plan. In most of these cases friends or family members are not available, and thus it falls on the nurse to both care for and comfort the patient. Another population to pay particular attention to is your younger hospital staff members—the medics, nursing assistants, operating room techs, etc. It is easy to forget that what seems routine to an experienced trauma surgeon or nurse can be emotionally devastating to an 18-year-old medic who is suddenly thrust into the chaos of combat medicine. Having a shared "debriefing" or "team huddle" after these events to discuss what happened, identify areas for potential improvement, and share any concerns or grief can work wonders in terms of your team's emotional well-being [1].

Editor's note: COL Matthew Martin, M.D., is currently serving on Active Duty in the US Army stationed at Fort Lewis, Washington, where he serves as the Trauma Medical Director and Director of Surgical Research. He has completed four combat deployments, where he served in various leadership roles including Chief of Trauma in Baghdad, Iraq, and Commander of a Forward Surgical Team in Afghanistan.

MAJ Matthew Eckert is an Active Duty surgeon serving in the US Army. He completed a fellowship in Trauma and Surgical Critical Care at Vanderbilt University, and now serves as the Associate Trauma Director at Madigan Army Medical Center. Dr. Eckert has served as the Commander for a Forward Surgical Team, and has deployed to Afghanistan in support of Operation Enduring Freedom.

<u>Sample Expectant Care Order Set</u>

Patient Name: ID Number:
Admit to: Expectant Care Area
Diagnosis:
Status: DNR/DNI
Physician: Pager number:

<u>Medications:</u>

1. Morphine sulfate 5mg/10ml   (100 mg in 200 ml)
    step 1: 5 mg iv push q5 minutes until comfort or respiratory rate < 20
    step 2: Start drip, hourly rate at the dose required to achieve comfort in step 1
    step 3: If pain or distress, return to step 1 and treat anxiety as in #

2. Midazolam (Versed)
    step 1: 2-4 mg iv push q30 minutes for anxiety/agitation
    step 2: if continued agitation or frequent dosing, start drip at 4mg/hr and titrate

3. Haldol 5-10 mg q10 minutes for continued agitation

4. Albuterol nebulizer q2 hours for wheezing
5. Scopolamine patch 1.5 mg topically BID as needed for secretions
6. Glycopyrrolate 0.1 mg iv q1 hrs as needed for secretions

<u>Treatments:</u>

1. Titrate oxygen for sats > 92% with maximal support of non-rebreathing mask
2. If intubated, extubate when pain and agitation control achieved as above
3. Stop any previously ordered labs or blood draws
4. Stop any previously ordered radiologic studies
5. Change IV fluids to Normal Saline at 10-20 cc/hr as a driver
6. Remove any unnecessary tubes or lines – nasogastric tube, central lines, etc.
7. Turn off all monitor alarms in the patient's room or area
8. Discontinue visiting hours, family/friends to be present as requested
9. Maintain comfortable environment – quiet, temperature, lighting, positioning
10. Call MD for resp rate > 30, discomfort, agitation, or anxiety not controlled by medications
11. Notify chaplain or other religious support as requested by patient or attendants
12. Notify physician and Patient Administration of patient death

Fig. 4.6 Standardized order set for the management and comfort care of expectant patients at a US Combat Support Hospital. With kind permission from Springer Science+Business Media: Rush R, Martin M. Expectant and end of life care in a combat zone in front line surgery: a practical approach. Martin MJ, Beekley A eds. Springer, New York; 2011

Conflicts of Interest The authors have no conflicts of interest to declare and have received no financial or material support related to this manuscript.

Disclaimer The results and opinions expressed in this chapter are those of the authors, and do not reflect the opinions or official policy of the US Army, the Department of Defense, or any other governmental agency.

References

1. Martin MJ, Beekley A. Front line surgery: a practical approach. New York: Springer; 2011.
2. Frykberg ER. Medical management of disasters and mass casualties from terrorist bombings: how can we cope? J Trauma. 2002;53(2):201–12.

3. Jones N, White ML, Tofil N, et al. Randomized trial comparing two mass casualty triage systems (JumpSTART versus SALT) in a pediatric simulated mass casualty event. Prehosp Emerg Care. 2014;18(3):417–23.

4. SALT mass casualty triage: concept endorsed by the American College of Emergency Physicians, American College of Surgeons Committee on Trauma, American Trauma Society, National Association of EMS Physicians, National Disaster Life Support Education Consortium, and State and Territorial Injury Prevention Directors Association. Disaster medicine and public health preparedness. 2008;2(4):245–6

5. Janousek JT, Jackson DE, De Lorenzo RA, Coppola M. Mass casualty triage knowledge of military medical personnel. Mil Med. 1999;164(5):332–5.

6. Martin M, Oh J, Currier H, et al. An analysis of in-hospital deaths at a modern combat support hospital.

J Trauma. 2009;66 Suppl 4:S51–60. discussion S60–51.

7. Lairet KF, Lairet JR, King BT, Renz EM, Blackbourne LH. Prehospital burn management in a combat zone. Prehosp Emerg Care. 2012;16(2): 273–6.

8. Stout LR, Jezior JR, Melton LP, et al. Wartime burn care in Iraq: 28th Combat Support Hospital, 2003. Mil Med. 2007;172(11):1148–53.

9. Barillo DJ, Cancio LC, Hutton BG, Mittelsteadt PJ, Gueller GE, Holcomb JB. Combat burn life support: a military burn-education program. J Burn Care Rehabil. 2005;26(2):162–5.

10. Taylor S, Jeng J, Saffle JR, Sen S, Greenhalgh DG, Palmieri TL. Redefining the outcomes to resources ratio for burn patient triage in a mass casualty. J Burn Care Res. 2014;35(1):41–5.

Removal of Unexploded Ordinance

5

John S. Oh

5.1 Introduction

In April 2006 in Afghanistan, our Forward Surgical Team was alerted that we would receive multiple casualties. The troops were still engaged in combat; therefore, we waited anxiously for them to arrive. One of the medics from our battalion aid station ran messages to our surgical facility from the operations center. The description of one patient stood out. He was a young specialist who was "impaled." With what, we did not know at the time, but his vital signs were obviously deteriorating. I started my triage plan before any casualties even arrived. With only one general surgeon and one operating room table, I decided ahead of time that this casualty would be triaged as an "urgent surgical" case. This meant brining him immediately into the facility to begin resuscitation and hemorrhage control. The others were stable, so they could be moved on to another facility.

Hours later, the medical evacuation helicopter finally arrived with the casualties. We immediately took the patient that was "impaled" into our surgical facility. He was covered in massive amounts of gauze dressings and sheets. There was a bulge around his pelvis underneath the dressings. His skin was pale, cold, and diaphoretic, obviously in shock. He was barely conscious. When we moved him inside, we immediately began removing the sheets and cutting away the bandages to see what the extent of his injuries were. He was impaled across his pelvis with a rod, the tail end of which was protruding from the left side of his pelvis. The opposite end of this foreign body went clear across the other side, but did not quite break through the skin.

The tail end of the foreign body had stabilizing fins, immediately recognizable as rocket-propelled grenade (RPG). This was quite a shock. Up to this point in the war in Afghanistan, there had been no accounts of victims who had survived being impaled with an RPG. We realized, since the patient was still alive and otherwise in one piece, that we had an unexploded ordnance (UXO) situation. Realizing that we did not know the explosive potential of the UXO and that we needed to immediately treat the patient or he would rapidly die of shock, I proceeded to don my body armor, and evacuated all nonessential personnel from the surgical facility. The bomb disposal team was summoned, and we immediately went to work. I explained to everyone who was left that this could explode at any time, and everyone left in the room was a volunteer and free to leave. To my surprise (and great relief), everyone stayed. What follows is a description of lessons learned and best practices to follow in this most unusual circumstance.

J.S. Oh, M.D., F.A.C.S. (✉)
Department of Surgery, Walter Reed National
Military Medical Center, 8901 Wisconsin Ave,
Bethesda, MD 20905, USA
e-mail: john.s.oh.mil@mail.mil

© Springer International Publishing Switzerland 2016
C.R.B. Lim (ed.), *Surgery During Natural Disasters, Combat,*
Terrorist Attacks, and Crisis Situations, DOI 10.1007/978-3-319-23718-3_5

5.1.1 Background

Worldwide, landmines and UXOs are a substantial health risk. As of 1998, there are approximately 60–70 million landmines scattered over approximately 70 countries [1]. In Afghanistan alone, there are an estimated 5–7 million landmines as of 1997 [2]. Afghanistan leads the world in landmine and UXO casualties with a case fatality rate of 50–55 % [1]. While many of these were placed in the 1980s during the Soviet occupation, the current conflict between Taliban and Allied forces has resulted in increased numbers of mines and UXOs in Afghanistan [3]. Rarely, as a result of combat, a victim may become impaled by military ordnance. A case series published in 1999 described 36 patients from World War II to through the Somalia conflict that were impaled with a UXO [4]. All of these casualties were impaled with a missile-type projectile. Half of the injuries were caused by M79 grenade launched 40 mm rounds, 12 by mortars (48–82 mm), and four by RPGs. A 2.76 in. rocket and a pen flare caused one injury each. In this series, four patients died before operation. Of the remaining 32 patients, all were operated on and survived without any injuries to any of the treatment staff. Of note, no comprehensive database for these types of injuries existed prior to 2006; therefore the true case fatality rate is most likely underreported. However, this case series investigated and recommended best practices for removal of UXO in a combat hospital setting. These recommendations included triage to a delayed surgical category, appropriate assemblage of personnel and protective equipment, avoidance of electrocautery, defibrillation, and other equipment that may transmit an electrical or magnetic current, isolation of the patient, and minimal manipulation of the UXO. In addition, they recommended an explosive expert, such as a military explosive ordnance specialist or civilian bomb squad personnel, be consulted as early as possible. These recommendations were codified in the War Surgery Manual and used in military medical training scenarios [5].

There have been three cases reported in Afghanistan since 2006. One case involved an approximately 2.75 in. rocket embedded in the scalp. The remaining two cases involved combat-ants that were impaled with an RPG, one in the lower extremity and one intra-abdominal. In all cases, the UXO was successfully removed and the patients survived. In the cases involving an RPG, the large caliber and high-velocity nature of these rounds resulted in large amounts of soft tissue damage and hemorrhage. In all three cases, the UXO was successfully removed during the operation and none of the treatment personnel or equipment was damaged. Each case was unique in the type of munition, severity of injuries, and operational setting. Therefore, significant amounts of flexibility and ingenuity were also required in each case. The fundamentals of management as described in the US Army Institute of Surgical Research Clinical Practice Guideline for Unexploded Ordnance Management dated 7 March 2012 are outlined in detail below [6]. Understanding these fundamentals leads to successful outcomes. These include proper transportation and triage, early identification of the type of ordnance the potential triggering mechanism involved, basic trauma assessment and resuscitation techniques, judicious anesthesia, and expeditious surgery.

5.2 Transportation and Triage

If the patient requires transportation with the ordnance in place, it is essential to properly ground the patient to avoid static electricity from causing the ordnance to trigger and explode. This is particularly important during rotary- or fixed-wing transportation. Aircraft can generate static electrical charges that must be dissipated, particularly prior to landing. It is essential to communicate the clinical scenario with the flight crew to ensure that the static charge is dissipated properly, according to aviation safety regulations. When positioning the patient, they should be extracted and positioned the same way they were found, if possible, to minimize disruption of the ordnance and the trigger mechanism.

Safe removal of unexploded ordnance requires significant coordination with local authorities and the emergency management system. The patient should be transported to a cordoned area, preferably a minimal safe distance (at least 10 m) from the main hospital, if possible. All nonessential personnel should move outside of the cordoned area. The local authorities should be informed that a patient with a UXO is under surgical care at the surgical facility or is due to arrive if prior notification is given, and that a bomb disposal team needs to be notified.

It is imperative that bomb disposal team be contacted and physically participate as part of normal coordination to establish safe distances and landmarks. Furthermore, they will dispose of the UXO after it is removed. Safe routes for transportation of the patient and the UXO once it is removed should be determined as early as possible.

Most importantly, the bomb disposal team will provide their opinion on the likelihood of detonation. This likelihood, in addition to the likelihood of survival, is factored into a risk–benefit analysis for proceeding to surgical intervention. In the author's personal experience, the EOD technicians also directly assisted in removal of the ordnance during surgery. They actively provided input into safe handling and directly provided safe transportation of the UXO after removal.

If possible, triage of the patient should be done outside the actual surgical facility. Ideally, this will be done nearby the main surgical facility but at a safe standoff distance. Safe removal of the UXO should be accomplished in an ancillary surgical site when the risk of detonation is high. This is done to avoid bringing the ordnance into the main operating room and through populated areas. In one instance during US military operations in Afghanistan, the UXO was removed by EOD personnel outside of the operating facility prior to completion of the definitive surgical procedure with an excellent outcome.

In a mass casualty scenario, a patient with an impaled UXO could potentially endanger staff and damage the main surgical facility. A risk–benefit analysis based on the number of casualties and severity of injuries may require that the patient with an impaled UXO be triaged to a delayed or even an expectant category. In cases where the patient is moribund, comfort care should be provided in a safe area away from the main surgical facility. A medical provider should provide adequate sedation and pain relief under the supervision of an explosives specialist.

If an ancillary surgical site could be established outside the main surgical facility, this site should be well lighted and have the necessary anesthetic and surgical equipment available. The floor should be level and large enough to place the operating table or gurney and to position portable X-ray equipment. Once the UXO has been removed, the patient can quickly be moved to the main operating room.

5.3 Ordnance Triggering Mechanisms

A basic understanding of triggering mechanisms for different types of projectiles will allow the surgeon and surgical team to inadvertently avoid causing detonation. As evidenced by previous reports of unexploded munition impalement, the impaled round was a propelled explosive device. These rounds basically consist of a propulsion system, a trigger mechanism, and a main explosive charge.

Triggering mechanisms vary by the type and variety of ordnance and may even vary within the same type of ordnance depending on where the ordnance was manufactured. The trigger, generally located at the tip of the main explosive charge, activates a firing mechanism that impacts onto a percussion cap which activates a detonator. The detonator explodes, thereby igniting the main explosive charge. In cases where the detonator or main explosive charge has not triggered, assume that a malfunction occurred causing the ordnance not to explode on impact. An inadvertent bypassing of the safety or the malfunction can cause the ordnance to explode. All retained ordnance should therefore be considered "armed" or activated to a degree that final triggering of the fuse would cause the ordnance to explode.

The ordnance becomes armed through a variety of mechanisms. One mechanism, typically used in 40 mm tube-launched (M79 or M19) grenades and tube-launched mortars, is based on the number of rotations or spins the grenade completes after leaving the launching tube. Upon impact, a naillike device located in the tip or nose of the device is pushed down into a fissile explosive that then detonates the main explosive charge. Pressure on the nose or tip of the device may trigger the device to explode.

Another trigger mechanism utilizes a piezo-electric crystal. This is most commonly employed in a rocket propelled grenade system. The rocket has a propulsion device and stabilizing fins for flight. The trigger utilizes a piezoelectric crystal which generates an electric charge on impact. This charge ignites the detonator which explodes the main charge. This crystal may be light, electrical, or heat sensitive. These mechanisms mean that either reorienting the patient or shining direct sunlight as well as providing a direct electric current to the device can cause it to fully trigger and explode.

5.4 Assessment and Resuscitation

Once the decision to proceed to treatment is made, the basic trauma assessment and resuscitation routine is followed. During this time, care is taken to protect the treatment team. Minimize traffic and personnel in contact with the patient. In addition to the routine personal protective equipment and sterile technique, ballistic protection must be used when possible. In the military setting, this consisted of a ballistic helmet, eyewear, and vest. In the civilian setting, this would have to be provided by a bomb or explosive disposal team.

Plain radiographs are considered safe with respect to potential inadvertent triggering of the UXO. The patient should not be reoriented to obtain the films, if possible, as any movement can inadvertently complete the triggering mechanism and cause an explosion. Portable radiograph machines should be utilized so the patient does not travel through the hospital. The effects of ultrasound and computed tomography scan on unexploded ordnance are not well documented in the literature [5, 7]. Therefore, the use of these imaging modalities should be delayed until the UXO is safely removed.

5.5 Anesthesia and Surgery

In most cases, general anesthetic will be used for these operations. For stable patients where the ordnance is impaled in an extremity, a nerve block is an acceptable alternative. For intubation, consider avoiding the use of non-depolarzing neuromuscular blockade to avoid the muscle twitches that accompany its administration. Use of supplemental oxygen during the operation should be limited as much as possible to eliminate this as a combustible source in case of detonation and fire.

Adjuncts such as electrical cautery should be avoided due to the transmission of an electrical charge or heat to the trigger mechanism. Likewise, any adjuncts that require an electrical source such as mechanical saws should be avoided in favor of manual saws. Use of mechanical blood warmers, monitors, blood pressure gauges, infusers, or pumps should also be minimized in order to reduce the risk of electrical static discharge [8].

Only utilize personnel that are deemed essential for the safe removal of the UXO. Additionally, all necessary equipment could be laid out in advance of the operation, thereby eliminating the need for an operating room technician. An assistant surgeon should be used only if it is absolutely necessary and the safe removal of the UXO could not be safely accomplished without this assistance or additional expertise.

Final selection of the surgeon(s) to conduct the operation should be left up to the lead surgeon in charge of the operation. It is imperative that the lead surgeon make every effort to limit and eliminate the need for additional staff, thereby minimizing the risk to the surgical team, particularly during a mass casualty scenario. The primary surgical principle is the removal of the UXO by the most expedient means possible. This may require "en bloc" resection of the tissue around the ordnance with amputation of the affected limb above the ordnance if necessary to save the life of the patient and minimize the risk to the treatment team. Simultaneous damage control operation for other injuries should be limited to life and limb preservation surgery. Definitive surgery should be delayed until after the ordnance has been removed.

5.6   Conclusion

This is a rare scenario that is associated with the additional stress of imminent danger to both the patient and the treatment team. Management decisions and priorities are all currently based on case series and expert opinion. Chances for optimal outcomes can be maximized by recognizing the principles of safe munition transportation, handling, operating theater safety, and expeditious surgery. Above all, remain calm. Personnel are your most valuable resource, and they will need firm, steady leadership.

Editors note: COL John Oh, MD is currently on Active Duty in the United States Army. He has served three tours in support of Operations Iraqi and Enduring Freedom. He and an orthopedic surgeon successfully removed the RPG in this patient. There were no injuries or casualties to the surgical team or the helicopter medical evacuation team. The injured soldier received a Purple Heart; and he worked hard at rehabilitation so he could walk to the podium to get it, as he did not want to receive it while in bed or in a wheelchair. His story can be read on his website.

References

1. Injuries associated with landmines and unexploded ordnance. Afghanistan 1997–2002. MMWR. 2003; 52(36):859-862
2. Giannou C. Antipersonnel landmines: facts, fictions, and priorities. BMJ. 1997;315:1453–4.
3. http://www.hrw.org/backgrounder/arms/landmines-bck1011.htm.
4. Lein B, Holcomb J, Brill S, Hetz S, McCrorey T. Removal of unexploded ordnance from patients: a 50-year military experience and current recommendations. Mil Med. 1999;163(3):163–5.
5. Cubano M, Lenhart M. 2013 Weapons effects and war wounds. In: Emergency war surgery manual. 4th edn. Chapt 1. 15–6. Borden Institute, Fort Sam Houston, TX.
6. http://usaisr.amedd.army.mil/clinical_practice_ guidelines.html
7. Schlager D, Johnson T, McFall R. Safety of imaging exploding bullets with ultrasound. Ann Emerg Med. 1996;28(2):183–7.
8. Schwaitzberg SD. Evolution and revolutions in surgical energy. In: Feldman LS, Fuchshuber P, Jones DB, editors. The Fundamental Use of Surgical Energy (FUSE) manual. New York, NY: Springer; 2012.

Hostage Rescue Surgery

6

Michael R. St. Jean

This chapter provides insight into a topic that we all assume to be fortunately rare and *Unusual*. The audience for this particular chapter by definition remains selective. However, the exponential growth of domestic and international terrorism, along with narcotic and human trafficking, has influences in every continent, every major country, down to the level of most major metropolitan centers. The likelihood that the community-based surgeon may someday be faced with challenges of providing resuscitative surgical interventions on a "hostage" rescue victim, on the surface, would seem minuscule. For the moment, if we expand the inclusion criteria, though, the odds percentages begin to creep up. My original perception of the application of this chapter would be for those surgeons in military or government service or surgeons affiliated with relief organizations traveling to politically charged areas as the ones who are likely to be called to assist in the event of a hostage rescue scenario. Upon further reflection, the advent of the continuous satellite national newscast is replete with instances that would meet an expanded, more inclusive

definition of "hostage." Webster's Dictionary full definition of the word "hostage" is:

1. (a) a person held by one party in a conflict as a pledge pending the fulfillment of an agreement, (b) a person taken by force to secure the taker's demands.
2. One that is involuntarily controlled by an outside influence.

A terrorist hostage or prisoner of war would fulfill the categorical definition, but what about the abducted or carjacked motorist? How about the kidnapped spouse or child in a domestic dispute that has gone horribly wrong? What of the illegal alien abandoned in a transit vessel or remote storage container? These are but a few examples of situations that at first glance appear to be cinematic fiction until one attune themselves to the national stage of pervasive violence that touches all aspects of our society. On their own merits, each one of these examples fulfills aspects of Webster's definition. Now the narrow aperture of view in the chapter title expands beyond the first inclinations of distant troubled lands like Iraq, Afghanistan, Syria, or Somalia. Border cities, major port of entry cities, even rural America are witness to these definitions. So with our newly defined patient population we can begin to dissect the pertinent aspects of how treating these patients provides challenges while at the same time, I believe, special privileges.

M.R. St. Jean, M.D., F.A.C.S. (✉)
Eastern Maine Medical Center, Northeast Surgery of Maine, Suite 330, Webber East 417 State Street, Bangor, ME 04401, USA
e-mail: mstjean@emhs.org

© Springer International Publishing Switzerland 2016
C.R.B. Lim (ed.), *Surgery During Natural Disasters, Combat, Terrorist Attacks, and Crisis Situations*, DOI 10.1007/978-3-319-23718-3_6

By way of professional courtesy, let me assure my fellow colleagues that any medical literature investigation, regardless of service, that searches "Hostages and Surgery" or any variation of such, is pointless. Fortunately, the instances of individuals in these particular scenarios requiring surgical resuscitative measures are rare. The Federal Bureau of Investigation (FBI) maintains a database of hostage and barricade incidents. According to the Hostage Barricade Database System (HOBAS), 96 % of the incidents requiring the response of law enforcement agencies do not include a hostage being taken [1]. The Crisis Negotiation Unit (CNU) of the FBI manages the information-rich database. In the 4 % of incidents involving a hostage being taken, approximately 80 % result in no injuries, with 47 % of incidents resulting in the hostage having an influence on the perpetrator(s) to resolve the situation [1]. Crime statistics collated by the FBI for the calendar year 2011 support the notion that metropolitan areas may not be the previously believed mecca for hostage type crises. Of the 5086 bank crimes committed in 2011, only 46 % occurred in metropolitan centers whereas the majority occurred in small cities, towns, and rural areas. Over two hundred acts of violence were performed during these crimes resulting in over thirty hostages being taken. [2] Although geographically these incidents appear to violate our preconceived notions of bucolic suburban society, the resultant injury rates remain thankfully low in comparison. In contrast, the resurgence of extremist ideologies into the previously safeguarded Western societies has proven it to have a more devastating effect. Unfortunately, the outcomes are often tragic as the world was recently witness to in France, as well as in unsuccessful rescue attempts in Somalia and Yemen this past year.

Prior to any discussion on Pre-Rescue preparations, I would be remiss not to address the topic of qualifications for participation as author. In June of 2011, I closed the chapter on my military career that encompassed 25 years of active service in the US Army. The majority of those years were as a community military hospital-based surgeon. As with most of my military surgeon colleagues, I was deployed numerous times to various combat and humanitarian theaters of operations. Over the course of these deployments, I was afforded unique exposure and experience to operations involving our chapter subjects, i.e., *Hostages*. My insight, for lack of a better term, is the result of personal involvement and participation in several scenarios, the majority of which never, thankfully, matriculated to the point of surgical involvement. However, those incidents that resulted in successful rescue and repatriation offer the matrix for this chapter. Being witness to these events alone stirs emotions to this day. Thus the privilege I alluded to above.

By way of retrospective example, the rescue of Private Lynch offers insight into approaches as well as possible lessons learned during the ordeal. I will attempt to revisit this particular rescue as an advisory example through the course of our discussion. Surveillance methods used, as well as pre-rescue planning, centered on technologies that in 2003 were state of the art military grade. Twelve years removed, a quick jaunt through the local electronics supply wonder store would outfit the novice with an array of audiovisual recording/drone module applications to outfit a private clandestine service. These advances are mirrored by similar progress in the level of medical information data storage. Electronic medical record filings in conjunction with global satellite internet or cellular access provide the most remote of providers with a wealth of potential patient specific data to access.

In the preparation phase of her rescue, the lack of background medical data as well as rudimentary intelligence on her condition provided vague details to rescuers. The Task Force presumed the worst and prepared accordingly. The facts as we knew them were that we had a young female in a known state of health and fitness prior to her capture. Now, eight days removed from an ambush and motor vehicle collision. She was also exposed to profound psychological stressors, disoriented, marginal nutrition and hydration support with limited medical interventions of dubious proficiency. Compounding these factors was the overshadowing possibility of mental, physical, and/or sexual abuse, which had been experienced by prior Coalition prisoners of war during the Gulf War. Intelligence gathered from sources prior to launch of the rescue mission offered little in the way of specific injury planning.

Contingency planning like any major surgical intervention revolved around possible complications, unexpected findings and the necessary reactions to said potential variances. Our similarities between military or aviation pre mission planning and perioperative safety have been adopted to foster the paradigm shift in risk recognition reduction strategies present in current surgical theaters. The medical contingency planning for hostage rescue scenarios can be compared to prolonged "Final Verification" or "Time Out" procedures for any major surgical intervention. Utilizing this model allows us to frame the actions around an extreme patient scenario in the contexts that are readily cogent to any current practicing community surgeon. Similarly, the advent of Tactical Emergency Medical Services (TEMS) arose from the application of military principles to the civilian sector by a core group of former military medical providers [2]. The result has been the development of a unique specialty over the last two decades which has resulted in much greater integration of immediate medical resuscitative support personnel into the planning of civilian and military special operations. These personnel are designed to be highly trained and specially equipped to deliver on or near "target" decisive interventions [3–6].

Proximity to the hostage/captive area is utilized as a corollary to risk, denoting decreasing risk with increasing distance from captive area to orient support personnel [5]. Different references may be utilized such as *SAFE/WARM/KILL* zones or *COLD/WARM/HOT* coding [6, 8]. The *COLD or SAFE zone* may relate in the surgical sense to the Pre-op Holding area, the area where information gathering and pre-surgical preparations may occur with the least hindrance. The *WARM zone* would likely relate to the scrub sink—the area where final planning and preparation measures are reviewed in detail for rehearsal before final committal to actions on objective. Lastly, the operational *KILL/HOT zone* would

equate to crossing the threshold into the surgical suite for engagement. Now we can proceed to highlight the necessary objectives of each zone with an eye towards maintaining the operational atmosphere of the tactical scenario.

6.1 Safe/Cold Zone

Perspective allows one to place their surroundings into context. The ability to objectively prepare for an intervention with reduced distractions is a routine occurrence for the average surgeon. Pre-mission planning or crisis intervention negotiations performed in this zone should be centered on information gathering, tertiary center support coordination along with resource consolidation in a safe, sterile, and unencumbered environment. Prior to 1 April, 2003, safe and sterile would be unlikely adjectives for the bomb crater littered airfield we occupied as our pre-mission *COLD zone* site. However, cold was an appropriate although undervalued assessment of the frigid March Iraqi nights. A scorching sun, scurrying scorpions and the odd Fedayeen mortar fire rounded out the list of distractions we faced in coordinating rescue rehearsals. Coordination with a co-located Combat Support Hospital allowed us the luxury of having a tertiary care facility with which to insure adequate medical material supply as well as opportunity for subspecialty consultation if the need presented itself.

Current-day TEMS missions function in the same arena with timely on scene communications to local tertiary medical centers to predetermine mission specific needs or facility specific protocols to allow for unhampered access. These communications are vital to avoid unnecessary command and control conflicts that might arise with the sudden arrival of various tactical, medical, and media personnel during or immediately following rescue efforts. This prerequisite along with the quantum progressive leap in military medical theater support was to be reinforced to me repeatedly during my career.

Over 7 years later, I was standing in a tertiary evacuation hospital in Afghanistan preparing for another hostage rescue mission. The scenery could not have been more diverse from the airfield outside Nasiriyah, Iraq in 2003. The trauma resuscitation area was state of the art with all the amenities of a current Level III accredited trauma center. Indeed the facility had undergone recent renovations and to the casual observer would appear to be a suburb of Denver except for the replacement of the Rocky Mountains with the Hindu Kush. The young female surgeon on call appeared more perplexed by the myriad of dignitaries, media, and security contractors in attendance than by the prospect of potential casualties. No scorpions, no dust and no freezing cold tonight, just a cornucopia of government agencies, relief organizations and reporters. Michael Durant, the helicopter pilot captured by Somali insurgents during the Battle of Mogadishu, referred to these individuals in his book "In the Company of Heroes" as stone touchers [9]. People more enamored with the idea of being around the former hostage than invested in his well-being. As is the case in most trauma resuscitation efforts, the necessity for proximity to the victim needs to be coordinated prior to arrival. Standard operating procedures outlining definitive responsibilities carry over to care of the hostage in the immediate post rescue evaluation and resuscitative efforts. Predetermining the role of all medical personnel involved as well as limiting unnecessary distractions to the team is the trauma director/surgeon's primary initiative.

In regards to viewing the *COLD/SAFE zone* priorities, the ability to gather information as it relates to the hostage condition will require the bulk of effort. Lack of direct access to the hostage prevents accurate health assessments; therefore, alternate means of extrapolating the most up to date condition becomes a multidisciplinary investigation. Psychologists, social workers, crisis negotiators, and even current law enforcement officials may prove invaluable to the medical planning. In recent years, the FBI has begun utilizing specially trained psychologists as integral parts of rescued hostage's repatriation and reintroduction efforts both in USA and overseas [10]. Access to these resources provides the medical team with insight into expected as well as unex-

pected reactions victims might display through the course of their rescue or treatment.

Some of the data required may be readily available—having access to hostage medical records or family members, whether in hand or by electronic access, this can eliminate potential delays in treatment if required urgently. The hostage's current condition may be elucidated through review of recent photo or video releases with the assistance of forensic analysis if available. Known factual elements such as length of captivity may provide little actionable intelligence unless they are augmented by hostage-specific related details. Is the hostage injured? If so, how severely? Is the hostage being fed and given adequate hydration regularly? What are the conditions of their captivity—sensory deprived, isolated, beaten, or tortured? What is their emotional state? Have they been victims of violence or abuse in the past that may indicate their ability to sustain these conditions? What is the hostage's impression or outlook on their condition? All of these factors will play some role in the successful post rescue treatment and eventual rehabilitation of the hostage victim. Approaching all of these questions and others with a coordinated multidisciplinary team maximizes the likelihood of uneventful post rescue transition with victim-focused recovery.

As stated earlier, the incidence of physical trauma in the majority of hostage scenarios is relatively low [5, 7]. Recent terrorist related incidents overseas have seen tragic endings with no role for surgical or medical intervention. With this in mind, how does the injured hostage who is successfully rescued represent an unusual situation for the community or military surgeon? As surgeons, we are all highly trained and compassionate to our patients. We all want our patients to experience minimal discomfort as well as speedy recoveries from our procedures or interventions. However, what we are least prepared for or capable of mitigating is the extreme emotional and psychological rollercoaster that these particular patients have endured prior to our introduction. Despite our best efforts at identifying these stressors prior to rescue, the full complement of their impact on the victim may not manifest until well after the physical recovery.

Prior to rescue or release, some semblance of the potential for psychological impact may be apparent. In the Gulf War, video releases depicted captured pilots with significant signs of physical abuse as well as the associated signs of psychological trauma. In depth analysis was not required to appreciate that the level of psychological impact of their treatment would outlast the temporary nature of their wounds. Similarly with Private Lynch, the details of her physical state, although rudimentary in nature, were overshadowed by concerns for potential physical, psychological, or sexual abuse. Psychologists specifically trained to interact with victims of hostage-taking or protracted physical and sexual abuse were not readily available on the battlefield in 2003 as they are integrated now into special operations or TEMS. Being able to anticipate the reaction of a hostage who has persevered through untold indecencies is a quandary but may play an integral role in the preparations of rescue forces tasked with mitigating that reaction in the midst of a chaotic rescue.

In certain instances that reaction may be counterproductive to the mission at hand or jeopardize law enforcement efforts. Depending on the nature of the hostage–perpetrator relationship, the tactics for resolution may place officials or operators in unique circumstances. The phenomenon of the Stockholm Syndrome would be an often cited but equally misunderstood parameter to the hostage crisis resolution. The exact influence of this condition, as well as the incidence of occurrence, is frequently debated but the nature of the dynamic between the hostages versus hostage taker leading to its development are pertinent to our discussion. The syndrome as we have come to understand it today arose as the result of a botched bank robbery in Stockholm, Sweden in 1973 [11]. During the course of the incident the perpetrators and hostages were co-located within the bank vault for several days. As negotiations with law enforcement persisted, the hostages became increasingly sympathetic to the robbers' plight. This persisted beyond the resolution of the

incident with hostages testifying on behalf of the robbers at trial as well as becoming romantically involved in the case of one of the robbers and hostages. Over the course of study of this case, the definition of the syndrome has evolved to require specific criteria. In general terms, the syndrome can be categorized as a paradoxically positive relationship between the hostage and the perpetrators that may appear irrational based on the potentially violent nature of the incident [12, 13]. Commonalities do tend to exist when these cases are reviewed. Typically, victims were kept isolated, directly threatened in some way, had opportunities to either escape or be removed from captivity but failed to do so, and demonstrated sympathy towards their captors post incident [11].

In 1995, Graham expounded a set of four inclusion criteria after reviewing nine various groups of victimized individuals: (1) that there exists a perceived threat to survival and belief that the threat will be carried out, (2) that the captives perceive some small kindness from the captor in the context of terror, (3) that the hostage experiences isolation from perspectives other than those of the captor, and (4) that the hostage has a *perceived* inability to escape [14]. In the event of prolonged captivity, the sensory deprivation of isolation in conjunction with continued exposure to unhygienic conditions, dehumanization, threats of death or physical abuse leads to behaviors aimed at mitigating the wrath of the captors [15].

The development of the Stockholm Syndrome may in fact have its origins in an evolutionary survival adaptation. Research in male chimpanzees has shown that the behaviors of entrapped individuals may be biologically based in the need to preserve the group dynamic. Male chimpanzees live in small bachelor groups for life with strict dominance hierarchies. A dominant male challenging a subordinate may be met with aggressive resistance but this will only lead to further retaliation. The subordinate is trapped in the group lest he be banished and unable to enter into another foreign bachelor group. Likewise other members of the group would be unwilling to offer comfort to the subordinate at the expense of retaliation from the dominant male. Thus the only course of action for the subordinate is to seek refuge in the company of his tormentor. A conditional reconciliation results with the subordinate's *reverted escape* to the lesser role and posturing of submission [16]. Identifications of these appeasement behaviors among humans would seem unlikely given the contrasting nature of a society marked by a larger, dual-sex, multigenerational dynamic with an eye towards social equality. However, in the isolation of a hostage scenario, the hostage may have reverted escape to their oppressors as the only *perceived* option. Attempts to do otherwise or seek solace amongst other hostages may spawn further retaliation [16]. So with these criteria in mind, a more accurate determination of the likelihood of the incidence of this syndrome in hostage scenarios would logically lead one to believe the occurrence to be common.

Actually, the incidence would appear to be less common and more dependent on the emotional intensity of the scenario rather than the protracted captivity as a variable. Along with a lack of physical abuse the emotional intensity combines to create a favorable environment for the development of the syndrome [13]. So on the surface, the development of these types of paradoxical relationships would appear to be at odds to the ultimate goal of safe hostage recovery. In fact, the basis of its development portends that the hostage would be more likely to be released or rescued unharmed. Crisis negotiators view this as a positive movement despite the fact that the hostages often display emotions of distrust, anger or resentment towards law enforcement similar to their captors. In order for the hostages to develop positive feelings towards their captors, the captors by definition must initiate some *perceived* kindness towards the hostages. In so doing the captors begin to humanize the hostages. This provides the crisis negotiators with the psychological ammunition to exploit the captors by furthering their own feelings towards the hostages. Identification of the hostages, referring to them by name or family associations increases the hostage's chances of survival [13]. Whether this be through positive reinforcement with the captors or providing a critical moment of hesitation that would allow doubt to prevent a harmful act against their hostages.

As reviewed above, the likelihood of this syndrome developing would have to be inverse to the rate of violence perpetrated against the hostages. In the 1985 hijacking of TWA Flight 847, the passengers were subjected to repeated death threats and beatings, which resulted in the death of one passenger, unceremoniously dumped on the tarmac. After eventual rescue 10 days later, the majority of the passengers expressed no signs of Stockholm Syndrome but rather relief at their rescue as the violence of their captors reinforced their belief that their survival would be dependent on the authorities.

The assimilation of all these factors is given independent merit in the pre-mission planning. Understanding the mental and emotional stability of the hostage prior to rescue affords the team with advantages the captors may not appreciate. These factors need to be risk stratified in any rescue operation plan as often they may alter the rescue team's actions unless considered as an integral part of the preparations.

6.2 Warm Zone

In all actuality this represents the final position of any surgical assets or response elements. In modern TEMS applications and all but the most extreme military units, this zone is for final staging and preparations. Surgical support either through civilian tertiary care or forward surgical assets on the battlefield will reside in this zone to provide needed surgical lifesaving interventions. Ideally this should be within a radius of extraction of under 60 min from the *HOT/KILL zone* to provide lifesaving interventions related to penetrating trauma in the civilian sector [6, 11]. Military medical doctrine in theater typically aimed for overlapping areas of surgical coverage to be within one hour flying evacuation time to a surgical facility from point of injury. Insuring adequate surgical support on location through coordination of local facilities, i.e., blood bank, transportation or specialty care availability prior to mission launch are paramount during this phase. All information gathered to this point is of little value without the capability to provide appropriate timely surgical support. With regard to Private Lynch, intelligence gained during the *SAFE zone* planning allowed the pre staging of necessary equipment and resources to insure no delay with extraction or if immediate surgical intervention was needed that access surgical suites would not be hindered.

Similarly, physically protecting the hostages during the rescue needs to be considered. For instance, providing ballistic eyesight and hearing protection to hostages during course of rescue needs to be coordinated at this zone. In an urban civilian environment this may be of little consequence as resources will be readily available. However, if in a remote foreign location, that is additional gear that may need to be carried in by rescue operators, contingency planning for actions or complications during the conduct of the operation may require additional extraction capabilities to be configured. Is the hostage physically able to support themselves through the process? Is the hostage ambulatory or bed ridden due to injury or cumulative deconditioning? Small details for an urban special operations unit may be of minor consequence given the proximity to additional personnel. For a military or government entity coordinating the release or rescue from a remote foreign mountainside or desert, the result may be a risk multiplier.

Communication with the medical personnel entering the *HOT zone* will be priority during these final rehearsals. Comfort in their capabilities as well as understanding the role they play in any treatment options that may arise during the operation. Clarity in defining options for the responders or paramedics will alleviate hesitation on their part that would otherwise potentially jeopardize an injured hostage. On the 1 April 2003 rescue, the option for more robust surgical presence was negated by command concerns for tactical capability and safety. Here is where the advent of TEMS and the maturation of military medical resuscitation have created a paradigm shift in the survivability of patients with penetrating trauma over the last decade. The benefits of a

generation of surgeons being trained and vetted in the auspices of military triage, damage control surgery and rapid extraction along the continuum of care have pressed beyond the borders of military medicine. Major metropolitan trauma centers throughout the country have embraced these individuals and their collective lessons learned. I can personally recall over half a dozen prior military surgeons who now serve in these centers as chief of trauma services that employ these concepts successfully. The benefits expand to the evacuation realm as well.

The identification of rapid evacuation out of military theater hospitals to medical centers in Europe or the USA, often within a matter of days after the injury, was key and helped to reduce the rates of wounded mortality. This resulted in the expansion of civilian-based globally capable evacuation companies. In the 2003 mission, we had the luxury of dedicated evacuation platforms out of a relatively intact military airfield. Today there are companies with services offered to insure medical, security, or combined extraction from across the globe with 24/7 online or telephonic medical support by trained paramedics and allied to the finest medical universities in the country.

The extraction phase of any rescue operation often presents the greatest risk. The adrenaline of an emotionally charged rescue is abated by an emotional hangover that robs the senses of the acuity and attention to detail that fostered the success. Metropolitan and suburban communities have access to dedicated ambulance and critical care capable aircraft. Companies like Global Rescue (www.globalrescue.com) and Ripcord (www.ripcordtravelprotection.com) can provide disaster planning, medical evacuation, and/or security rescue for corporate, business, or casual travelers from nearly any point on the globe to a hospital of their choice. These companies are staffed by highly qualified, specially trained former special operations soldiers and sailors with real world experience in the aspects of this chapter. Coordination prior to travel with medical clearance and support services insure a level of security that is utilized by the likes of National Geographic, the US Ski Team and numerous globally active organizations. Similarly, the FBI has begun forward deployment of victim advocacy associates along with psychologists trained in the management of high stress conflicts to assist with repatriation efforts [10]. Given that they no longer reside within the realm of government encumbered military resources, these companies offer individuals a level of security assurance that did not legally exist in the previous decade.

6.3   Hot Zone

Surgical intervention within the rescue *HOT zone* will require coordination with first responders on target. These lifesaving procedures can be performed by these individuals with the Hippocratic intent adapted to the tactical world of Do Not Allow Further Harm! Securing the hostage as primary goal. Stabilization if injured by whatever field expedient Advanced Trauma Life Support intervention while simultaneously distancing the hostage from the *HOT zone*. The presence of dedicated surgical capabilities within the *HOT zone* compounds the risk while creating logistical handicaps for the tactical commander. Extraction to predesignated locations within the *SAFE zone* affords the surgeon with the ability to become patient focused with no inherent concerns for the tactical environment.

As has been mentioned previously, the likelihood of serious injury requiring dedicated damage control surgery historically has been rare. More commonly the rescue operators and the perpetrators represent the highest likelihood for serious injury. The application of damage control surgery principles has been well established for multitudes of traumatic injuries and is beyond the scope of this chapter [17]. Pertinent to this chapter is the appreciation of the holistic nature of response to the injured or non-injured hostage recently rescued/released. Pre mission planning may have identified the need for specific specialty availability such as grief or sexual abuse counselors, victim advocates, psychologist and psychiatrists trained in repatriation debriefing. Family members and friends cannot be over-

looked for their inherent security profile to the hostage. Disorientation compounded by a loud chaotic rescue may result in a hostage being unable to acknowledge their own security despite their removal from a previously hostile environment. A simple gesture, a quick phone call, a familiar face may be the impetus to the sudden emotional realization that their ordeal has been relieved. In the still photograph attached to this chapter, the folded America flag presented to Private Lynch at the moment of her rescue is clutched vigorously. In Afghanistan years later, the stalwart gentleman unharmed throughout his ordeal and rescue broke into tears at the sound of his family on cellular phone. Their ordeals were over, their rescues complete, their healing initiated at the point of that recognition. The surgeon's role, much like that in the operating theater, is to be the facilitator of healing and insuring that whether surgery is required or not the checklist for successful resolution and repatriation has been verified.

6.4   Discussion

As surgeons we are faced with varied and often complex patient presentations on a daily basis. The methodology we utilize to insure quality surgical care delivery revolves about a series of interconnected information pathways. We review radiologic, laboratory, and physical data pertinent to each individual. We adapt our surgical procedural plan to the idiosyncratic nature of the specific patient to insure reproducible high quality of care outcomes. We analyze input from other specialists, providers and family members to formulate a plan or approach that they are comfortable with in regards to patient care. Along the course of the patient's perioperative care it is the surgeon acting as navigator or conductor. Subtle changes in course or condition are adjusted according to various data changes. The application of these principles is the hallmark of sound surgical care. It is that very application that allows the modern surgeon to adapt to the most unusual of situations. The subject of this chapter is yet another albeit infrequent and fortunately unlikely situation that requires the same principle applications. The tenets of a hostage rescue scenario:

1. Prior assessment of the hostage's health, physical conditioning, mental capacity, and degree of injury set into motion a series of preparations.
2. Preparations should be designed with the goal of securing physical well-being for the hostage while targeting reversal of the toxic stimuli they have been exposed to along the course of care. Pre-mission identification of key personnel and resources tasked with protecting the hostage during rescue operations.
3. Pre-mission recognition of the hostage's level of sustained emotional or psychological trauma. Development of cogent treatment plan to expedite their return to a caring environment where they are able to resume a prior "normal" state of health.

This unusual situation when viewed through the analogy of a surgical patient navigation appears very common to the practicing surgeon. Carl Dickens, a former military behavioral psychologist with the FBI's Office of Victim Advocacy believes most hostages have the ability to tap into personal strengths during captivity. "Recovered victims are not broken or damaged," he said. "They are just normal people who have gone through an abnormal situation. It's important for families to recognize that their loved ones may be weak and shaken when they come home—but they are not broken" [10].

6.5 Epilogue

The passage of time, along with this project, has allowed the opportunity to reflect on this scenario with a more circumspect view. Although trained to treat patients of various trauma afflictions, the prospect of interacting with a patient recently traumatized in such a unique fashion posed daunting personal quandaries. "What would I do if …?" "How would I react to …?" These questions filled my mind the hours prior to the rescue mission being launched. Our forces had been brought together in rapid fashion and despite the fact that my medical cohorts were well-rehearsed in our roles, this was in essence the first potential for our interaction in a casualty setting since the onset of the invasion. Being uprooted and given short notice for missions was what we were trained to accomplish at a high standard. In the hours prior to mission launch, we reviewed and game-planned multiple scenarios. Integral for this process was the support of our command. The years have dulled the exact words in my memory but the piercing gaze and frank directive of the rescue mission commander to me that afternoon are still diamond clear. Paraphrasing—"Doc, do whatever it takes but get her home!" With the support of all the assets arrayed and the Task Force commander's directive, there was no mention of media assembled or to be involved. Quite the contrary—the presence of cameras surprised me as well as those immediately present after rescue. We all knew to give them a wide berth. Nothing good could come from an inadvertent comment made in the haste of an adrenaline-charged moment.

One of the most rewarding aspects of that mission would serve as an impetus for future growth and professional development on my part. In April of 2003, I had up until that time only sparse interactions with the operators. Sitting in the stifling sunlight of an Iraqi midday, our team fielded questions from the operators in regards to conditions, as well as possible scenarios during the rescue, as they may affect Private Lynch. As we talked and reviewed intelligence reports, I was struck by the focus and professionalism of these elite operators. Highly trained to unrelenting standards. Mission-focused, but all adept at improvisation on the fly in life-or-death situations, they exhibited the same qualities we strive to achieve as surgeons. Over the years as my privileged interactions expanded with these individuals, a mutual trust and respect was developing. My opinion was valued and regularly sought out during mission planning as well as training exercises back in garrison. Lifelong friendships were forged along the way while developing tactical trauma resuscitation paradigms that have been validated in combat repeatedly. Owing to the relationships that were fostered by my colleagues and myself, the interactions of our tactical medical support planning were integral to future hostage rescue missions. In retrospect, these relationships would have served me better in 2003 when my comfort level with the operators was in its infancy. At the time, the idea of having a surgeon or similarly skilled provider "on target" would have been roundly dismissed. However, in 2015 the role of physicians, including surgeons, in TEMS scenarios has become much less controversial. Indeed, the special operations communities, both military and civilian, have dramatically increased the percentage of medical involvement in both planning and execution of operations. The providers are valued as resources for their immediate on-site capabilities as well as the security of the operators' health. I have been privileged to participate in this latter aspect significantly throughout my career. The comfort of knowing that an individual you train with, sometimes live and share meals with on a daily basis, will be waiting to render lifesaving aid in case of disaster has been personally relayed to me countless times. Those are the memories that remain crystal clear despite the years.

Editor's Note: COL (ret) Michael St. Jean, M.D. served 25 years in the US Army. He served as a trauma surgeon on seven tours in Iraq and Afghanistan, 6 of them with the Joint Special Operations Command. He was one of the lead surgeons on the mission to rescue Private Jessica Lynch.

References

1. Thompson J. "Crisis" or "Hostage" negotiation? The distinction between two important terms. FBI Law Enforcement Bulletin. March 2014.

2. FBI Stats and Services Reports and Publications. Bank crime statistics. FBI Stats and Services Reports and Publications. 2011.

3. Young J, Sena M, Galante J. Physician roles in tactical emergency medical support: the first 20 years. J Emerg Med. 2014;46(1):38–45.

4. Ciraulo D, Barie P, Briggs S, et al. An update on the surgeons scope and depth of practice to all hazards emergency response. J Trauma. 2006;60(6):1267–74.

5. Vainionpaa T, Perajoki K, Hiltunen T, et al. Integrated model for providing tactical emergency medicine support (TEMS): analysis of 120 tactical situations. Acta Anaesthesiol Scand. 2012;56:158–63.

6. Rinnert K, Hall W. Tactical emergency medical support. Emerg Med Clin North Am. 2002;20:929–52.

7. Gildea J, Janssen A. Tactical emergency medical support: physician involvement and injury patterns in tactical teams. J Emerg Med. 2008;4:411–4.

8. Casualty Care Research Center. Counter narcotics and terrorism operational medical support medical director's course handbook. 2nd ed. Bethesda, MD: Casualty Care Research Center. 2012.

9. Durant M, Hartov S. In the company of heroes. New York: Penguin; 2003.

10. FBI Bulletin. Psychologist specializes in kidnapping, hostage cases. FBI Bulletin. April 2014

11. Namnyak M, Tufton N, Szekely R, et al. 'Stockholm syndrome': psychiatric diagnosis or urban myth? Acta Psychiatr Scand. 2008;117:4–11.

12. Cantor C, Price J. Traumatic entrapment, appeasement and complex post-traumatic stress disorder: evolutionary perspectives of hostage reactions, domestic abuse and the Stockholm syndrome. Aust New Zeal J Psychiatr. 2007;41:377–84.

13. De Fabrique N, Romano S, Vecchi G et al. Understanding Stockholm syndrome. FBI Law Enforcement Bulletin. 2007;10–15.

14. Graham D, Rawlings E, Ihms K. A scale for identifying 'Stockholm syndrome' reactions in young dating women: factor structure, reliability and validity. Violence Vict. 1995;10:3–22.

15. Allodi FA. Post-traumatic stress disorder in hostages and victims of torture. Psychiatr Clin North Am. 1994;17:279–88.

16. Cantor C. Evolution and posttraumatic stress: disorders of vigilance and defence. Hove: Routledge; 2005.

17. Nessen S, Lounsbury D, Hetz S. War surgery in Afghanistan and Iraq. A series of cases, 2003–2007. Washington, DC: Office of the Surgeon General; 2008.

Awake Tracheostomy in an Austere Setting

7

Yong U. Choi

7.1 Case Presentation

In the summer of 2003, a young 25-year-old male was involved in an explosion. The explosive device was homemade with various objects placed inside the explosive. One of the projectiles was a large metal fragment that became lodged in the right jaw of the patient. The fragment was protruding from the side of the face and measured approximately 10 in. in length. He was brought to a combat support hospital in the middle of the desert. The hospital was constructed with multiple connecting tents and thus was a very austere environment. The hospital did not have a computed tomography scanner and was outfitted with only plain X-ray equipment. As he was brought in for triage in the emergency department, everyone was surprised at the state of the patient. He was calm and alert. He did not seem scared or worried about his injury. In fact, he seemed to wear the large fragment protruding from his face as a badge of honor. On initial appearance, the injury seemed devastating. However, the patient was very lucky. Remarkably, he did not have any other severe injuries. In fact,

Y.U. Choi, M.D., F.A.C.S. (✉)
Department of Surgery, Dwight D. Eisenhower Army Medical Center, DDEAMC, General Surgery Clinic, 300 Hospital Road, Fort Gordon, GA 30905, USA
e-mail: yuchoi11@gmail.com

he was able to communicate with the medical staff using nonverbal methods. Through this method of communication, he was able to convey the fact that he did not feel pain anywhere else. He was awake and alert and was spontaneously breathing. His vital signs were stable. He had no other obvious injuries on secondary examination aside from a few small lacerations on the arms and face.

A focused abdominal sonography for trauma was performed using a handheld ultrasound device, which was negative. We all commented on the fact of how truly lucky this individual was to only have suffered the injury to his jaw. Due to the large fragment in the right jaw, anesthesia personnel could not obtain a clear view for intubation. The metal fragment was not removed due to the fear of massive bleeding from the vessels. With the fragment in place, there was no extensive bleeding from the injury site. Part of the metallic fragment could be seen inside the oral cavity. A thorough discussion with all the medical personnel ensued. In order to remove this fragment, the patient would have to be put under general anesthesia, but with the piece of metal in his mouth, he could not be intubated in the usual manner. So most of the discussion centered on the different options we had to obtain a definitive airway. After all options were weighed, it was decided that we would perform an awake tracheostomy in order to put the breathing tube into his trachea. The thought of using local anesthetic and placing a tracheostomy tube on an awake individual seemed odd to some. However, thinking outside the box was necessary in this situation. The operating room was alerted and prepared for a procedure.

The patient was significantly counseled about the procedure and all questions were answered. He communicated with us through written text. We wanted to make the surrounding as calm as possible so the patient would not be too anxious. As time passed, the excitement in the emergency room decreased and it went back to business as usual. As he was a young male, he seemed more excited than nervous with a sense of the adventure of it all. In fact, he wanted the medical staff to take a picture of him with the metal fragment protruding from the side of his face so that he could show his mom and family. Obviously, we declined his request. We played music for him in the operating room in an effort to make him more comfortable. He was placed supine on the operating table and the bed positioned in a "beach chair" position with the head and back elevated. The patient was given a suction device and was told to use it as needed to clear his oral cavity of any secretions. He had to be kept upright due to the risk of aspiration. The neck was than prepped and draped with towels. The proposed site of the incision was marked and local anesthetic was injected in the area. Every 2–3 min during the procedure, we had to stop and allow the patient to suction his oral cavity with the suction device. It was a little interesting to have the patient suction his own mouth during the surgery. However, we felt that this would give him some sense of control and relieve the anxiety he might have felt. Even though he did not show it on the outside, we assumed he would be very nervous about surgeons in gowns and masks injecting needles and cutting into his neck while he was fully awake.

A transverse skin incision was made approximately 3 cm superior to the sternal notch. Next, careful dissection was performed down to the strap muscles. The strap muscles were then divided at the midline. Careful dissection was performed to not injure the anterior jugular vein. Again the patient remained cognizant throughout the entire procedure. Local anesthetic was injected as needed during the dissection. Once

the trachea was visualized, anesthesia personnel was alerted because we were ready to put the breathing tube into his trachea and timing was crucial. They injected medication to put the patient to sleep. Once he was asleep, we had to move very quickly to secure his airway. The trachea was elevated using the trachea elevator and quickly entered with a scalpel. The opening was then dilated. A cuffed tracheostomy tube was inserted into the trachea and connected to the ventilator. The balloon of the cuff was inflated to ensure good seal of the tracheostomy tube. Next, end-tidal CO_2 monitor was connected and this was verified along with equal breath sounds bilaterally. The tracheostomy tube was then secured with sutures to prevent dislodgement during the remainder of the procedure and for evacuation after the procedure.

Once the airway was controlled and the patient was under general anesthesia, the patient was turned over to the oral maxillofacial surgeon for the removal of the large metal fragment and management of the fractured jaw. The fragment was removed without complications. None of the large vessels were injured and minimal bleeding was encountered during the removal of the fragment. The wound was copiously irrigated with normal saline and the fractured mandible was stabilized. The patient tolerated the procedure well and was kept on the ventilator. He was recovered in the post-surgery unit. Subsequently, he was evacuated to the next level of care. He remained intubated and evacuated to a fixed facility.

7.2   Discussion

In all trauma situations, the physician is taught that airway should be assessed and addressed first. Both Advanced Trauma Life Support and Basic Life Support courses stress the importance of airway. The wars in Iraq and Afghanistan have taught us a great deal on head and neck trauma and airway management. Thousands of soldiers have suffered from craniomaxillofacial (CMF) battlefield injuries during Operation Iraqi Freedom (OIF) and Operation Enduring Freedom (OEF) [1]. In OIF, there were a higher percentage of head and neck traumas due to the effectiveness of body armor that shielded the chest and abdomen but left the head and neck exposed [2]. This significantly changed the patterns of injury seen by the medical staff. Brennan et al. reported on 196 patients who presented with airway compromise requiring either intubation or a surgical airway over a 30-month timeframe. Within these 196 patients, 46 % had penetrating face trauma and 31 % had penetrating neck trauma [3]. The most common mechanism of injury for the head and neck was from an explosion of the improvised explosive device (IED) [4]. These usually occur at close range and are high-velocity injuries [5]. Such injuries result in massive bleeding and tissue loss. With this mechanism of injury, airway management can be very challenging.

Pre-hospital airway management is paramount to maximize survival of trauma patients. Goedecke et al. emphasized that providers in the field need to recognize the importance of ventilation and the risks of failure to ventilate the lungs [6]. An analysis of battlefield cricothyrotomy by Mabry revealed the success of pre-hospital cricothyrotomy in Iraq and Afghanistan was dependent on the experience of the provider. In the military, pre-hospital treatments are provided by trained medics. However, they have a varying degree of experience. The military medics had a 33 % failure rate for emergent cricothyrotomy compared to 15 % for physicians and physician assistants [7]. Even with appropriate management, a large percentage of these patients do not survive due to severe gunshot wounds to the face and neck along with explosion-related injuries [7]. All these patients would be classified as difficult and challenging airway patients.

In a controlled setting, the ideal airway management would be endotracheal intubation. However, in MASCAL settings with severe head and neck injuries, endotracheal intubation may not be feasible due to significant trauma and bleeding causing poor visualization. The difficult airway is defined as a situation where a trained anesthetist has difficulty with mask ventilation and/or tracheal intubation [8]. There are various factors that contribute to a difficult airway. Massive trauma to the head and neck definitely would fall under the category of a difficult airway.

Depending on the extent of injury, there are various methods to address the challenging airway. These include awake intubation, fiberoptic intubation, retrograde intubation, and intubation under anesthesia [9].

Awake intubation is more time-consuming and is less pleasant than intubation under anesthesia. However, it is safer due to the patient maintaining spontaneous breathing and pharyngeal/laryngeal muscle tone [7]. Awake fiberoptic intubation is the technique of choice by most experts in a difficult airway. The patient has to be well informed and a trained operator with appropriate equipment is needed [7]. Retrograde intubation consists of a guidewire being placed in the trachea through the cricothyroid membrane via a cannula and needle. The wire is retrieved with forceps and brought out through the mouth. The endotracheal tube is then placed over the guidewire into the trachea [7].

However, there are times when the above options are not feasible due to either lack of equipment or the severity of the injury. If a patient has an impending airway compromise and endotracheal intubation is not feasible, an emergent tracheostomy or cricothyroidotomy should be performed. Bell et al. reviewed their experience with civilian low-velocity penetrating neck trauma. In their review, 14 % of patients required a tracheotomy [10]. Therefore, a surgeon, no matter what type or setting of practice, needs to be familiar with the various options for elective and emergent airway control.

In the case of the patient described at the beginning of this chapter, the large metallic fragment precluded the ability to perform the above-described methods. All surgeons and anesthesia personnel were consulted. After discussing the various options available, it was decided that an awake tracheostomy was the best course of action. Due to our austere conditions, no fiberoptic equipment was available. Since the patient was breathing spontaneously, it was safe to proceed with an awake tracheostomy with local anesthetic.

Initially, tracheostomy was seen as a very dangerous procedure with high mortality rates. However, the techniques and indications were standardized by Chevalier Jackson in the early twentieth century. This reduced the rates of morbidity and mortality and the prevailing attitudes toward tracheostomy changed [11]. In this day and age, tracheostomy is seen as one of the preferred methods for airway control during an airway emergency. The majority of these procedures are done during a code where the patient is unconscious. Otherwise, the patient may get a tracheostomy after being intubated for a prolong period of time in an intensive care unit setting and thus will be under general anesthesia. A recent literature search did not reveal many descriptions or publications about an urgent awake tracheostomy.

Yuen et al. performed a retrospective review of 73 adult patients who underwent a tracheostomy under awake conditions. These patients all had impending airway obstruction and a nonmalignant cause of airway obstruction was the most common indication. Other causes of airway obstruction included deep neck infections and malignancy [12]. Surgical access was successful in all patients with airway compromise due to hemorrhage. Overall, they concluded awake tracheostomy is a life-saving procedure for those with impending airway obstruction [12].

In this day and age, surgeons may find themselves in a very austere environment. This can be on the battlefield overseas or in small rural community. If surgeons are faced with a disaster or a MASCAL scenario, airway control may be difficult due to facial injuries and trauma. In that case, an option available to the surgeon is an awake tracheostomy. It has been shown to be safe by Yuen et al. [12]. The true scenario described at the beginning of this chapter is also an indication that awake tracheotomy works and may be the only option in certain situations.

Editor's Note: COL Yong Choi, MD is currently on Active Duty in the United States Army. He has served in four deployments to Iraq and Afghanistan including one as the Commander of the 555th Forward Surgical Team.

Disclaimer The views expressed are those of the author(s) and do not reflect the official policy of the Department of the Army, the Department of Defense, or the U.S. Government.

References

1. Lew TA, Walker JA, Wenke JC, Blackbourne LH, Hale RG. Characterization of craniomaxillofacial battle injuries sustained by United States service members in the current conflicts of Iraq and Afghanistan. J Oral Maxillofac Surg. 2010;68:3–7.
2. Owens BD, Kragh JF, Wenke JC, Macaitis J, Wade CE, Holcomb JB. Combat wounds in Operation Iraqi Freedom and Operation Enduring Freedom. J Trauma. 2008;64:295–9.
3. Brennan J, Gibbons MD, Lopez M, Hayes D, Faulkner J, Eller RL, Barton C. Traumatic airway management in Operation Iraqi Freedom. Otolaryngol Head Neck Surg. 2011;144(3):376–80.
4. Brennan J. Head and neck trauma in Iraq and Afghanistan: different war, different surgery, lessons learned. Laryngoscope. 2013;123:2411–7.
5. Champion HR, Holcomb JB, Young LA. Injuries from explosions: physics, biophysics, pathology, and required research focus. J Trauma. 2009;66:1468–77.
6. Goedecke A, Herff H, Paal P, Dorges V, Wenzel V. Field airway management disasters. Aesth Analg. 2007;104(3):481–2.
7. Mabry RL. An analysis of battlefield cricothyrotomy in Iraq and Afghanistan. J Spec Oper Med. 2012;12(1):17–23.
8. Practice guidelines for management of difficult airway: an updated report by the American Society of Anesthesiologists Task Force on Management of Difficult Airway. Anesthesiology. 2003;98:1269–77.
9. Lavery GG, McCloskey BV. The difficult airway in adult critical care. Crit Care Med. 2008;36:2163–73.
10. Bell RB, Osborn T, Dierks EJ, Potter BE, Long WB. Management of penetrating neck injuries: a new paradigm for civilian trauma. J Oral Maxillofac Surg. 2007;65:691–705.
11. McWhorter AJ. Tracheotomy: timing and techniques. Curr Opin Otolarynngol Head Neck Surg. 2003;11:473–9.
12. Yuen HW, Loy AHC, Johari S. Urgent awake tracheotomy for impending airway obstruction. Otolaryngol Head Neck Surg. 2007;136:838–42.

Pediatric Emergencies in the Combat or Austere Environment: As Easy as A, B, C!

8

Matthew J. Martin, Zaradhe M.S. Yach, and Matthew J. Eckert

8.1 Setting and Background

The material and cases described in this chapter were derived from the experiences on multiple combat deployments of the authors in support of Operation Enduring Freedom and Operation Iraqi Freedom. These included a deployment to Forward Operating Base Ghazni, Ghazni Province, Afghanistan, where author Z.Y. served as the Senior Medical Officer of a US Provincial Reconstruction Team and author M.M. served as Commander of the 655th Forward Surgical Team.

M.J. Martin, M.D. (✉)
Department of Surgery, Madigan Army Medical Center, 9040 Fitzsimmons Avenue, Tacoma, WA 98431, USA

Trauma and Acute Care Surgery Service, Legacy Emanuel Medical Center, Portland, Oregon
e-mail: matthew.j.martin16.mil@mail.mil

Z.M.S. Yach, B.S., M.S.
Mercy Medical Group, 2110 Professional Drive, Suite 120, Roseville, CA 95661, USA
e-mail: Zaradhe@hotmail.com

M.J. Eckert, M.D., F.A.C.S.
Department of Surgery, Madigan Army Medical Center, Tacoma, WA, USA

Trauma and Acute Care Surgery Service, Legacy Emanuel Medical Center, Portland, Oregon
e-mail: matthew.j.eckert.mil@mail.mil

8.2 Introduction

The basic tenet of the urgent trauma care of both adults and children is to proceed with a rapid and prioritized process of initial evaluation and urgent interventions for life-threatening pathology. This has been promulgated worldwide among physicians by the Advanced Trauma Life Support (ATLS) course and among pre-hospital personnel through the similar Pre-hospital Trauma Life Support (PHTLS) course. Both courses teach the "A, B, C" approach to evaluation, which focuses on identifying life-threatening problems involving the airway, breathing, or circulatory systems. The initial evaluation and care of pediatric patients with significant traumatic injuries or surgical pathology should take this same approach, but with considerations given to some of the key unique anatomic and physiologic differences in children that can lead to disaster if not anticipated and managed appropriately.

An appreciation of the specialized staffing, training, and equipment that is required to provide optimal emergent pediatric care has long been recognized by the American College of Surgeons and other organizations that regulate the certification of hospitals as pediatric trauma centers. However, the reality is that severely ill or injured children will often present to a facility that is not specialized and equipped for

© Springer International Publishing Switzerland 2016
C.R.B. Lim (ed.), *Surgery During Natural Disasters, Combat, Terrorist Attacks, and Crisis Situations*, DOI 10.1007/978-3-319-23718-3_8

Fig. 8.1 Chapter author (Z.Y.) during a Provincial Reconstruction Team mission, surrounded by Afghani children while discussing the need for a local clinic and assessing the healthcare needs of the local families. Photo courtesy of US Air Force 1st Lieutenant Katherine Roling

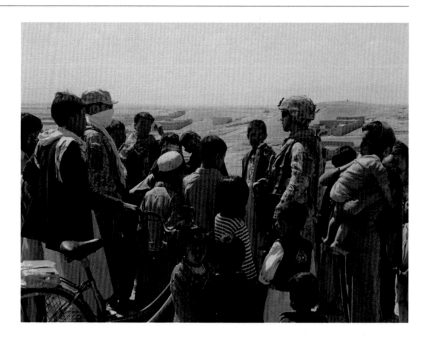

high-level pediatric care, but still require immediate evaluation, interventions, and resuscitation. This has been particularly true in the austere environment of the modern battlefield, where forward military medical treatment facilities (MTF) have continuously been called upon to treat large volumes of severely injured children despite not being primarily equipped or staffed for pediatric care. Children represent a particularly vulnerable population to traumatic injury, and this is greatly magnified during times of war (Fig. 8.1). Childhood mortality in countries at war rises steeply, and is attributable to both wartime trauma and medical/infectious disease coupled with a significant degradation or even collapse of the countries countries' healthcare infrastructure. Although this topic is certainly relevant to military physicians, the same principles and lessons will hold true in many civilian settings, such as natural disasters, MASCAL events, or even in remote rural locations with no nearby tertiary care or pediatric referral center.

This section focuses on practical advice for the health care provider faced with a pediatric emergency that requires fast decision making and urgent focused intervention. This will often be done without access to a full complement of pediatric supplies, a situation that is challenging but that can be overcome with some modification of standard adult equipment or improvisation with whatever is immediately available. The flow of the chapter follows the standard A, B, C approach, focusing on a challenging airway case first, followed by an emergent breathing issue and concluding with a life-threatening circulatory problem. Each area is illustrated by an actual case from the authors' experiences during combat deployments, and although the cases represent unique and uncommon pathology or injuries, the underlying principles behind their management are universal. Our first piece of advice is to remember that even though you and your facility may not be the ideal person and place for a pediatric emergency, never forget what a small group of dedicated and like-minded individuals can accomplish when faced with a challenge under adverse conditions.

8.3 Airway Emergencies in Children

8.3.1 Case 1

A 3-year-old Iraqi female was brought to a military treatment facility with increasing stridor and dyspnea, as well as intolerance to oral intake for several days. Her history was remarkable for a large congenital cystic hygroma of the face/neck that was resected a year earlier at a different military MTF. In addition, she had diffuse lymphangiomatosis of the tongue that had progressively increased in size and was now causing airway obstruction and the inability to swallow solids or liquids (see Fig. 8.2). On presentation she was awake and mildly agitated, was moving minimal amounts of air with inhalation and had loud

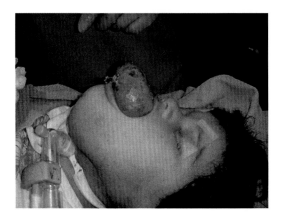

Fig. 8.2 Iraqi child with massive lymphangiomatosis of the tongue who presented with near-complete airway obstruction

stridor and gurgling with each breath. An adequate airway needed to be established urgently. Direct visualization or suctioning of the posterior oropharynx was not possible due to the massive tongue. She was hemodynamically stable but had an oxygen saturation of 86 % on a non-rebreather mask. An attempt at placing a nasal airway and then assisted breathing via BVM was made, but was unsuccessful in increasing inspiratory airflow. At this point it was decided to proceed with a surgical airway, and the patient was quickly moved to the OR table. A standard open tracheostomy was performed via a midline cervical incision, with creation of an inferiorly based tracheal flap (see Fig. 8.3) and inertion of a#4 Shiley tracheostomy device. The patient recovered uneventfully, subsequently underwent a hemiglossectomy at our facility, and had the tracheostomy successfully removed several weeks later (see Fig. 8.4).

8.3.2 Discussion

Pediatric airway emergencies are among the most challenging problems to face any practitioner, whether in the austere environment or at a Level

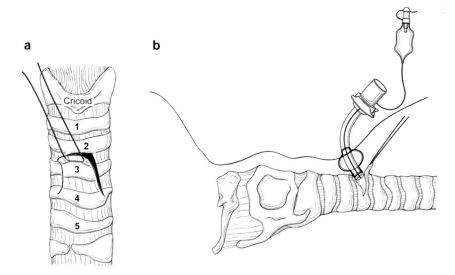

Fig. 8.3 Operative technique for modified Bjork tracheostomy involves creation of an inferiorly based (upside-down "U" shape) tracheal flap (**a**) which can then be elevated and used to guide the tracheostomy into position (**b**). Reprinted with permission Viehweg, T.L., "Face, Eye, and Ear Injuries," in Martin M, Beekley A. *Front line surgery: a practical approach.* New York: Springer Publishing Inc., 2011

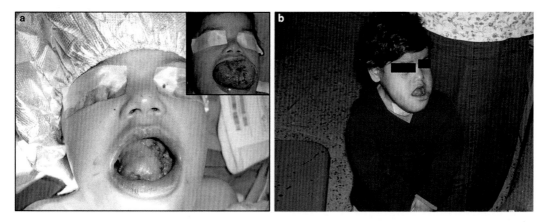

Fig. 8.4 (**a**) Intraoperative photograph showing completed hemiglossectomy, with preoperative photo for comparison inset. (**b**) Postoperatively the patient was able to resume oral intake and the tracheostomy has been removed

1 pediatric trauma center. In addition to all of the well-known concerns in adult adults, there are several key anatomic and physiologic factors in children that make this area fraught with potential danger if not fully anticipated and appreciated. These will also vary by age, and the level of difficulty or potential complications is roughly inversely correlated with age. While the adolescent or teenager can generally be treated similar to an adult, younger children must be approached with a higher level of anxiety and respect for the very real and potentially fatal complications that can arise from failure to recognize and treat an airway emergency, or from delayed recognition of complications secondary to an airway intervention [1]. The best way to improve chances for successful management of a pediatric airway emergency is to be as prepared as possible, including adequate equipment and supplies, training, and support. Even if you are not an active pediatric trauma or tertiary referral center, if there is any reasonable chance that an acutely ill or injured child will be brought to your facility then you should ensure you have the minimal necessary supplies for the initial management and stabilization of that patient. Arguably the most important piece of equipment is an up to date Broselow tape that will serve as a guide to most medications and supplies required to handle the common airway, breathing, and circulation emergencies.

There are multiple important anatomic differences between children and adults with respect to the airway that should be appreciated and considered. Children have large heads and tongues as well as foreshortened airways. This makes airway occlusion due to the tongue a much larger issue in the pediatric patient population, particularly if there is an altered level of consciousness from an associated brain injury, sedation, or shock. The neutral or "sniffing" position in children is obtained with less neck extension than in adults, and over-extension can actually worsen your view of the airway during attempts at intubation. On direct laryngoscopy the airway and vocal chords are in a more anterior position, requiring more anterior traction for adequate visualization. If a clear view of the vocal chords is still elusive, then gentle cricoid pressure may help move the chords into view. The cross-sectional area of the airway is also significantly less than in an adult, and can easily become obstructed by edema, blood clots, foreign/ingested objects, dislodged teeth, or extrinsic compression from an adjacent hematoma or significant soft tissue swelling (classically seen with cervical spine fractures). The trachea is very short, making right mainstem intubation and inadvertent extubation very common events. Verify the correct position of the tube, and then SECURE it tightly. Remember that the difference between a properly placed endotracheal tube and an inadvertent extubation or mainstem intubation in a small child may be only 1–2 cm, so a simple piece of tape securing the airway may not be enough protection from dislodgment. Have someone dedicated to manually holding the airway as well as maintaining the head/neck in a stable position during all patient movements (such as logrolling) and during any patient transport. The safest posture is just to assume that the worst will happen during transport, and have adequate airway equipment and replacement endotracheal tubes to perform reintubation with the patient at all times.

There also should be great respect and appreciation paid to the physiologic differences between children and adults with respect to the airway. Babies and small children are rapid shallow breathers, so it may be difficult to differentiate respiratory distress from simple agitation or even a normal baseline breathing pattern. Unlike adults, children have very little respiratory reserve (lower tidal volumes and functional residual capacity) and an inability to maintain oxygenation with prolonged periods of apnea. Even short periods of apnea or hypoventilation can lead to rapid atelectasis and desaturation, and is often followed quickly by bradycardia and then full cardiopulmonary arrest. Babies also are obligate nasal breathers and can develop respiratory distress with no obvious source of oropharyngeal airway pathology if the nasal passages become obstructed. This should also be considered when administering supplemental oxygen; use either nasal cannula or a facemask that covers both the nose and mouth to deliver oxygen in spontaneously breathing infants and small children.

The approach to an acute airway emergency in a child should follow a stepwise approach of maneuvers with rapid escalation if the initially chosen approach is not effective [2]. A rapid search for the source of airway compromise can help guide the optimal intervention, but should not take precedence over establishing a definitive airway if there is active or impending respiratory distress or airway loss. In addition to trauma, the most common other causes of airway emergencies in children will be infectious, anatomic or congenital anomalies, foreign body (typically ingested), burns/inhalation injury, or allergic/anaphylactic reactions. In the acute setting of respiratory distress, there is little initial diagnostic work-up required beyond a focused physical exam to look for signs of impending respiratory arrest or airway compromise, identify any obvious signs of an anatomic or traumatic cause, and obtain a brief history if possible. Supplemental oxygen should be administered immediately and then quickly followed by suctioning of the oropharynx to remove any blood or debris. If there are signs of an obstructed airway then positioning with a chin lift or jaw thrust maneuver can be attempted, as well as insertion of an oral or nasopharyngeal airway. Preparations for intubation or even a possible surgical airway should be made by gathering all available equipment (preferably already prepositioned on an airway cart) and the necessary personnel to assist with airway management.

One of the common mistakes the authors have witnessed during these often chaotic situations is forgetting the simple maneuver of bag-valve-mask (BVM) ventilation of the patient. Unless the airway is physically obstructed by either a large foreign object or severe displaced facial fractures, BVM ventilation can provide fully adequate oxygenation and ventilation in virtually all pediatric patients, and can turn a rushed emergency intubation or surgical airway into a more deliberate and less urgent procedure. One of the common mistakes among inexperienced personnel is pressing the mask down onto the face in an attempt to get a tight seal—this often compresses the midface and tongue and worsens airway obstruction. Proper BVM technique should be thought of as trying to lift the face up into the mask, rather than pressing the mask down onto the face. An additional unique consideration in pediatric patients undergoing intubation is the risk for bradycardia, which can occur from increased vagal tone during induction and direct laryngoscopy or from hypoxia during attempts at intubation. We recommend administering atropine (0.1–0.5 mg IV) during rapid sequence induction, or at least having it standing by. We would also strongly recommend having a well-stocked cart or designated area with equipment for the "difficult airway." This would include pediatric laryngoscopes and preferably a video laryngoscope with pediatric blades, various size bougies and stylets, a bronchoscope, and alternative airway devices such as a laryngeal mask airway (LMA) or a dual-esophageal/tracheal intubating tube (i.e., King airway or Combi-tube). There are various formulas promoted for estimating the appropriate size of endotracheal tube (ETT) to use in children, with the most common being $4+(age/4)$ for children 2 years or older [3]. Alternatively the diameter of the 5th digit or the width of the fingernail on the 5th digit can provide a reliable estimate of the proper ETT diameter required [4]. Finally, the traditional practice of using uncuffed endotracheal tubes in pediatric patients has given way to widespread acceptance of cuffed tubes in all ages (with the exception of select neonates) [3].

In the event that the above measures fail or are not available, then a surgical airway should be rapidly established. This is a difficult procedure even in many controlled and elective settings, and should not be taken lightly under any circumstances. However, a solid knowledge of the anatomy and anatomic variations in children, as well as some of the "tricks of the trade," can make these procedures significantly less stressful with a high success rate. There are several available options for placing a surgical airway, and the choice should take into account the patient age and size, presence of neck trauma or pathology, the training and comfort level of the surgeon or provider performing the procedure, and the relative urgency of the need for a surgical airway. Although cricothyrotomy is taught as the standard first-line surgical airway in adults, it is a less attractive option in pediatric patients, particularly in younger age children [2]. In fact, many experts consider an age of 5 years or less to be a relative contraindication to attempting a cricothyrotomy, due the small size of the cricothyroid space and its proximity to the vocal chords. Attempts at a "crich" may fail due to the inability to get an adequate sized tube into the cricothyroid space, or may result in damage to the airway from attempting to introduce a larger tube than the space can handle. In addition, the close proximity to the vocal chords can result in significant injury to these structures, or to inadvertent placement of the tube above the level of the chords. An often described but rarely performed alternative is the

"needle cricothyrotomy," which entails placement of a 14-gauge IV catheter (or similar sized tube) percutaneously through the cricothyroid membrane [5]. What is not as often spelled out is what to do next with this catheter once it is in the airway. One option is to connect it to tubing carrying high-flow oxygen, cut a side hole in the tubing, and then use a finger to alternate covering and releasing the side hole, providing an inhalation phase with high-flow oxygen and then an exhalation phase with release of the high flow pressure. Another option is to connect a 3 or 5 cc syringe (with the plunger removed) to the IV catheter, and this will serve as an appropriate sized adaptor to connect to an Ambu bag and provide bag ventilation. It should be noted that this method can provide very good short term oxygenation, but will not provide adequate ventilation and should only be utilized as a temporizing maneuver while preparing to establish a more definitive airway [6, 7].

The most definitive surgical airway is a properly placed and secured tracheostomy tube. Although this surgical procedure is relatively straightforward in both adults and pediatric patients in the elective setting, it can be a daunting task in the emergency situation with poor lighting, inadequate retraction and exposure, ongoing bleeding, and distorted or injured anatomy. The two most important adjuncts to success with an emergent surgical airway are (1) proper lighting and (2) having an assistant provide adequate retraction and exposure. We prefer a vertical skin incision for emergencies, as it can easily be extended superiorly or inferiorly if the initial incision location was not optimal or to provide improved exposure if visualization is inadequate. Common errors that can occur are being too cephalad and entering the cricothyroid space instead of a tracheal interspace, dissecting into the thyroid gland which typically results in significant bleeding, and dissecting off to the side of the trachea rather than down onto the midline. These errors can be avoided with some simple maneuvers; most importantly, keeping the trachea firmly grasped between two fingers and maintaining dissection straight down onto the midline will avoid missing the midline and will also help prevent additional bleeding by staying in the avascular median raphe of the strap muscles. In addition, have the assistant use a tracheostomy hook (or a makeshift hook can be made by bending an 18-gauge needle to form a hook) to lift the trachea up into the field rather than struggle to dig deeper into the low neck. Depending on the size of the child and the trachea, a horizontal incision into the trachea may be adequate to allow passage of the tracheostomy tube. In younger children this may be inadequate, in which case an H-shaped incision or alternatively an inverted U-shaped incision (see Fig. 8.3) can be made to divide the tracheal rings and allow passage of an appropriately sized tube. If no pediatric tracheostomy tubes are available, then a properly sized endotracheal tube can be placed but should be very well secured to avoid inadvertent dislodgment during patient movement or transport. Finally, although we consider a cuffed endotracheal tube to be the best "definitive" airway, remember that it is hard to improve upon a patient airway with adequate spontaneous breathing. Do not rush to intubate just because an injury looks "bad"; a normal patent airway with adequate ventilation is possible in many injury types, including massive facial trauma with multiple fractures.

8.4   Breathing Emergencies in Children

8.4.1   Case 2

A 4-year-old Iraqi male was brought to a US Army Combat Support Hospital after thoracic trauma secondary to a dog bite. The patient was injured during the pursuit of a suspected insurgent by US military forces, including a military working dog. When the suspect ran into a house occupied by the patient and his family, the military dog was sent in after him ahead of the soldiers. The dog quickly cornered the suspect, but as the dog lunged to bite down on the suspect's arm, he grabbed the child and used him as a human shield, placing him into the jaws of the dog as he was biting down. The dog bit down on the child's left chest and then shook him several times before releasing him. On arrival to the hospital the patient was awake but agitated, crying, and tachypneic. He had multiple puncture wounds on his left chest in a semicircular pattern consistent with a dog bite (see Fig. 8.5), and had audible air movement into the largest puncture wound with inspiration. There were decreased left-sided breath sounds, as well as left chest crepitus and audible air movement through the

Fig. 8.5 Preoperative photo showing multiple small puncture wounds on left thorax after the child was used as a human shield against a military working dog attempting to apprehend a suspected insurgent. Although the wounds appear relatively minor, the patient had an open pneumothorax as well as a traumatic lung hernia

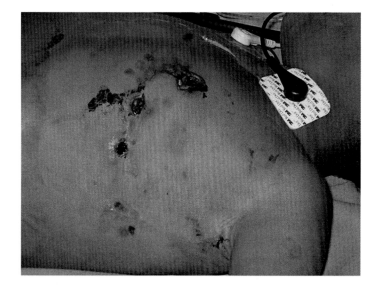

largest puncture wound with each inspiration. He had visible asymmetry of his chest wall (left > right) that increased during his initial evaluation, and his oxygen saturation was 80 % by pulse oximeter. A diagnosis of tension pneumothorax was made and a 20 French left tube thoracostomy was placed with an immediate large rush of air and improvement in the patient's vital signs and oxygen saturation. The "sucking chest wound" was covered with an occlusive dressing and the patient was taken to the operating room to explore the wounds and perform irrigation and possible closure. On surgical exploration there was noted to be an internal degloving of a large section of skin and subcutaneous tissue from the underlying chest wall in the area of the dog bite, as well as a 6 cm linear laceration through the intercostal muscles of the 6th intercostal space with a small segment of lung herniated through the rib space. The lung herniation was reduced and the intercostal muscles were reapproximated in two layers with absorbable suture, followed by irrigation and debridement of the skin wounds and then partial wound closure over a negative-pressure vacuum dressing. The child made an uneventful recovery, had his wounds closed and chest tube removed 3 days later, and was discharged to home with his family.

8.4.2 Discussion

Airway and breathing emergencies in children are often intimately related, and sometimes it may be difficult to determine whether the primary problem is related to airway obstruction/insufficiency or due to a thoracic or pulmonary process. Examination by inspection, palpation, and auscultation can often determine the source and even the exact pathology resulting in breathing dysfunction, but the examination can also be limited by the surrounding noise and chaos, the presence of other distracting injuries, crying or screaming of the child, and lack of cooperation with the exam. As discussed above for airway, it may also be difficult to determine if a rapid shallow breathing pattern is due to a significant injury or is due to fear/pain/agitation. Another

key point to remember is that children tend to swallow larger volumes of air, particularly when crying/screaming or being given supplemental breaths by BVM. This often results in massive gastric distension that can actually cause respiratory compromise, and should prompt immediate gastric decompression via a nasogastric or orogastric tube.

The diagnostic work-up for a suspected breathing emergency should be rapid, focused, and prioritized. This means that only immediately life-threatening pathologies should be ruled out initially, and the remainder can be evaluated in the secondary survey and additional diagnostic studies. The primary pathologies of concern in this area include tension pneumothorax, open pneumothorax (aka "sucking chest wound"), hemothorax, and flail chest/pulmonary contusion. Although cardiac tamponade is traditionally considered under the C-circulatory category, it can result in respiratory distress and decompensation manifesting as a B-breathing problem. The diagnostic workup required to identify these problems is relatively simple, and should include a focused exam, a portable chest X-ray, and a FAST (focused assessment with sonography for trauma) exam. A normal chest X-ray essentially rules out pneumothorax and hemothorax as a cause of respiratory distress, and a negative pericardial view on the FAST exam similarly rules out a large effusion with tamponade effect. Alternatively, ultrasound can be extended beyond the standard FAST exam to encompass evaluation of the chest for pneumothorax and hemothorax as well as tamponade. Ultrasound has actually been shown to be superior to chest X-ray in detecting thoracic pathology, and this skillset can be acquired rapidly with basic focused hands-on training [8, 9].

In this case, the child presented after a very atypical mechanism that resulted in a combination of blunt (crush) and penetrating (canine bite) injury to the thorax. Although there were only several small puncture/lacerations visible externally and no active bleeding, the children presented in respiratory distress requiring a rapid assessment to identify the exact cause. The exam was also notable for audible air movement into the chest with inspiration, confirming the diagnosis of an open pneumothorax or "sucking chest wound." These types of wounds have gained widespread fame in combat settings, but may still be seen in both blunt and penetrating civilian trauma. The most important concept to understand and properly treat these injuries is that the sucking wound itself is not the primary problem, so dressing or sealing the wound may not result in any significant improvement if the patient has already developed respiratory distress. The classic teaching for immediate care of a sucking chest wound involved trying to create a "three-sided" dressing that would leave one side open for air to exit the wound, but not allow additional air to enter the chest. We have found this to be difficult to achieve, particularly in the pre-hospital setting. The current recommendation from the military Tactical Combat Casualty Care course is to cover the wound with a completely occlusive dressing and monitor for signs of tension pneumothorax, with removal of the dressing to relieve tension if it occurs [10]. Also of interest in this case was the presence of a traumatic lung hernia (also known as "traumatic ribcage hernia"). These are rare hernias that may be seen after penetrating thoracic injuries or with major blunt chest wall trauma. Unless they are immediately visible through a laceration or open wound, they can be difficult to diagnose by physical exam or plain X-ray studies. The majority are identified with computed tomography (CT) of the chest (see Fig. 8.6), which also provides information about associated injury to the lung, ribs, and chest wall muscular and fascial layers. In this case the defect was a penetrating linear laceration of the intercostal muscles that was amenable to primary reapproximation. In cases with larger soft tissue injuries, primary repair may be impossible and thus reconstruction may require prosthetic or biologic mesh. In blunt trauma these are often also associated with multiple rib fractures, and reconstruction of the bony thoracic wall with rib plating may be required to allow adequate closure and stabilization.

When dealing with an open pneumothorax, respiratory distress will typically be from either the development of a tension pneumothorax or less commonly from underlying injury to the lung such as a large laceration or pulmonary contusion. The focus on immediate intervention and treatment should be on treating any tension physiology if present, or preventing the development of a tension pneumothorax. This is done by placement of a well-positioned and functioning chest tube, or alternatively by decompression

Fig. 8.6 CT scan example of herniation of a portion of the left lung (*arrow*) through a traumatic defect in the chest wall

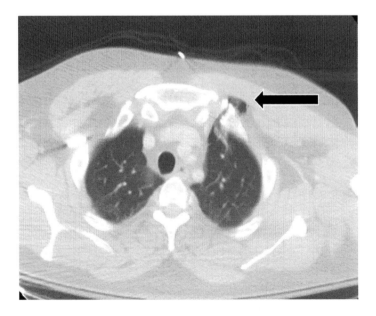

with a needle thoracostomy until a chest tube can be placed. Once this has been done, attention can then be turned to the chest wall defect which can now be addressed as a non-emergent problem. Initial care of the wound should only require placement of an occlusive dressing that covers the defect along with adequate irrigation and debridement of devitalized tissue as needed. The definitive management of the chest wall defect will depend on the size of the defect and the amount/type of injury to surrounding soft tissues and bone. Most of these defects can be closed primarily by suture reapproximation of the intercostal and chest wall muscles/fascia, but larger defects can prevent significant reconstructive challenges. Another good option that has been used extensively in forward military treatment facilities is to place a negative-pressure therapy device such as a Wound Vac (KCI Inc., San Antonio, TX). This will often achieve complete coverage of the wound, prevent any further air entrainment, evacuate any residual air or fluid through the wound, and promote significantly faster healing and wound closure. It also is ideal for grossly contaminated or high-risk wounds that are not amenable to immediate primary closure.

The management of other common causes of post-traumatic respiratory distress in children (typically due to a pneumo and hemothorax) is similar to adults, with two additional challenges. The first is selecting an appropriate sized chest tube. Very small tubes are fine if you only have air to evacuate, but larger tubes (at least 20 French) should be used to evacuate blood and reduce the chance of clogging of the tube by small blood clots. The second challenge in placement is tube location. For infants and small children it is physically impossible to put your finger or even a Kelley or tonsil clamp into the pleural space to assist in directing the tube during placement. Most small tubes come with trocars to assist in placement; we recommend removing the trocar if you are not familiar and comfortable with it. If using the trocar we still recommend a cut down technique as most surgeons are far more familiar with that method than the percutaneous chest tube placement. To assist

with accurate placement, pull the trocar back 1 cm so that the point is located within the tube and then perform cut down on top of the rib as normal. The trocar can then be used as a steering mechanism to guide the tube into any part of the thoracic space desired. However, it is still possible to injure the lung or mediastinal structures during tube placement so the trocar should only be advanced enough to guide the tube but not enough to damage intra-thoracic structures [11]. Another key point to remember is that for a tension pneumothorax, the life-saving treatment is not the placement of the tube; it is the opening of the pleural space and evacuation of trapped air. Once this has been done (usually by puncturing the pleura with a blunt clamp or curved Mayo scissors, and then widening the opening by spreading the instrument), then placement of the chest tube can be delayed if there are other life-threatening issues that require your attention. Finally, always remember that chest tubes can kink, clog, or be malpositioned so that they do not effectively evacuate air or blood. Do not assume that because a chest tube is present that there cannot be a developing pneumothorax or ongoing major bleeding. Tube position should be confirmed with a post-placement chest X-ray and then follow-up imaging as dictated by the underlying pathology. In addition, frequent checks of the tube and the suction/canister system to confirm adequate function should be routinely performed.

8.5 Circulation Emergencies in Children

8.5.1 Case 3

From 2009 to 2010, I (author Z.Y.) was deployed as the Senior Medical Officer of a Provincial Reconstruction Team (PRT) in Ghazni, Afghanistan. Our PRT was a combined team of military, Department of State, and US Agency for International Development members, and our mission was to collaborate with the Afghan leaders to promote and fund projects in sectors of government including health care. Our PRT was

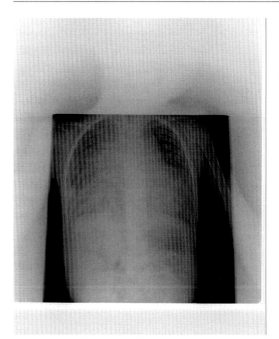

Fig. 8.7 Chest X-ray demonstrating enlarged cardiac silhouette consistent with either cardiomegaly or large pericardial effusion effusion

assigned to Forward Operating Base (FOB) Ghazni. We were lucky to have both a first-aid station (which we used as a clinic for "sick call") and a Forward Surgical Team (FST) co-located on this base. The mission of the FST was to provide emergent trauma care to all coalition soldiers, injured combatants and civilians, as well as urgent general and orthopedic surgical care. However, it was very common that "mission creep" would occur and both the PRT and the FST would provide both urgent and semi-elective humanitarian type care to local nationals who had few other alternatives.

The PRT's medical mission included running a local national clinic within the walls of the base which treated Afghans who didn't otherwise have access to care. One of these patients was a 3-year-old girl brought in by her father for worsening fatigue and shortness of breath. They initially sought care for her fever, cough, and shortness of breath at the provincial hospital in Ghazni City. There she had a chest X-ray, which showed an enlarged heart silhouette (Fig. 8.7). The doctor there deemed that her symptoms were related to

cardiomegaly and told her father that nothing could be done about it. Despite the family's lack of financial resources, her father proceeded to seek help at several other hospitals. During one of these visits a cardiac ultrasound was performed that demonstrated a large pericardial effusion, but due to the father's inability to pay they were referred to a public hospital where the patient was treated with intravenous antibiotics and had a sputum study that reportedly was negative for tuberculosis. She was discharged following the completion of the antibiotics but without intervention for the effusion. Her father then consulted with a different hospital, but this facility required 100,000 Afghanis (equivalent to $2190 USD) in advance. One of the doctors there knew of our PRT and advised them to seek us out for possible care.

Upon physical exam the patient was notably small for her age. She was coughing frequently, and could only walk short distances without becoming dyspneic. She had visible intercostal and substernal retractions. She was tachypneic and her heart sounds were muffled with no murmurs or other abnormal heart sounds. She preferred sitting upright and leaning forward (Fig. 8.8), and became agitated with any attempt to place her supine. She was tachycardic and borderline hypotensive with a systolic blood pressure of 80 mmHg. I consulted the Forward Surgical Team on our base that was commanded by my coauthor (M.M.). He gave immediate approval to bring her into the facility where we performed an ultrasound which showed a large pericardial effusion with signs of early cardiac tamponade (see Fig. 8.9). After additional discussion with our anesthesia provider, we decided to proceed with an urgent pericardiocentesis and placement of a percutaneous drain into the pericardial space. This was performed under Ketamine conscious sedation and using an 8 French cordis central line kit. Approximately 300 cc of bloody fluid was aspirated with immediate relief of tamponade by ultrasound and relief of her tachypnea and shortness of breath. The patient was started on a course of antibiotics and an anti-tuberculosis regimen, part of which had to be purchased at a local bazaar due to the lack

Fig. 8.8 Three-year-old patients with cardiac tamponade. These patients will prefer sitting upright and leaning forward, and typically become agitated with any attempts to place them supine

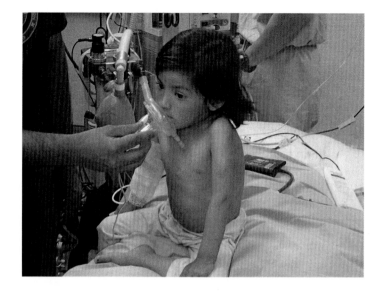

Fig. 8.9 Preoperative bedside echocardiogram showing massive pericardial effusion and evidence of tamponade

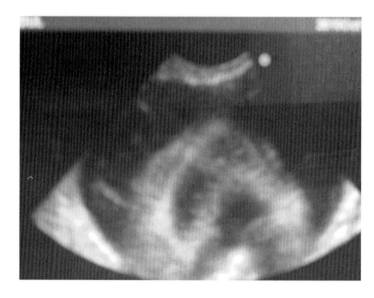

of any well-stocked pharmacies or clinics in the area. The drain output declined steadily and was removed at a 2-week follow-up visit. However, the patient was brought back the following week with recurrent symptoms and an ultrasound confirmed reaccumulation of the pericardial fluid with evidence of early tamponade. At this point a decision was made to proceed with a more definitive drainage procedure, and the patient was taken to the operating room of the FST and underwent wide opening of the pericardial sac with partial percardiectomy and placement of a closed-suction drain in the pericardial space, all done via a subxiphoid approach (Fig. 8.10). The patient recovered well from this procedure and had the drain removed 2 weeks later. She was seen several times over the next 3 months with no recurrence of the effusion on echocardiogram (Fig. 8.11) and with complete resolution of her symptoms (Fig. 8.12). Although we were unable to send the pericardial fluid or pericardial tissue for any microbiologic or mycobacterial analysis, she was given a full course of treatment for presumed tuberculous pericarditis.

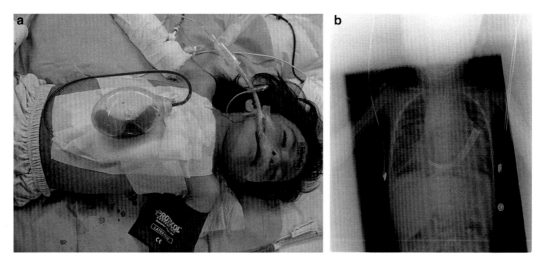

Fig. 8.10 (**a**) Immediate postoperative photo after subxiphoid partial pericardiectomy and placement of closed suction pericardial drain. (**b**) Postoperative chest X-ray shows improved cardiac silhouette and drain in pericardial space

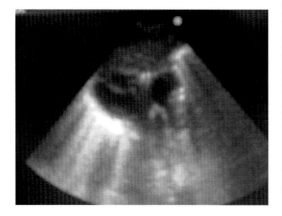

Fig. 8.11 Postoperative echocardiogram shows complete resolution of pericardial effusion

8.5.2 Discussion

Although this case of presumed infectious pericarditis with a giant effusion and tamponade is extremely uncommon, particularly in the USA, it highlights several key points about the evaluation and management of circulatory insufficiency in pediatric patients. To rapidly assess circulation in a pediatric patient, the first step is an overall visual exam and assessment of general mental status. An awake, alert, or even crying child with normal skin color indicates an acceptable minimum level of perfusion and blood pressure. A

pulse exam should also be immediately performed, and we prefer first assessing the femoral pulse rather than attempting to identify peripheral pulses (which can be difficult even when present and normal in infants and small children). In addition to the strength and character of the pulse, assessing the heart rate is of much greater importance in children than adults. Tachycardia in a child, particularly in the absence of any severe pain or agitation, is an ominous sign that may be the only warning prior to cardiovascular collapse. Children have excellent compensatory mechanisms and vasomotor tone that helps to maintain systemic blood pressure even in the face of large volume hemorrhage, cardiogenic shock, or hypovolemia. Thus, hypotension occurs much later in these scenarios in children compared with adults, leaving little time for interventions to reverse the cause of shock. The common final sign of either cardiovascular or respiratory collapse in children is frequently bradycardia, and should prompt immediate initiation of ACLS protocols and resuscitation. Simultaneous with the circulatory exam is a rapid survey for any signs of active hemorrhage with immediate intervention as indicated. Among pediatric trauma victims, cardiovascular instability should always be assumed to be due to hemorrhage until proven otherwise. Other possible causes such as tension pneumo- or hemothorax, cardiac tamponade, and

Fig. 8.12 The patient and her father (with the chapter authors) at her final follow-up visit with resolved effusion and resolution of all symptoms

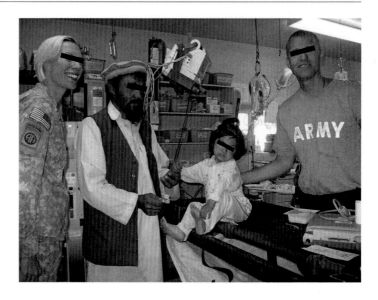

spinal cord injury should be readily identified during the primary survey. Figure 8.13 demonstrates an algorithm for the rapid assessment of all the potential sites of exsanguinating hemorrhage and the several common alternative causes of hemodynamic instability among pediatric trauma victims. Although the standard ATLS teaching is to prioritize airway and breathing before assessing circulation, current military doctrine has made assessment of the circulation and control of active hemorrhage the top priority for both adult and pediatric combat trauma victims [12, 13]. This is based on the well documented fact that most of the potentially preventable early deaths from trauma are due to hemorrhage and not to airway or breathing issues [14–16].

Resuscitation of the pediatric patient with cardiovascular instability should be performed simultaneously with the rapid focused diagnostic assessment outlined above, and not delayed while waiting to identify the underlying etiology. One of the most important aspects of trauma resuscitation that has been developed and validated during the recent conflicts in Iraq and Afghanistan is the concept of "damage control resuscitation" (DCR). Although commonly thought of as just giving early plasma along with packed red blood cells, DCR represents a paradigm shift in resuscitation that includes balanced ratios of blood

products to provide needed clotting factors and platelets in addition to red blood cells, minimizing large volume crystalloid administration, and immediate aggressive interventions to attain early hemorrhage control [17–19]. Rapid or massive transfusion protocols developed for children have generally been similar to those being established in adults. A 1:1:1 ratio of PRBCs to FFP to platelets is becoming standard, although there continues to be a lack of controlled data in pediatric trauma patients and some data suggesting that the benefit in this population may be significantly less than what has been demonstrated in adults [20, 21]. What is significantly different are the volumes that are used in creating these ratios. The volumes are all weight based and calibrated in milliliters, not units of blood. As an estimate 80 ml/kg is considered one total blood volume in a child. Remember that while 200–400 ml blood loss in an adult is not of major concern, in a small child this can represent near exsanguination (see Fig. 8.14). A key concept for surgeons, and particularly adult surgeons who are not routinely performing pediatric surgery is to *pay close attention to your blood loss, including lap sponges, and don't get behind!* What may seem like relatively small volumes of hemorrhage can constitute a large portion of the circulating blood volume, particularly in infants and younger children. Begin by administering products in boluses

Fig. 8.13 Approach for rapid identification of the cause of shock in the unstable pediatric patient. Algorithm for the rapid evaluation of the pediatric patient with suspected hemorrhagic shock. Figure modified with permission from Martin, M, "To Operate or Image (Pulling the Trigger)," in Martin M, Beekley A. *Front line surgery: a practical approach.* New York: Springer Publishing Inc., 2011

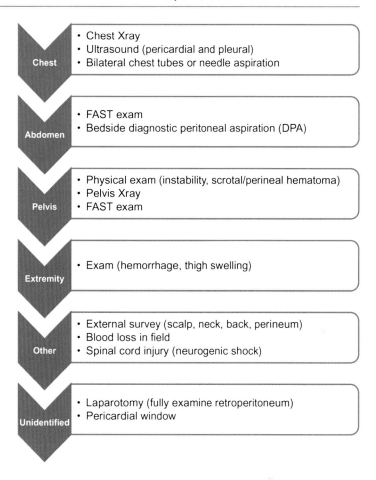

Chest
- Chest Xray
- Ultrasound (pericardial and pleural)
- Bilateral chest tubes or needle aspiration

Abdomen
- FAST exam
- Bedside diagnostic peritoneal aspiration (DPA)

Pelvis
- Physical exam (instability, scrotal/perineal hematoma)
- Pelvis Xray
- FAST exam

Extremity
- Exam (hemorrhage, thigh swelling)

Other
- External survey (scalp, neck, back, perineum)
- Blood loss in field
- Spinal cord injury (neurogenic shock)

Unidentified
- Laparotomy (fully examine retroperitoneum)
- Pericardial window

Fig. 8.14 Graph showing the relative circulating blood volumes of patients by age. Note the sharp decline in blood volume as age decreases, and contrasted to volume in a standard can of soda at the far right

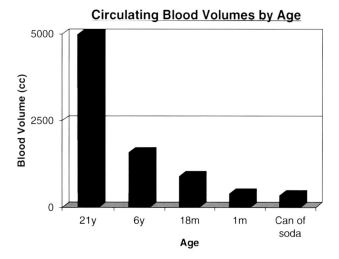

Circulating Blood Volumes by Age

of 10 ml/kg for both packed red blood cells and plasma. Platelets can be administered at 10–15 ml/kg or one single donor unit per 10 kg of body weight [11]. In the exsanguinating and coagulopathic child there has been little data on the role of pharmacologic adjuncts to treat or reverse components of the coagulation deficiency. There was a great deal of interest in recombinant activated factor VII (Novoseven) as an adjunct to reverse the acute coagulopathy of traumatic shock, but this was later tempered by lack of efficacy in controlled trials and concerns about increased thrombotic events [22, 23]. Another promising agent that is becoming widely utilized is tranexamic acid (TXA), an anti-fibrinolytic agent that was found to decrease mortality in a large prospective randomized trial of adult trauma victims [24]. In addition, several retrospective series of battlefield trauma victims have described improved survival associated with TXA administration in adults [25, 26]. More recently, the first published series of TXA use in pediatric trauma patients similarly identified a possible mortality benefit, but further study is clearly warranted in children to clarify indication, dosing, and efficacy [27].

In this case, the cardiovascular instability was found to be secondary to a giant pericardial effusion that was non-traumatic in origin. A pericardial effusion occurs when fluid fills the fibroelastic sac surrounding the heart known as the pericardium. This creates pressure in a tightly enclosed space and, depending on how quickly it develops and how much stretch the sac can accommodate, leads to elevated trans-mural pressures on the heart chambers. For acute pericardial effusions, tamponade can occur with relatively small volumes of fluid in the pericardial sac (<100 ml). Larger volumes of effusion can be seen in chronic effusions that build up more slowly as seen in this case. As the pressure on the heart muscle increases, it impacts the ability for the heart chambers to fill (decreased preload) and ultimately results in a similar decrease in cardiac output that can lead to cardiogenic shock due to cardiac tamponade. Early tamponade can be identified by several clinical signs including muffled heart sounds, jugular venous distension, hypotension, pulsus paradoxus, and equalization

of cardiac filling pressures. Although this condition can be difficult to diagnose during its earlier phases, it can be readily and easily diagnosed by clinical exam and confirmed by bedside ultrasonography in most patients. Although ultrasound can miss very small effusions, it can readily identify an effusion of the size required to product any signs of tamponade or "pre-tamponade" physiology.

Pericardial effusion can be caused by a variety of conditions. The most common causes overall are: Acute pericarditis (viral, bacterial, tuberculosis, or idiopathic), autoimmune disease, postmyocardial infarction or cardiac surgery, sharp or blunt chest trauma (including a cardiac diagnostic or interventional procedure), malignancy (particularly metastatic spread of noncardiac primary tumors), mediastinal radiation, renal failure with uremia, myxedema, aortic dissection extending into the pericardium, and selected drugs [28–30]. The cause of pediatric effusions depends greatly on geography and the patient population, with infectious causes predominating in less developed countries. In this case, the pericardial effusion was likely triggered by an infectious process. Despite the report of a single negative sputum culture, the available history, clinical, and radiographic evidence (coupled with the known endemic incidence of tuberculosis in Afghanistan) made tuberculous pericarditis the most likely etiology and the patient responded to an appropriate TB treatment regimen. However, without definitive confirmatory serologic or microbiologic confirmation, the other common causes of pericardial effusion remain a possibility.

This patient evidenced classic signs of pericardial tamponade including tachycardia, muffled heart sounds and jugular venous distension, hypotension, and a preference for remaining in the seated upright position and leaning forward. This is another classic finding in patients developing tamponade, and the patient should be kept in the sitting position or hunched forward while preparations for intervention or surgery are being made (Fig. 8.8). There is often a perceived urgency to intubate these patients, but remember that this may precipitate hemodynamic decompensation due to the supine positioning as well as the lysis of elevated sympathetic tone and vasodilatory effects of medications used for intubation. If a surgical procedure or operation is emergently required and the patient is able to maintain spontaneous breathing, then it is often preferable to keep them awake through transport and positioning on the OR table, and only perform rapid sequence induction when the patient is prepped and draped and the surgical team is ready to begin the procedure. Alternatively, and as used initially in this case, a pericardiocentesis or percutaneous drain placement can be done in the field or emergency department (ED) setting with proper sedation and analgesia in select patients. This has the benefit of avoiding complete paralysis/deep sedation and the possible resultant rapid hemodynamic decompensation described above. Performing invasive or painful procedures on injured children almost always requires sedating agents. In the child who does not require intubation, ketamine is an excellent (and underutilized) fast-acting hypnotic that provides reliable short-term sedation for procedures such as laceration repair or fracture reduction/stabilization (dose 1–1.5 mg/kg IV, 4 mg/kg IM). We recommend giving a low dose of benzodiazepine also to minimize emergence agitation. Ketamine in children is a potent sialogogue; the use of atropine or glyco-pyrrolate can help decrease excessive oral secretions. Ketamine also does not have the vasodilatory effects of other analgesic or sedating medications, and thus it is an excellent choice in the patient with borderline or low blood pressure or concerns for ongoing bleeding [11].

Finally, the emergent management of a pericardial effusion with tamponade in an austere setting requires a rapid and logical approach to diagnosis and intervention, and may require improvisation with whatever supplies and equipment are immediately available. For a traumatic effusion the patient should be considered to have a cardiac injury and in most settings should proceed to a median sternotomy and cardiac repair. If the diagnosis is unclear on ultrasound, a subxiphoid pericardial window can be readily performed, with conversion to open cardiac repair if the effusion is confirmed to be due to hemorrhage. However, in a more austere setting and with non-traumatic effusions, the management should focus on relieving cardiac tamponade in

the simplest and least invasive manner, identifying the etiology, and initiating appropriate therapy to treat the underlying condition and prevent recurrence. Percutaneous drainage of a large effusion can be readily done in the emergency department environment, particularly with real-time ultrasound guidance. The guiding principles should be to remove enough fluid to resolve the tamponade effect, but if the fluid is clearly blood then continued aspiration should not be performed and preparations should be made for either immediate open surgical exploration or transfer to a better equipped facility. For non-traumatic effusions a percutaneous drain should be left in the pericardial space to provide continued drainage and prevent early recurrence of tamponade. In the austere environment you may not have commercially made percutaneous drain kits designed for this indication. One of the most versatile items that can be adapted to treat many of the Airway, Breathing, and Circulation emergencies is a central line kit. The kits typically contain the central line, a long guide wire, an access needle/syringe, and often a separate large angiocatheter. In this case an 8 French cordis kit was placed into the pericardial sac using a Seldinger technique. We have also used central line kits to serve as an improvised needle thoracostomy or even chest tube, as a needle cricothyrotomy or even temporary percutaneous tracheostomy, and to access the airway and place a retrograde wire as a guide for the endotracheal tube in difficult intubations.

8.6 Conclusions

This chapter has attempted to provide some insights and clinical pearls for the provider who is called upon to manage A, B, C emergencies in the pediatric patient, and several of these key points are summarized in Table 8.1. The management of emergent airway, breathing, or circulation problems in pediatric patients can be extremely difficult, particularly in a combat or austere environment without access to specialized equipment, supplies, and pediatric expertise. As with all emergent situations, an optimal outcome depends on the ability of the provider to perform a rapid and focused assessment

Table 8.1 Clinical pearls and pitfalls in managing pediatric airway, breathing, and circulatory problems

Airway

1. A patent airway is hard to improve upon—if the patient is moving air and maintaining oxygen saturation, don't rush to attempt intubation unless you are fully prepared

2. Don't forget simple maneuvers first—suction, chin lift/jaw thrust, and oral/nasal airway

3. Bag-valve-mask ventilation works great in almost all pediatric patients and can provide completely adequate temporary oxygenation and ventilation

4. Don't compromise exposure, evaluation, and ability to intubate due to c-spine concerns. Remove the collar and do what you have to do to secure the airway

5. Expect bradycardia with intubation, and either give atropine or have it ready

6. A surgical airway will fail without adequate lighting and a good assistant to retract/expose

7. A needle cricothyrotomy can buy you time with oxygenation but will not provide good ventilation. Avoid open cricothyrotomy in children if at all possible

8. Have a "difficult airway" cart prepared and available for airway emergencies

9. A Broselow tape is one of the most important aids to emergency pediatric care

Breathing

1. Assessment for breathing emergencies in children is challenging—look for tachypnea, nasal flaring, intercostal retractions, and abdominal breathing

2. Lung sounds can be present even with a significant pneumothorax, particularly in intubated patients receiving positive pressure ventilation

3. Suspected tension physiology should prompt immediate decompression with either a needle thoracostomy or chest tube

4. The treatment for a "sucking chest wound" is a chest tube first, then deal with the wound

5. A normal upright chest X-ray effectively rules out a pneumothorax or hemothorax as the source of any respiratory distress or hemodynamic instability

6. Ultrasound for pneumo and hemothorax is easily integrated into the FAST exam, and can be more reliable than even chest X-ray

7. Chest tubes can kink, clog, or be in the wrong position (or even wrong body cavity); always confirm position on X-ray and troubleshoot to endure adequate function

(continued)

Circulation

1. Hypotension is a very late finding in children with circulatory shock; do not rely on a normal blood pressure as a marker of stability

2. Marked or worsening tachycardia is a red flag that there is ongoing bleeding or volume losses

3. A rapid prioritized search for the source of shock can be completed in minutes (see Fig. 8.13)

4. Control of active bleeding is the top priority in combat trauma injuries

5. Bradycardia indicates the patient is about to arrest; intervene immediately

6. Start resuscitation in synchrony with the diagnostic workup for patients with signs of shock

7. A balanced resuscitation with plasma, PRBCs, and PLTs will help avoid major coagulopathy and may carry a survival benefit

8. Tamponade is readily identified with ultrasound, and should prompt either immediate drainage or open surgical exploration

prioritizing airway, breathing, and circulation issues, and then initiating life-saving interventions as needed. Excellent outcomes can be achieved through leadership, teamwork, preparation, and flexibility or improvisation to adapt to the situation and these challenging scenarios.

Editor's note: Colonel Matthew Martin is an active duty Army trauma surgeon stationed at Fort Lewis, Washington, where he serves as the Trauma Medical Director and Director of Surgical Research. He has completed four combat deployments, where he served in various leadership roles including Chief of Trauma in Baghdad, Iraq, and Commander of a Forward Surgical Team in Afghanistan.

Zaradhe Yach is a nurse practitioner working for Mercy Medical Group in the Sacramento area of California. She served 14 years on active duty and is currently a Commander in the Navy Reserves. She completed two deployments as a nurse practitioner—the first with Expeditionary Medical Facility (EMF) Kuwait and the second as the Senior Medical Officer for a Provincial Reconstruction Team (PRT) in Ghazni, Afghanistan.

Conflicts of Interest The authors have no conflicts of interest to declare and have received no financial or material support related to this manuscript.

Disclaimer The results and opinions expressed in this chapter are those of the authors, and do not reflect the opinions or official policy of the US Army, the US Navy, the Department of Defense, or any other governmental agency.

References

1. Jafarpour S, Nassiri SJ, Bidari A, Chardoli M, Rahimi-Movaghar V. Principles of primary survey and resuscitation in cases of pediatric trauma. Acta Med Iran. 2014;52(12):943–6.
2. van As AB, Manganyi R, Brooks A. Treatment of thoracic trauma in children: literature review, Red Cross War Memorial Children's Hospital data analysis, and guidelines for management. Eur J Pediatr Surg. 2013;23(6):434–43.
3. Taylor C, Subaiya L, Corsino D. Pediatric cuffed endotracheal tubes: an evolution of care. Ochsner J. 2011;11(1):52–6.
4. King BR, Baker MD, Braitman LE, Seidl-Friedman J, Schreiner MS. Endotracheal tube selection in children: a comparison of four methods. Ann Emerg Med. 1993;22(3):530–4.
5. Mace SE, Khan N. Needle cricothyrotomy. Emerg Med Clin North Am. 2008;26(4):1085–101. xi.
6. Graham CA. Needle cricothyrotomy. Br J Hosp Med. 1994;51(3):133.
7. Watanabe S, Iinuma Y. Emergency needle cricothyrotomy may not be useful in case of tracheal collapse. J Anesth. 1989;3(2):229–30.
8. Wilkerson RG, Stone MB. Sensitivity of bedside ultrasound and supine anteroposterior chest radiographs for the identification of pneumothorax after blunt trauma. Acad Emerg Med. 2010;17(1):11–7.
9. Monti JD, Younggren B, Blankenship R. Ultrasound detection of pneumothorax with minimally trained sonographers: a preliminary study. J Spec Oper Med. 2009;9(1):43–6.
10. Butler FK, Dubose JJ, Otten EJ, et al. Management of open pneumothorax in Tactical Combat Casualty Care: TCCC guidelines change 13-02. J Spec Oper Med. 2013;13(3):81–6.
11. Martin MJ, Bcckley A. Front line surgery: a practical approach. New York: Springer Publishing Inc.; 2011.
12. Butler FK. Tactical Combat Casualty Care: update 2009. J Trauma. 2010;69 Suppl 1:S10–3.
13. Butler Jr FK, Blackbourne LH. Battlefield trauma care then and now: a decade of Tactical Combat Casualty Care. J Trauma Acute Care Surg. 2012;73(6 Suppl 5):S395–402.
14. Eastridge BJ, Mabry RL, Seguin P, et al. Death on the battlefield (2001-2011): implications for the future of combat casualty care. J Trauma Acute Care Surg. 2012;73(6 Suppl 5):S431–7.
15. Holcomb JB, McMullin NR, Pearse L, et al. Causes of death in U.S. Special Operations Forces in the global war on terrorism: 2001-2004. Ann Surg. 2007;245(6):986–91.
16. Kotwal RS, Montgomery HR, Kotwal BM, et al. Eliminating preventable death on the battlefield. Arch Surg. 2011;146(12):1350–8.
17. Borgman MA, Spinella PC, Perkins JG, et al. The ratio of blood products transfused affects mortality in patients receiving massive transfusions at a combat support hospital. J Trauma. 2007;63(4):805–13.
18. Holcomb JB. Damage control resuscitation. J Trauma. 2007;62 Suppl 6:S36–7.
19. Holcomb JB, Jenkins D, Rhee P, et al. Damage control resuscitation: directly addressing the early coagulopathy of trauma. J Trauma. 2007;62(2):307–10.
20. Nosanov L, Inaba K, Okoye O, et al. The impact of blood product ratios in massively transfused pediatric trauma patients. Am J Surg. 2013;206(5):655–60.
21. Hendrickson JE, Shaz BH, Pereira G, et al. Implementation of a pediatric trauma massive transfusion protocol: one institution's experience. Transfusion. 2012;52(6):1228–36.
22. Dutton RP, Parr M, Tortella BJ, et al. Recombinant activated factor VII safety in trauma patients: results from the CONTROL trial. J Trauma. 2011;71(1):12–9.
23. Monpoux F, Chambost H, Haouy S, Benadiba J, Sirvent N. Recombinant activated factor VII in paediatric practice. Universal hemostatic agent? Arch Pediatr. 2010;17(8):1210–9.
24. CRASH-2 Trial Collaborators, Shakur H, Roberts I, et al. Effects of tranexamic acid on death, vascular occlusive events, and blood transfusion in trauma patients with significant haemorrhage (CRASH-2): a randomised, placebo-controlled trial. Lancet. 2010;376(9734):23–32.
25. Morrison JJ, Ross JD, Dubose JJ, Jansen JO, Midwinter MJ, Rasmussen TE. Association of cryoprecipitate and tranexamic acid with improved survival following wartime injury: findings from the MATTERs II study. JAMA Surg. 2013;148(3):218–25.
26. Morrison JJ, Dubose JJ, Rasmussen TE, Midwinter MJ. Military application of tranexamic acid in trauma emergency resuscitation (MATTERs) study. Arch Surg. 2012;147(2):113–9.
27. Eckert MJ, Wertin TM, Tyner SD, Nelson DW, Izenberg S, Martin MJ. Tranexamic acid administration to pediatric trauma patients in a combat setting: the pediatric trauma and tranexamic acid study (PED-TRAX). J Trauma Acute Care Surg. 2014;77(6):852–8. discussion 858.
28. Kuhn B, Peters J, Marx GR, Breitbart RE. Etiology, management, and outcome of pediatric pericardial effusions. Pediatr Cardiol. 2008;29(1):90–4.
29. Browne GJ, Hort J, Lau KC. Pericardial effusions in a pediatric emergency department. Pediatr Emerg Care. 2002;18(4):285–9.
30. Hoit BD. Diagnosis and treatment of pericardial effusion. 2013. www.updtodate.com/contents/diagnosis-and-treatment-of-pericardial-effusion. Accessed 2 Jan 2015.

The Oklahoma City Bombing

David W. Tuggle

On Wednesday, April 19, 1995 at 9:02 a.m., Timothy McVeigh set off a bomb housed in a rental truck in front of the Alfred P. Murrah Federal Building in downtown Oklahoma City. The bomb most likely consisted of over 4000 pounds of ammonium nitrate fertilizer with additional explosives added. This explosion caused the partial collapse of the north face of this 9-story building. There were 15 federal agencies and three non-federal agencies in this building. The article by Mallonee et al. [1] provides a comprehensive summary of the injuries involved and will be referenced extensively. More than 500 people were employed in this building. In addition, there was a day care center on the first floor and another one diagonally across the street in the YMCA.

I was helping an intern through an inguinal hernia repair at the Children's Hospital of Oklahoma when the operating room charge nurse came into the room and asked if I knew where I was supposed to be. A bomb had gone off in downtown Oklahoma City. I replied that I did. I assumed that this was a disaster drill, since our hospital typically arranged for disaster drills in April and October in the middle of the week.

A few moments later she came back and said that a bomb really had gone off in downtown OKC and asked what we needed to do. I finished the case and went to the front desk to see how many Operating Rooms (OR) were running. I told the charge nurse to cancel all electives from that moment on and send the pre-op patients home immediately. I also asked her to contact the eight attendings who had cases scheduled that day and ask them to check in to the OR to be available for stat cases. This was necessary because there was not a single trauma center in Oklahoma City at the time and therefore no surge response had been drilled or implemented. I then went to the emergency department, as my role was typically the surgical triage officer during disaster drills. The medical and nursing response was much better than any drill we had ever had, because everyone knew it was not a drill. Within 30 min the first patient to arrive had a wound of the forehead with exposed brain. We dressed the wound lightly while I called neurosurgery. They were already in the OR waiting for patients, so this child was in the Emergency Department for less than 10 min before he was transported to the OR.

Within ten minutes other children arrived including one with a vascular injury and my partner, William P. Tunell MD took him to the OR for a vascular repair. As we waited for more patients, we listened to the county disaster command radio net. The communications were poor however we could tell that there was a considerable amount of

D.W. Tuggle, M.D. (✉)
Department of Trauma, Dell Children's Medical Center of Central Texas, 1301 Barbara Jordan Blvd, Ste 400, Austin, TX 78723, USA
e-mail: davidtuggle@gmail.com

© Springer International Publishing Switzerland 2016
C.R.B. Lim (ed.), *Surgery During Natural Disasters, Combat, Terrorist Attacks, and Crisis Situations*, DOI 10.1007/978-3-319-23718-3_9

radio traffic about the children in the 2 day care centers. We later were told that the county-wide communication was poor, due to the fact that only 3 of 15 hospital ED radios were functional [2]. Our radio was one of the functional ones.

J. Andy Sullivan MD was the Chief of Pediatric Orthopedics at the time, and was in the ED as the orthopedic triage officer. As we listened we decided that there was chaos and inadequate transportation available for the children at the scene. We asked a police Captain stationed in our ED to escort us to the bomb site to see if we could provide further aid, which he did.

We approached the southern face of the Murrah building and were instructed that this was a crime scene. My first impression was that there were numerous volunteer rescue workers, and none had protective equipment. I asked our police escort if he could go to the nearest construction site and acquire all of the hard hats he could find, which he did. Once Dr. Sullivan and I had hard hats, we entered the building with fire department personnel. At this point there were three live victims left entrapped in the building. On the first floor, we watched the firemen removing debris from around a woman whose left arm and leg were entrapped. Dr. Sullivan and I agreed that she would most likely be extracted successfully. Then the firemen took us to the basement. One fireman was leaning with his hand against a large cement pillar in the basement and I asked him what he was doing. He replied he had been told to feel the pillar and if it moved, he was to order the evacuation of the entire building. We approached the young woman trapped beneath a similar pillar farther into the basement. We debated whether we could raise this pillar without having the remainder of the building come down, and in consultation with the fire department decided there was no way to move the pillar without more building coming down. The pillar was on the mid shaft of the woman's right tibia, and the knee was accessible. She was awake and we spoke with her, reassuring her we were working to get her free. The third patient was undergoing extrication and would likely be freed.

At that moment, we were told to evacuate the building, as a bomb sniffing dog had detected explosives and the police were concerned there was a second explosive device. We were led 2 blocks away from the building, and there we formulated a plan. We agreed that the only way to rescue her would be to amputate her leg. Dr. Sullivan went back to the hospital to acquire amputation equipment and analgesic medication. I had a mobile phone I had brought with me and would call him with any other additional needs once the all clear was given to re-enter the building. Approximately 45 min later I was allowed to return and went to examine our patient. She appeared to be hypothermic and hypotensive by physical examination. In discussion with the fire department there was no option to move the pillar. I called Dr. Sullivan and asked him to come with the equipment and medications. When he arrived we both went to the basement with ten firemen and two paramedics to assist. Despite numerous attempts by Emergency Medical Technicians and myself, we could not establish an IV for medication delivery. Dr. Sullivan had brought midazolam and morphine, along with an amputation set. Our patient was responsive enough to give verbal consent for amputation after a discussion of the situation. I gave her 4 mg of midazolam by direct internal jugular vein injection. Morphine was not given to avoid respiratory depression that could lead to respiratory arrest. A tourniquet was placed at mid thigh for approximately 10 min. Oxygen was supplied by mask. The entry way into the space where she was trapped was about 2 feet wide and slanting down at a 45° angle. It would only allow one person to be next to her at a time. After placement of the tourniquet, Dr. Sullivan performed a right through the knee amputation virtually standing on his head, with multiple disposable scalpels and an amputation knife which I passed to him as needed. After completing the amputation the patient was extracted from the entrapment site and I obtained direct vascular control of her popliteal vessels. After I had clamped and tied her vessels, she was taken up the stairwell by the fire department and paramedics and loaded into an ambulance that we had waiting. I rode with her and the paramedics to the University Hospital ED where she was resuscitated, and then taken to the operating room for formal closure of her amputation wound [3].

Under the direction of the Oklahoma State Commissioner of Health at the time, Jerry Nida, the Oklahoma Department of Health was ordered to catalog the injuries and mortalities associated with the bombing. According to Mallonee et al., 759 people sustained injuries. This included 167 people who died (22 %), 83 survivors who were hospitalized (11 %), and 509 people who were treated and released (67 %). Fifty-seven percent were female. The median age of the injured was 39. One volunteer rescuer was injured by falling debris, sustaining an unrecognized epidural hematoma, which ultimately caused her death. While most of the injured were taken to six hospitals located closest to the bomb site, 18 hospitals in the metropolitan area treated 511 adults and 38 children. An additional 233 persons were treated in physicians' offices or clinics.

Nineteen children, 16 of whom were in the day care center, died as a direct result of the blast. The injury patterns among the 19 dead children included a 90 % (17 of 19) incidence of skull fractures, 15 of those with cerebral evisceration (skull capping); 37 % with abdominal or thoracic injuries; 31 % amputations; 47 % arm fractures, 26 % leg fractures; 21 % burns; and 100 % with extensive cutaneous contusions, avulsions, and lacerations. Forty-seven children sustained non-fatal injuries with only seven children requiring hospitalization. The injuries sustained by the seven hospitalized children included two open, depressed skull fractures, with partially extruded brain, two closed head injuries, three arm fractures, one leg fracture, one arterial injury, one splenic injury, five tympanic membrane perforations, three corneal abrasions, and four burn cases [4].

Of the 592 survivors, 83 were hospitalized, 351 were treated in an ED and released, and 158 were treated by a private physician and did not go to an emergency room. Of the 506 victims with a soft tissue injury, the most common locations were extremities (74 %), head and neck injuries (48 %), face (45 %), and chest (35 %). There were 18 survivors with potentially fatal injuries including five with carotid artery or jugular vein

lacerations, three with facial or popliteal artery lacerations, eight with severed nerves, tendons, or ligaments, and two with deep lacerations with bone injury.

Four patients had the onset of Acute Respiratory Distress Syndrome (ARDS), six patients had a pneumothorax (four closed, one open, and one hemopneumothorax). Three patients were noted to have pulmonary contusions. Four patients had abdominal injuries. One had a partial bowel transection. Another had both a spleen and renal injury; and another one patient had a liver laceration. The fourth abdominal injury was the final patient we treated that day at my hospital.

I was still on call that evening when I was called to the ED to see the last patient evacuated from the building at about 9 p.m. The patient was a 14-year old girl who had burns and a tender abdomen. She was hypotensive and hypothermic. We resuscitated her with crystalloid and blood, but she remained hypotensive, therefore I took her to the OR and performed a splenectomy, and dressed her burns. She did not require skin grafting and was discharged about a week after the bombing.

A total of 210 (35 %) of survivors sustained musculoskeletal injuries. Twenty-two (37 %) of 60 persons with fractures and dislocations had multiple fractures. The most common sites of fractures and dislocations were extremities (legs, 40 %; arms, 38 %), face and neck (37 %), and back, chest, or pelvis (25 %). The most common sites of injury for the 150 persons with musculoskeletal strains and sprains included the chest and back (53 %), neck (29 %), and extremities (legs, 27 %; arms, 9 %). One person sustained an incomplete spinal cord injury with transient neurologic deficits. Another person had to have a leg through the knee amputation to be extricated from the building basement [3].

Of 80 persons diagnosed with a head injury, 35 (44 %) were hospitalized. Eight persons sustained severe brain injuries (AIS head 4 or 5), including four who had open skull fractures, two who had subdural hematomas, and two who had depressed skull fractures. Among 72 persons with mild or moderate head injury (AIS head 1, 2, or 3), the most prevalent diagnoses included 33 persons (46 %) with concussions and 25 persons (35 %) with closed head injury. Of the 59 victims with ocular injuries, nine had ruptured globes, including four who also had detached retinas; one other person had a detached retina. The most frequent eye injuries among the 36 persons not hospitalized were corneal or scleral abrasions (15, 42 %) and lacerations, contusions, or glass in the eye (6, 17 %).

Nine persons had thermal burns covering up to 70 % of their body surface area, including seven who were hospitalized. The seven persons hospitalized, including four children younger than 5 years, were located in the Murrah Building near the point of bomb detonation. One person was burned inside a car stopped next to the Murrah Building; another person sustained burns in the doorway of an adjacent building. The face and neck regions were the most frequent sites of burns (67 %). All of these patients had partial-thickness burns, except for two people who had full-thickness burns to less than 10 % of total body surface area.

Among survivors, 210 (35 %) were reported to have sustained auditory damage. However, for 132 (63 %) of these persons, a formal medical diagnosis was not documented. Among the 78 persons with medical diagnoses of auditory damage, the most frequent diagnoses were as follows: hearing loss 31 (11 sensorineural, 1 conductive, 1 mixed type, and 18 unspecified); bilateral or unilateral tympanic membrane perforation (22); acoustic trauma (13); and tinnitus, vestibular injury, and otalgia (12). Among the 83 hospitalized patients, 14 % were documented to have sustained tympanic membrane rupture.

A total of 167 persons died as a direct result of the blast; 162 persons died at the scene, three persons were dead on arrival at an emergency department (2 died of multiple trauma and 1 died of head trauma), and two persons were hospitalized and died 2 days after admission (head trauma) and 23 days after admission (multiple injuries with resulting sepsis, acute respiratory distress syndrome, and multiorgan failure). Three pregnant women died. The Office of the Chief Medical Examiner determined the probable cause of death was multiple injuries for 122 persons (73 %), followed by head trauma (24 persons), chest trauma (13 persons), head and neck trauma (3 persons), traumatic shock (3 persons), and fractured cervical spine (2 persons).

The rescue and recovery effort spanned a total of 16 days from immediately after the blast to May 4, 1995. Eighty-eight bodies (53 %) were recovered during the first week, 51 (31 %) during the second week, 25 (15 %) during the remaining 3 days, and three were recovered after implosion of the building on May 23, 1995. Sixty-one percent of the bodies were identified less than 1 day following recovery, 24 % were identified within 24–48 h following recovery, and 15 % were identified 72 or more hours following recovery. Among the 163 persons who died in the Murrah Building, 118 (72 %) were employed in the federal building, 15 (9 %) were children in the day care center, and 30 (18 %) were visitors, including four children. Three additional persons died in two buildings (Athenian, Water Resources) directly across the street from the Murrah Building, and one person died in the outdoor parking lot across the street.

A building occupant survey determined that 361 persons were in the Murrah Building at the time of the blast and 88 % were injured. Ninety-eight percent of persons killed and 26 % of persons who sustained nonfatal injuries were located in the Murrah Building. Mallonee and colleagues provide some statistical analysis of the injured. People who were located in the collapsed region of the building were significantly more likely to die (153/175, 87 %) than persons in the uncollapsed region (10/186, 5 %) (RR, 16.3; 95 % CI, 8.9–29.8). This difference was more pronounced on the upper floors (4–9) than on the lower floors (1–3). On the upper floors, 72 (97 %) of 74 persons in the collapsed area died, compared with 2 (2 %) of 105 persons in the uncollapsed area (RR, 51.1; 95 % CI, 12.9–201.7); on the lower floors, 81 (80 %) of 101 persons in the collapsed area died, compared with 8 (10 %) of 79 persons in the uncollapsed area (RR, 7.9; 95 % CI, 4.1–15.4). Survivors in the collapsed region were significantly more likely to require hospitalization (18/22, 82 %) than survivors in the uncollapsed region (32/176, 18 %) (RR, 4.5; 95 % CI, 3.1–6.5).

Injury rates in the four adjacent buildings ranged from 38 % in the Journal Record Building to 100 % in the Athenian Building. Survivors in the uncollapsed part of the Murrah Building were significantly more likely to require hospitalization (32/176, 18 %) than survivors in the other four buildings combined.

President William J. Clinton signed Public Law 105-58 on October 9, 1997. This law created the Oklahoma City National Memorial as a unit of the National Park System. The Outdoor Symbolic Memorial was dedicated on April 19, 2000, the fifth anniversary of the bombing. President Clinton joined more than 20,000 people to dedicate the site. President and Mrs. George W. Bush dedicated the Memorial Museum on Presidents' Day, February 19, 2001 [5].

9.1 Conclusion

Based upon this experience, and subsequent mass casualty events involving tornados in Oklahoma, I think that chaos is the rule, not the exception, in mass casualty events of any type. Having plans and drills are good, but having disaster drills with chaotic events inserted are better. When planning disaster drills, always think about inserting irrational and unexpected events into the process. This will help responders at all levels to think about how to fix any problem in the moment. In addition, I think the following concepts are important to consider when dealing with a situation similar to the Oklahoma City bombing:

1. Surgery in the field is a very rare event.
2. Keeping a team ready is not practical.
3. What is useful is knowing who in the group is ready and willing to respond.
4. There was no fallout from cancelled cases in this hospital. People understood.
5. 6 ORs were running at the time of the bombing; but the cases were quick and did not impact operating on victims.

Editor's Note: Dr. David Tuggle practices in the Austin, Texas area. The patient described in this chapter survived her amputation but her current status is unknown. The Oklahoma City bombing remains the deadliest attack on United States soil by a United States citizen. This year marks the 20th anniversary of that bombing.

References

1. Mallonee S, Shariat S, Stennies G, Waxweiler R, Hogan D, Jordan F. Physical injuries and fatalities resulting from the Oklahoma City bombing. JAMA. 1996;276(5):382–7.
2. Maningas PA, Robison M, Mallonee S. The EMS response to the Oklahoma City bombing. Prehosp Disaster Med. 1997;12(2):80–5.
3. Raines A, Lees J, Fry W, Parks A, Tuggle D. Field amputation: response planning and legal considerations inspired by three separate amputations. Am J Disaster Med. 2014;9(1):53–8.
4. Quintana DA, Parker JR, Jordan FB, Tuggle DW, Mantor PC, Tunell WP. The spectrum of pediatric injuries after a bomb blast. J Pediatr Surg. 1997;32(2):307–10.
5. http://www.oklahomacitynationalmemorial.org/index.php. Accessed 3 Jan 2015.

The Experience of Disaster Response in Sri Lanka: From Reaction to Planning the Future

10

Rochelle A. Dicker and Julie E. Adams

10.1 Introduction

On December 26, 2004 at 7:58 am there was a powerful 9.0 magnitude earthquake off the coast of Indonesia. The catastrophic tsunami that followed hit the coast of Indonesia 15 min after the earthquake and reached Sri Lanka just 2 h later. Though warnings were issued to nations in the Pacific Ocean, no such alarms were raised for nations of the Indian Ocean as there was no comparable system in place [1]. The attention of the world was immediately captured and international efforts began at every level from individuals donating skills, time, or money to large nations coordinating together to provide help. Unfortunately for many, there was no chance for help; the estimated mortality in Sri Lanka was greater than 30,000—it was the second most affected country. In addition, more than 500,000 people were displaced from their homes in Sri Lanka. Most deaths, an estimated 82 %, occurred on the day of the tsunami. The remainder occurred within the following 7 days, significantly limiting the window in which meaningful life-saving aid could be provided. Deaths were secondary to drowning or tsunami-related crush injuries [2, 3].

At the time of the tsunami in Sri Lanka, the country was more than two decades into an armed conflict between the Liberation Tigers of Tamil Eelam (LTTE or Tamil Tigers) and the Sri Lankan military. A ceasefire had been negotiated and signed in 2002, though the Eastern Province remained under the control of the LTTE. This region of the country was hard-hit by the tsunami with more than 60 % of the damage occurring in the north and east.

Upon learning of the destruction from the tsunami that day, we felt an immediate compulsion to respond to what appeared to be a mass casualty event. The definition of a MASCAL event is when "the number of patients and the severity of their injuries exceed the capability of a facility to deliver care in a routine fashion" [4]. The Tsunami's effect on the people and the health care facilities in northeastern Sri Lanka clearly met the defined criteria. Not only were health care facilities overwhelmed, many of them were damaged or destroyed. The result was that human suffering was beyond the capacity of the system to manage it. It can be argued that the ability of that system, *pre*-tsunami was also perilously inadequate to manage daily surgical disease and trauma. There was a chronic factor that played an even greater role in the state of care of

R.A. Dicker, M.D. (✉)
Department of Surgery, UCSF at San Francisco
General Hospital, 1001 Potrero Avenue, Ward 3A,
San Francisco, CA 941100, USA
e-mail: Rochelle.Dicker@ucsf.edu

J.E. Adams, M.D.
Department of Surgery, University of Vermont
Medical Center, 111 Colchester Avenue, Burlington,
VT 05401, USA
e-mail: Julie.adams@uvmhealth.org

© Springer International Publishing Switzerland 2016
C.R.B. Lim (ed.), *Surgery During Natural Disasters, Combat,*
Terrorist Attacks, and Crisis Situations, DOI 10.1007/978-3-319-23718-3_10

surgical disease and trauma in many regions of Sri Lanka in 2004: low- and middle-income countries chronically suffer from poor access to care, inadequate numbers of trained personnel, and under-resourced surgical infrastructure. The tsunami just served to peel back the scab. In addition, though it occurred during a ceasefire between the government of Sri Lanka and the LTTE, this was tenuous and further complicated delivery of personnel and goods to civilians most affected. During the days following the tsunami, mass casualty care *and* routine health care, both surgical and non-surgical, were severely compromised. Years after the tsunami, populations still lack access to proper care for prevention and treatment of communicable and non-communicable diseases alike.

Triage refers to "sorting of patients according to their need for treatment and the available resources" [4]. The ultimate goal is to turn a mass casualty event into a *multiple casualty event*, defined as an event in which "many patients receive treatment as required simultaneously" [4]. Triage is a mechanism by which this can occur. Figure 10.1 illustrates a typical mechanism by which triage is conducted. Surgeons often play a critical role in primary or secondary triage, leadership at the incident command center, and provide clinical care. However, in low- and middle-income countries, a disaster plan may not exist. Lack of infrastructure, poor communication mechanisms, limited personnel and consumable resources further limit the capacity for response. Certainly, the 2004 tsunami on the shores of northeastern Sri Lanka overtook the health care system that existed at that moment, and for months in its aftermath.

Sri Lankans are not alone in the effect armed conflicts have had on their health systems, and this can be difficult to quantify. We personally experienced significant delays in reaching the region we intended to serve with all of our donated supplies. We left the United States 6 weeks after the Tsunami. Once in Columbo, Sri Lanka with 200 kg of surgical gear and consumables, we headed to Kilinochchi, 250 miles to the northeast. The trip along the contested A9 highway took 12 h as we crossed multiple governmental and LTTE checkpoints along treacherous roads (Figs. 10.2 and 10.3). The situation had been even worse in years prior. The A9 highway had been closed from 1990 until the very fragile ceasefire of 2002, depriving the region of basic health care and welfare needs. There were also an estimated 1.5 million land mines present in the north and east, making travel hazardous. Prior to the tsunami, child malnutrition rates in the northeast region were twice the national average [5].

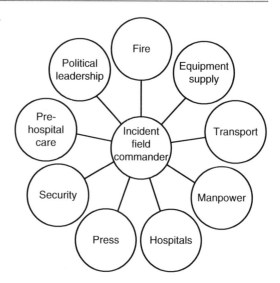

Fig. 10.1 Components of disaster response

10.2 Expectations Versus Reality

Given our arrival 6 weeks after the tsunami, we anticipated playing a role in providing care for people with infected wounds, degloving injuries, and perhaps surgical diseases that were put on the "back burner" during the surge of tsunami-related injuries. We found a situation very different than anticipated. Our encounters were simply that of a typical scenario plaguing many low-income countries today regarding surgical disease and trauma: surgical disease in many places in the world, including the northeast portion of Sri Lanka, is neglected and under-resourced.

Victims of the tsunami fell into four main categories: those who were swept out to sea and drowned, those who were fatally injured or

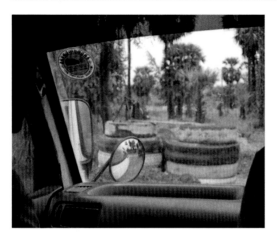

Fig. 10.2 Militarized checkpoint on A9 highway

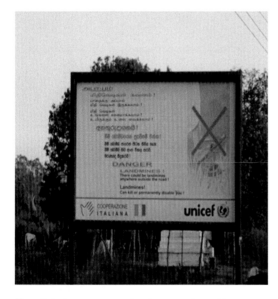

Fig. 10.3 It was thought that the tsunami would put more people at risk for landmine injuries

crushed from hitting objects on land (such as trees), those who suffered from minor soft tissue injuries, and finally those who experienced major psychological trauma from loss in the setting of an already war-torn community. There was a tremendous amount to be done for surgical disease and trauma care, representing a chronic backlog, but little for tsunami-related injuries. Psychological trauma was everywhere. We met families who fled the area due to war, returned during the ceasefire in 2002, only to lose everything again during the tsunami.

Surgical disease has been described by Dr. Paul Farmer as the "neglected stepchild of global health." Injury alone kills more people than TB, malaria and HIV *combined*, however, as of yet, it has not garnered the resources commensurate with the burden [6]. Recently, research including field surveys [7], hospital surveillance studies [8–12], and accounts of workforce distribution has raised more awareness of the magnitude of surgical disease. Also encouraging is the statement by the World Health Assembly in May 2007 urging member states to "identify a core set of trauma and emergency-care services" [13]. Finally, at the time of writing this chapter, the Lancet Commission for Global Surgery report has just been released, further advocating for research focused on capacity building for surgical care in low- and middle-income countries [14].

Emergency and essential surgical care is a concept recognized by the World Health Organization (WHO). The vision of the WHO is to provide leadership and guidelines for establishment of universal access to high-quality emergency and essential surgical services. The Emergency and Essential Surgical Care Programme was established to address challenges and take the lead-in efforts to reduce the burden of surgical disease [15]. As stated by the WHO, this can be done by strengthening education and training, establishing standards for care, implementing quality assurance programs, and developing and adopting evidence-based policies. The cornerstone of these principles is an understanding of needs by region, and the region's current capacity to care for the population.

This background has great relevance to our experience after the Tsunami. We arrived too late to play a key surgical role in a MASCAL response and at a time when a very short visit could have some unintended negative consequences. First, people arriving to these events outside of a well-trained, coordinated organization presents burden itself; we needed food, shelter, and transportation. All of this is in short supply during times of a MASCAL. Lack of training and preparedness. Lack of training and preparedness can turn the best intentions into liabilities. Furthermore, treating patients without a plan for postoperative management after a medical visit could compromise patient care. Although we brought much of our own supplies, short medical missions by well-intentioned individuals also may ultimately burden resource-strained setting in the use of staff, consumables, security personnel (at times), and infrastructure necessary for surgical care.

As we recognized these potential consequences, we shifted the focus during our short time there; our primary driver then became the vision of someday seeing the development of systems to deliver daily essential surgical care. A lack of infrastructure for such essential surgical care makes implementation of a MASCAL protocol essentially impossible.

With these concepts in mind, we put down our stethoscopes and knives and picked up our notepads and pens. The following is a report that we compiled based on our own observations and the sentiments of the local stakeholders.

10.3 Kilinochchi Public District Hospital

This is an extremely busy public hospital serving approximately 200,000 people. Though the official inpatient capacity is 120, there were 400 inpatients there during our visit. While this area was not directly hit by the tsunami, as it is not on the coast, it was the major referral hospital for the northeast after the tsunami.

While the hospital serves all medical needs, it is important to note, both for visitors as well as health officials monitoring the region, the very high number of patients admitted daily with snakebites (approximately five per day). These are generally from cobras and vipers. There is a hospital protocol to obtain a clotting time and monitor for local as well as general neurotoxic symptoms to evaluate the need for antivenom. All patients who we saw required antivenom to treat life-threatening symptoms. The week prior to our arrival an aid worker was bitten and evacuated, with an uncertain health outcome.

10.3.1 Physical Plant

1 Operating room.

1 Small procedures room.

Plain X-ray machine—we saw many films which were of good quality.

No surgical pathology capacity.

ICU with four beds but no ventilators.

Intermittent problems with water supply and dimming, unreliable electricity.

Very crowded wards with many patients on mats (not mattresses) on the floor.

10.3.2 Supplies

Some basic, many borderline functional surgical instruments.

Vicryl and nylon suture primarily.

Very few numbers of drapes and gowns (one appropriately draped patient would sacrifice much of the day's supply of drapes and towels putting the patients at risk of infectious complications).

There is a functioning autoclave.

10.3.3 Anesthesia Capacity

Automated blood pressure, pulse oximetry, and cardiac monitoring in OR.

For general anesthesia: ketamine and atracurium; also spinal anesthesia.

No ventilator (general cases are handbag ventilated currently if the patient requires intubation).

10.3.4 Human Resources

No surgeon (visiting plastic surgeon from UK during our visit, who limited his practice to facial and extremity injuries/burn contractures).

There is a Sri Lankan ob-gyn surgeon (we were under the impression this was a temporary posting for 6 months).

Two persons capable of giving anesthesia: District Medical Officer (DMO) Dr. Satha and his brother Dr. Sivamurthy.

Surgical assistants for most procedures though there was some difficulty in communication due to language barrier.

Approximately six medical officers totally caring for hospital population.

Nursing:patient ratio of 1:40–60.

10.3.5   Accommodation for Visiting Doctors

The CHC Guesthouse was quite limited with only intermittent running water, absent electricity between 12 and 5 a.m. (and thus no functional fan), and no food on site. There was mosquito netting provided over each bed. A woman assisting prior visitors with accommodations at the site left during the week of our stay, and this may have had some impact.

10.3.6   Some Supplies We Donated Included

Approximately 100 instruments including straight scissors, mosquito and mayo clamps, tooth and non-tooth forceps, heavy needle drivers.

Vicryl suture 2-0, 3-0, 4-0, 5-0.

Many other medical/surgical supplies such as sterile and non-sterile gloves, bandages, needles, syringes.

10.3.7   Needs

Full-time Surgical capacity; 24 h trauma capacity.

Pathology capacity for this region (as all specimens currently are sent to Colombo or Jaffna with months of waiting).

10.3.8   Physical Plant

More consistent running water and power.

Another operating room if possible (we often had to do two procedures at once in the same room).

10.3.9   Human Resources

Full-time general surgeon also capable of orthopedic surgery OR a rotating system of perhaps local and international surgical personnel.

Increased number of nurses for operating room and wards.

10.3.10   Supplies

Note: the DMO has a detailed list of surgical needs on the Kilinochchi website www.kilimedical.com which we found to be generally quite accurate in terms of the actual needs there.

Anesthesia machine with inhaled anesthetic and training on use of machine.

Oxygen concentrator.

Lidocaine (1 %, 2 % and lidocaine mixed with epinephrine)—there are many minor procedures which can be done with local anesthesia and this is essential.

More sterile drapes and gowns.

More operating room boots.

Bandage and supplies for minor surgical procedures.

Betadine and alcohol preps.

Examination table/operating room table cleaning reagents.

Suture: silk/nylon/vicryl/prolene especially 2-0, 3-0 and for prolene, 0.

10.3.11   Training

More education on emergency/trauma and postoperative care.

10.3.12   Summary Statement for Kilinochchi

First, in terms of security and travel, even with documentation from the CHC, there was a long wait at the first army checkpoint (2–3 h) and several of our boxes were searched though nothing was removed. Additional documents from donating organizations were scrutinized by both police and army officials. By comparison, we had no trouble at the LTTE checkpoint or in registering with the LTTE office in Kilinochchi. We rarely observed any weapons in the north.

After arrival, we were put immediately to work and shown our first several patients with very chronic large inguino-scrotal hernias. We performed one of these herniorrhaphies the next morning as well as an appendectomy the first day. This patient would have had to be transferred to Jaffna if we had not been present. This poses a significant risk to patients in cases of surgical emergencies in the northeast as the checkpoints close at 5:30 p.m., therefore transfer is impossible after that time (and there is no full-time surgeon in the region).

We evaluated 50–70 patients a day in 3 days of clinic and performed approximately 40 minor procedures (for acute and chronic problems) such as: repair of fresh lacerations and initial trauma care, excision of masses, evaluation and cleaning of chronically infected wounds, incision and drainage of acute infections, biopsies of masses (this was possible given a visiting pathologist at that time but is usually not possible), excision of thrombosed external hemorrhoids, etc. The DMOwas able to make a radio announcement about our presence to attract patients, but even the day before the announcement was made, we saw more than fifty patients. We were able to perform several biopsies due to the presence that week of a visiting pathologist who was able to do a touch prep and make diagnoses which immediately changed the management for those patients.

In summary, this hospital is chronically under-resourced both in terms of human resources and physical plant/supplies. The vast population there will always be in need of help. It was clear that hand-delivering supplies (Fig. 10.4) to this region is the best way to ensure that they arrive at the desired destination—this was confirmed by other individuals and groups working in the region, including hospital personnel who had significant delays and missing supplies sent from overseas, held up either in customs in Colombo or due to lack of authorization to get through the army checkpoint.

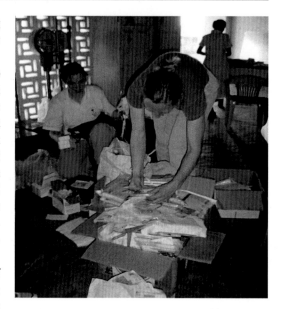

Fig. 10.4 Dr. Rochelle Dicker and Dr. Julie Adams delivering medical supplies in Mullaitivu

10.4 Kilinochchi Private (LTTE) Hospital

Generally, this hospital appeared to be better equipped for surgery with a full-time general/obstetric surgeon and general anesthesia capacity with an anesthesia machine. We were told that patients, if able, pay a nominal fee for care and for those unable to pay, the fee is waived.

Review of the OR log showed few procedures being done there: 1 in January, 12 in February, and most were sterilization and hernia repairs. The bed capacity is approximately 45, but there were few inpatients when we visited the site. We met a patient with esophageal cancer, clearly end-stage and cachectic, who had been sent back to Kilinochchi from Jaffna where it had been decided that he did not require therapy after a positive esophageal biopsy.

It was unclear to us how much sharing of resources existed between the two hospitals, but it generally seemed to be very minimal while we were there. We felt that this could be an opportunity for improvement.

10.5   Puthukkudiyiruppu Hospital (LTTE Private Hospital)

Puthukkudiyiruppu Hospital is the primary surgical referral center for the Mullaitivu District with a population of approximately one million.

10.5.1   Physical Plant/Anesthesia Capacity

Good running water and electricity.

Two operating rooms equipped with anesthesia machines including inhaled gas such as isoflurane.

Plain X-ray machine and ultrasound machine.

Air-conditioning for operating rooms.

10.5.2   Human Resources

Trained Full-time anesthetist.

Trained OR surgical technicians/nurses.

No surgeon.

10.5.3   Supplies

Suture and mesh for hernia repairs, generally well-supplied in terms of instruments and consumables.

Gowns/hats are single use and adequate in comparison to Kilinochchi.

10.5.4   Accommodation

Doctors' quarters is air-conditioned with two shower/toilets, adequate running water, three meals/day.

10.5.5   Needs

Full-time surgeon—they can certainly support this.

Sustained supply of consumables.

Education and training in trauma and surgical care.

10.5.6   Summary

This was by far the best equipped facility we visited—unfortunately we did not see many patients, as there was not a regular clinic day due to Good Friday and a Hindu festival. We did visit several camps, and the hospital in Mullaitivu, to announce our presence and services for referrals and to deliver supplies.

We treated one scalp laceration and performed one inguinal hernia repair with mesh. We had the good fortune of overlapping our stay with a very dedicated anesthesiologist from North America who brought the anesthesia machines to this hospital in the past (from Canada) and had trained the full-time anesthetist who works there. He was teaching the paramedic students in life support and checking the equipment in his short visit on this occasion. He was able to give spinal anesthesia for our operation. Clearly his sustained commitment has had an enduring impact on not only equipping the hospital, but also training the staff. We also left behind a significant supply of surgical instruments, consumables, suture, etc.

In the weeks prior, there had been a visiting orthopedic team from Malaysia operating around the clock. Additionally, there was a visiting ophthalmology team from Australia which set up their own facilities and performed many cataract surgeries, ophthalmologic evaluations, and also distributed glasses. It was clear that this hospital had supported many visiting overseas surgeons in the past.

We had the opportunity to teach parts of the Advanced Trauma Life Support curriculum to the paramedical students there, with an anesthesiologist functioning as a translator, though many of the students spoke English moderately well. We also left behind a substantial variety of surgical instruments, suture, and other related supplies.

Our assessment was that the physical plant and supplies were adequate there, but they lack a full-time surgeon. An ob-gyn surgeon (from the Kilinochchi Private Hospital) does occasionally visit and operate there performing some general surgery as well. If provided with sustainable human resources and advertisement as a referral center (especially until Mullaitivu hospital rebuilds), this hospital could support a lot of procedures and general surgical care. International surgical teams need to be coordinated to avoid overlap while providing continuity of care for patients. Planning ahead with community sensitization and outreach could serve a large population in a short time.

10.6   Mullaitivu Public Hospital

10.6.1   General Evaluation

There is a clinic area and waiting area.

Staffed with a DMO who has worked there since 1996, who is very dedicated—he is the only physician there.

10.6.2   Needs

Most of this hospital was directly damaged by the tsunami, and only the most basic clinical care was being provided upon our visit.

10.6.3   Summary

We left a significant amount of medical and surgical supplies here, including medications. Some of this will most likely be for future use when the new hospital becomes functional again. We appreciated the difficulty in getting supplies there given its status not only in the northeast, but as a higher-security zone within the LTTE-controlled areas. We, therefore, chose to leave a majority of basic supplies there. We had an escort from the LTTE on the ride both to Puthukkudiyiruppu as well as to Mullaitivu, and back to Kilinochchi. We were naïve to this escort arrangement prior to our leaving the US.

The DMO noted that almost all supplies they had received had been from international groups, not from the government. The DMO there (as well as the hospital director in Puthukkudiyiruppu) were very interested in advanced notice so they could organize lists of patients.

We did visit several camps of people displaced by the tsunami in Mullaitivu, as the hospital was coordinating medical team visits to these camps. We felt that there was a need for a more thorough evaluation of tsunami-related traumatic surgical problems such as chronically infected wounds or missed injuries, which might be in the camps but have been neglected. This would best be further evaluated through advanced notice to those displaced and allow for organized screening.

10.7   Batticaloa

10.7.1   General Situation

There is a public teaching hospital serving a population catchment area of about one million in the district. There were two full-time general surgeons at the hospital, one Sri Lankan, the other a visiting WHO surgeon. While we did not conduct a detailed needs assessment of the surgical capacity there, we met at length with the surgeon who explained that basic needs, in terms of anesthesia and surgical supplies/consumables, were being met. His greatest request was for a transurethral resectoscope for enlarged prostates. He had visiting surgeons work with him, and there were 3 surgeons from the Upstate New York medical team to assist that week in addition to a urologic surgeon from California.

10.7.2   Activities

We were asked to conduct mobile clinics in settlement camps and ran three half-day clinics with 80 patients at each site. We treated mostly primary care issues with the most common problems being:

1. A severely traumatized population, most of whom had significant family losses, material losses and stress symptoms that included appetite and sleep disturbance, sadness, and hopelessness. We provided psychological support, pharmacotherapy only in the form of sleep aids to some, and referrals to local groups such as the nongovernmental organization (NGO) SHADE, which had already

been providing psycho-social support to some villages in this region before the tsunami. For example, in pointing out one patient to them, SHADE explained that they had already been working with her and had taken her to a gravesite for grieving. While it was initially started as a foreign-based NGO 5 years ago, SHADE has been entirely locally run and staffed for the last year.

2. There was disruption in the care of common medical problems such as hypertension and diabetes for patients who lost their medications and had neglected these problems post-tsunami.
3. Diarrhea/Gastroenteritis as well as respiratory infections in children and adults.
4. Many skin infections (fungal and bacterial) and chronic neglected wounds.
5. We did make several surgical referrals for skin abscesses that required surgical drainages to the hospital.

Supplies for the mobile clinics were well stocked by the local CHC/TRO office. We stayed in a hotel while there for several nights. This region is generally heavily patrolled by the army and we were often stopped but not searched. There is a LTTE-controlled area in Batticaloa outside the city center as well; however, we had no trouble moving through the region.

10.8   Conclusions

In summary, our visit to Sri Lanka was not all that we expected. We entered a war-torn country with people in some areas, now internally displaced, chronically lacking access to health care; this, and not tsunami-related injuries, became the focus of our visit. Understanding the local challenges of such a population and performing a needs assessment are necessary tasks when working to build any system for health care delivery. Engagement of local partners is essential in understanding the needs of the population and the priorities. Short-term missions should be approached only by experienced people linked with well-established organizations. Injury is a public health issue of vast proportions. Development of systems of care can only come through diligent understanding of the burden of injury, the resources necessary, development of advocacy, and strong partnerships with countries most in need. A final political note: The LTTE has been defeated and no longer control the North.

Editor's Note: Rochelle A. Dicker, MD is currently a Professor of Surgery and Anesthesia at the University of California, San Francisco. The vast majority of humanitarian experience in global surgery is in capacity building with partners in Cameroon, Uganda, and India. She co-Directs the UCSF Center for Global Surgical Studies (global.surgery.ucsf.edu). Her experience in Sri Lanka opened her eyes to how she can best contribute to the field of Global Surgery as an academic surgeon. She has won numerous awards and has been recognized nationally for her work.

Julie E. Adams, MD travelled with Dr. Dicker to Sri Lanka after the tsunami to render surgical and capacity building assistance. She is currently the Program Director for General Surgery at the University of Vermont.

References

1. Li XH, Zheng JC. Efficient post-disaster patient transportation and transfer: experiences and lessons learned in emergency medical rescue in Aceh after the 2004 Asian tsunami. Mil Med. 2014;179(8):913–9.
2. Nishikiori N, Abe T, Costa DG, Dharmaratne SD, Kunii O, Moji K. Timing of mortality among internally displaced persons due to the tsunami in Sri Lanka: cross sectional household survey. BMJ. 2006;332(7537):334–5.
3. Nishikiori N, Abe T, Costa DG, Dharmaratne SD, Kunii O, Moji K. Who died as a result of the tsunami? Risk factors of mortality among internally displaced persons in Sri Lanka: a retrospective cohort analysis. BMC Public Health. 2006;6:73.
4. Dicker R, Schecter WP. Civilian Hospital Response to Mass Casualty Events. Editors: Asensio JA and Trunkey DD. Current Therapy in Trauma and Surgical Critical Care (pp. 67–73). Mosby/Elsevier, 2008 Philadelphia, PA.
5. Ozgediz D, Adams JE, Dicker RA. Trauma on trauma. Lessons from the tsunami and civil conflict in Sri Lanka. Pharos Alpha Omega Alpha Honor Med Soc. 2007;70(1):28–33.

6. World Health Organization. Injuries and violence: the facts. 2010. http://www.who.int/violence_injury_prevention/key_facts/en/. Accessed May 2015.

7. Mock CN, Gloyd S, Adjei S, Acheampong F, Gish O. Economic consequences of injury and resulting family coping strategies in Ghana. Accid Anal Prev. 2003;35(1):81–90.

8. Juillard CJ, Stevens KA, Monono ME, Mballa GA, Ngamby MK, McGreevy J, Cryer G, Hyder AA. Analysis of prospective trauma registry data in Francophone Africa: a pilot study from Cameroon. World J Surg. 2014;38(10):2534–42.

9. Juillard C, Etoundi Mballa GA, Bilounga Ndongo C, Stevens KA, Hyder AA. Patterns of injury and violence in Yaoundé Cameroon: an analysis of hospital data. World J Surg. 2011;35(1):1–8.

10. Jayaraman S, Mabweijano JR, Lipnick MS, Caldwell N, Miyamoto J, Wangoda R, Mijumbi C, Hsia R, Dicker R, Ozgediz D. Current patterns of prehospital trauma care in Kampala, Uganda and the feasibility of a lay-first-responder training program. World J Surg. 2009;33(12):2512–21.

11. Jayaraman S, Mabweijano JR, Lipnick MS, Caldwell N, Miyamoto J, Wangoda R, Mijumbi C, Hsia R, Dicker R, Ozgediz D. First things first: effectiveness and scalability of a basic prehospital trauma care program for lay first-responders in Kampala, Uganda. PLoS One. 2009;4(9):1–7.

12. Jayaraman S, Ozgediz D, Miyamoto J, Caldwell N, Lipnick M, Mijumbi C, Mabweijano J, Hsia R, Dicker R. Disparities in injury mortality between Uganda and the United States: a comparative analysis of a neglected disease. World J Surg. 2011;35(3):505–11.

13. World Health Assembly (WHA). Sixtieth World Health Assembly (May 2007). Health systems: emergency-care systems- WHA resolution 60.22. http://apps.who.int/gb/ebwha/pdf_files/WHA60/A60_R22-en.pdf. Accessed May 2015.

14. Meara JG, Leather AJM, Hagander L, et al. Global surgery 2030: evidence and solutions for achieving health, welfare, and economic development [published online April 21, 2015]. Lancet. http://www.thelancet.com/pdfs/journals/lancet/PIIS0140-6736%2815%2960160-X.pdf. Accessed May 2015..

15. World Health Organization (WHO). WHO Global Initiative for Emergency and Essential Surgical Care. http://www.who.int/surgery/globalinitiative/en/. Accessed May 2015.

A Surgical Response to the Haiti Earthquake 2010

11

Eileen M. Bulger and Susan M. Briggs

11.1 Introduction

Worldwide, it is estimated that earthquakes are responsible for approximately 1.87 million deaths in the twentieth century with approximately three times as many patients with serious injury [1]. A recent review of the human impact related to earthquakes between 1980 and 2009 reported an estimate of 372,634 deaths, 995,219 injuries and with 61 million people affected [1]. This review did not include the 7.0 earthquake which struck Haiti in 2010 with an estimate of 222,500 fatalities and the 8.9 earthquake with tsunami in Japan in 2011 with an estimate of 28,000 deaths. Injuries sustained as a result of earthquakes are largely due to structural collapse, resulting in penetrating and blunt traumatic injuries, many of which result in crush syndrome, compartment syndrome, and asphyxiation.

Management of patients with these injuries requires a prompt surgical response to minimize additional mortality and morbidity. Large earthquakes often lead to severe disruption of infrastructure and damage to the local hospitals, injury to healthcare workers or their families, and disruption of transportation, all of which result in increased difficulty in responding to the medical needs of the population.

A recent example of such a catastrophe was the 7.0 earthquake which struck Haiti in January of 2010 with over 33 aftershocks. The epicenter of the quake was approximately 25 km from the capitol city, Port au Prince and resulted in massive structural collapse in a highly populated area. In addition to the 222,500 fatalities, there was an estimated 300,000 injuries, and 1.5 million people displaced [2]. A recent population-based study reported the injury rate to be 40.2 injuries/1000 individuals [3].

Prior to the quake, Haiti was reported to be the poorest country in the western hemisphere with over 70 % of people living on less than two US dollars per day and gross national income per capita of $520 US. Unemployment was reported as high as 66 % and over 80 % of the population of Port au Prince was reported to be living in slum conditions. Poor building construction has been blamed for the widespread structural collapse following the quake. The healthcare infrastructure prior to the quake was also challenged with 60 % of the population lacking access to

E.M. Bulger, M.D. (✉)
Department of Surgery, Harborview Medical Center,
University of Washington, Box 359796,
325 9th Avenue, Seattle, WA 98104, USA
e-mail: ebulger@uw.edu

S.M. Briggs, M.D., M.P.H.
Department of Surgery, International Trauma and
Disaster Institute, Massachusetts General Hospital,
8 Hawthorne Place, Suite 114, Boston,
MA 02114, USA
e-mail: sbriggs@partners.org

© Springer International Publishing Switzerland 2016
C.R.B. Lim (ed.), *Surgery During Natural Disasters, Combat,
Terrorist Attacks, and Crisis Situations*, DOI 10.1007/978-3-319-23718-3_11

basic healthcare, 80/1000 children dying before age five, and a life expectancy of 61 years. Fifty percent of the population was children with high rates of malnutrition. The leading causes of death were infectious diseases including diarrhea illnesses, respiratory infections, malaria, tuberculosis, and HIV/AIDS. It was estimated that 5.6 % of the population between ages 15 and 49 years were HIV-positive.

Following the quake the healthcare system was quickly overwhelmed and relied on a broad international response, both through official government agencies as well as non-governmental agencies. Many of these organizations already had humanitarian missions in Haiti. USAID coordinated the relief efforts on behalf of the US government, which included deployment of search and rescue teams, emergency food and water assistance, and assistance with establishment of temporary shelters and sanitation. USAID has continued to provide support during the recovery and reconstruction phases [4]. The total USAID response cost is estimated at nearly $500 million US dollars with another $382 million in pledges to the international Haiti reconstruction fund [5].

Medical teams from the National Disaster Medical System (NDMS) were deployed along with the US Navy hospital ship, the USS Comfort. The US military frequently deploys for international missions to provide security for the medical teams and resources for patient evacuation. Military teams provided support at multiple sites in Haiti, including the US field hospital in Port-au-Prince.

This report will discuss the experience of the surgeons responding to this event on behalf of the US Government with the International Medical Surgical Response Teams (IMSuRT) which are managed by the National Disaster Medical System under the Department of Health and Human Services [6]. There are three IMSuRT teams based in the US. IMSuRT East is based in Boston, Massachusetts at Massachusetts General Hospital. IMSuRT South is based in Miami, Florida at the University of Miami's Ryder Trauma Center, and IMSuRT West is based in Seattle, Washington at Harborview Medical Center, University of Washington. The primary mission of these teams is to provide the full spectrum of surgical specialty care, non-operative and operative, especially in austere environments. These teams are composed of 50 members with flexible and mobile equipment and supplies (including pharmaceuticals and blood products) and a mobile field hospital [7]. IMSuRT teams are configured to provide sufficient medical personnel for acute care, definitive operative care, critical care, and evacuation. The National Disaster Medical System also provides Disaster Medical Assistance Teams (DMATs) that provide initial evaluation and triage capability. These teams may deploy with the IMSuRT teams or other assets of the NDMS system to augment the mission. All of these teams are comprised of federalized civilian health care providers who undergo advanced training in disaster medicine, including the Incident Command System, disaster triage, and gross decontamination.

11.2 The IMSuRT Response to the Haiti Earthquake

The on-call members of the IMSuRT teams were put on alert for deployment shortly after the quake, and members from all three IMSuRT teams were mobilized. Several DMAT teams were also deployed both to support the IMSuRT mission and to provide medical assessment teams across the affected region. Early after the quake there were significant challenges with transportation of the team and their equipment cache due to significant disruption of the Port au Prince airport. Upon arrival in Port au Prince, the team was staged at the US Embassy until a secure site for the field hospital could be identified and all equipment arrived. A site for deployment of the field hospital was identified at the former infectious disease treatment and research center known as Gheskio. While many of the buildings sustained damage as a result of the quake, the central courtyard was of sufficient size to construct the tent-based field hospital and the surrounding buildings provided the ability to establish a secure perimeter. The 82nd Airborne

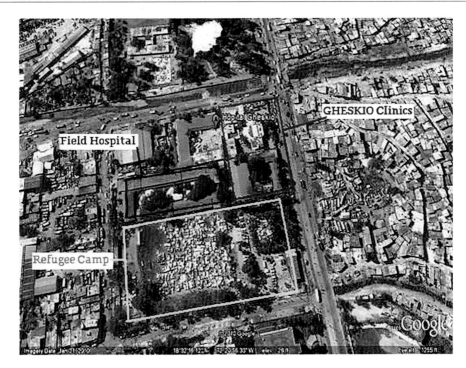

Fig. 11.1 Aerial view of the IMSURT field hospital at Gheskio, Port au Prince, Haiti, Jan 2010: courtyard with tents reflects the footprint of the field hospital with selec-tive use of surrounding buildings based on structural integrity. Lower part of image shows a refugee tent city that formed in an open field adjacent to the hospital

was tasked to provide security as the area was considered a "hot zone."

Figure 11.1 shows a Google map image of the field hospital at Gheskio. The upper part of the image shows a refugee tent city that formed immediately adjacent to the compound. Once the location was established, team members rapidly assembled the tents and equipment so they could begin seeing patients. Operating room and ICU capabilitywere quickly established as there was a significant demand for these services. Figure 11.2 illustrates the OR and ICUconfiguration. The field hospital began seeing patients 5 days after the quake. Personnel were deployed for 2-week rotations with the hospital fully operational for 6 weeks followed by a draw down period. At the conclusion of the deployment, all tents and remaining equipment were donated to the Haitian government.

Over the course of the deployment, the unit treated approximately 3000 patients of whom 300 required operative procedures. Of these, approximately 50 % of the procedures were related to orthopedic trauma and the other 50 %

a variety of general surgery and obstetrics issues. The most common operative procedure-swere revisions of amputations, placement of external fixators for fracture management, and wound debridements to clean and treat non-healing, chronic wounds. The team treated a wide variety of other surgical emergencies including acute abdomens from bowel obstructions or perforations, acute gunshot wound injuries, cesarean sections for complications associated with childbirth, and acute injuries resulting from car versus pedestrian crashes. Procedures were performed under both general anesthesia and conscious sedation. A daily wound care clinic was established for wounds that required ongoing debridement or complex dressing changes, which could be done with conscious sedation, largely with ketamine.

In addition to the expected surgical emergencies related to the earthquake, the unit quickly became a full service hospital with a large number of childbirth cases and patients with severe infectious disease complications,

Fig. 11.2 Operating room and intensive care unit, IMSURT Field hospital. (**a**) The OR set up; (**b**) the six- to nine-bed ICU which was attached to the operating room

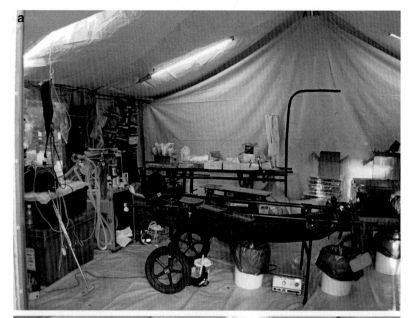

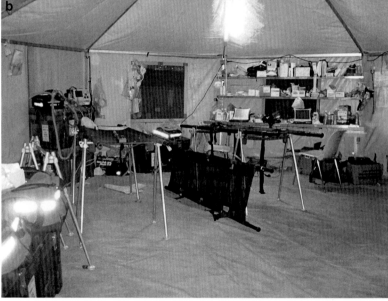

primarily children. Complications associated with childbirth included management of eclampsia and preeclampsia, amniotic fluid embolization, post-partum cardiomyopathy, and complex post-partum infections. The team had to adapt to provide neonatal care to high-risk infants and many infants with severe respiratory diseases. Severe cases of both neonatal and adult tetanus, meningitis, tuberculosis, and typhoid were also treated.

The unit had limited access to blood products and initially no imaging capability on site except for portable ultrasound. Four weeks into the deployment, a portable X-ray machine was obtained. Prior to that, only plain X-ray imaging was available during the day at an off-site facility. Transport to this area was dangerous due to gang activity so the facility was used sparingly for stable patients. The field hospital had ICU capability, including portable ventilators but did not have enough pediatric ventilators to support the increasing number of critically ill children. It was necessary to handbag many of the pediatric patients round the clock as no facilities were available for evacuation. The USS Comfort had limited pediatric ICU facilities and evacuation to other facilities in the US was limited and not available initially. In some cases the only option was expectant (palliative) care.

11.3 Management of Crush Injuries

One pattern of injury that is common in a post-earthquake scenario is the syndrome associated with crush injuries [8, 9]. This can result from a part of the body, commonly an extremity, being trapped for a prolonged period. The basic management principles include addressing the ABCs of injury care (Airway, Breathing, Circulation) along with aggressive fluid resuscitation to minimize renal injury and monitoring the extremity for compartment syndrome. The clinical signs of compartment syndrome include pain with passive motion of the extremity, parasthesias, pallor, and absent or diminished pulses. The absence of a pulse in the effected extremity is a late sign and suggests a high risk of permanent muscle injury. Pressure in the compartment can be measured if this equipment is available but is rarely utilized in mass casualty incidents. Treatment for suspected compartment syndrome involves fasciotomies of effected extremity. The decision to perform a fasciotomy hinges on the timing of the event to minimize muscle ischemia. Fasciotomy should be performed within 4–6 h of the development of compartment syndrome and many authors suggest that patients who present with more than 12 h of ischemic time already have irreversible tissue loss. Fasciotomy wounds at this time point may increase the risk of infection; and so these patients may be better served by an amputation.

Management of patients with trapped extremities may be very challenging. If the extremity has been trapped for more than 4 h, the patient should be given 1–2 l of intravenous normal saline to mitigate the reperfusion injury before release of the extremity. If that is not possible, a tourniquet should be applied to the limb immediately prior to extraction. Extraction of the patient should be managed by experienced search and rescue teams if possible. Field amputation should only be considered as a last resort.

Crush syndrome reflects the systemic manifestations of a crush injury. This includes reperfusion injury, which leads to third spacing of fluid and hypotension, myoglobinuria, which may progress to renal failure, and electrolyte abnormalities which may lead to cardiac arrhythmias. Treatment is aggressive fluid resuscitation (200–300 cc/hour) to maintain urine output and treatment of electrolyte abnormalities. The urine can be alkalinized by adding 2 ampules of sodium bicarbonate to 1 l of D5W and administered as a continuous infusion. It is unclear whether alkalization of the urine provides additional benefit beyond aggressive volume resuscitation. Despite aggressive therapy, many patients will progress to renal failure and so it is important to understand whether resources for dialysis are available.

11.4 Lessons Learned

There were several lessons learned by the surgeons who responded to this event that should be valuable for disaster responders in similar circumstances. These include:

1. *Be prepared to treat the full spectrum of injuries and illnesses, which may exceed your normal practice.*

   Surgeons responding to an earthquake event should recognize that they will be called upon to do far more than surgical intervention for injuries. Other common medical emergencies continue to occur, and the field hospital may be the only medical resource for the population. Surgeons should be prepared to manage routine and complicated obstetrics issues and common medical emergencies such as myocardial infarctions, asthma attacks, etc. [10]. Clinicians will also be called on to care for the full spectrum of ages from neonates to the elderly. Resources for pediatric drug dosing, such as the Broselow tape, are very valuable.

During this deployment, the surgeons provided the bulk of critical care services for a wide range of illnesses. The surgeon must be familiar with the medications carried in the pharmacy cache and how to manually calculate infusions when necessary (Fig. 11.3). The surgeon should also train with the equipment in the cache, including portable ventilators, monitoring systems, and use of the portable ultrasound as the primary diagnostic tool.

2. *Understand incidence and treatment of local endemic diseases.*

When deployed internationally, it is vital to understand the infectious diseases, which may be endemic to the region. These are diseases that may not be commonly encountered in the US and may prove challenging to diagnose and manage. One example of such a case from this deployment was a young man who developed systemic tetanus after a traumatic ankle

Fig. 11.3 ICU management. (**a**) The manual calculations of continuous infusions which were posted on the IV pole for nursing management. (**b**) The monitoring equipment and ventilators for the ICU patients

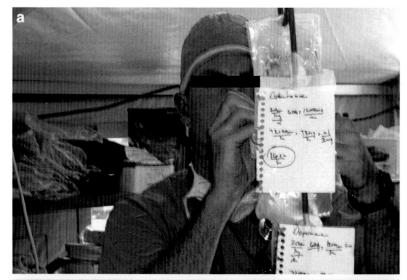
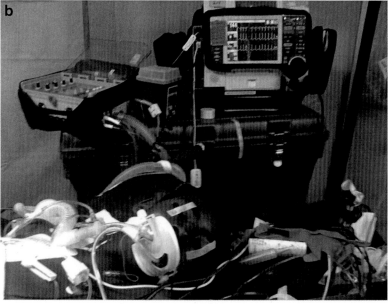

injury. His wound was managed with an acute amputation and debridement, and he was given tetanus immunoglobulin. He required extensive prolonged mechanical ventilation and sedation for management of the consequences of this infection. Ultimately this patient was evacuated to the US mainland for long-term care. Tetanus patients are highly sensitive to light and noise stimulation and so attempts were made to minimize excessive stimulation by covering his head with a box in this chaotic environment (Fig. 11.4). Afshar et al. have published a review of tetanus management in the disaster setting [11]. Another case involved a young boy who presented with what clinically appeared to be an acute abdomen, but was in fact an acute typhoid infection.

3. *Ensure you haveadequate security and resourcesto support the medical mission.*

The importance of security and logistics cannot be understated. Due to the high demand for medical care, security is needed to control access to the field hospital and provide protection for personnel. Desperation following a major earthquake can lead to widespread looting and chaos. During this deployment several patients were treated with gunshot wounds and stab wounds as a result of violence following the event. The advantage of deploying with a US Government team is that the US military is often available to provide security resources.

The logistics officer is a key member of the team who is responsible for ensuring the resources required for the mission. This includes an ongoing supply of food and water for the team as well as replenishing critical medical supplies. During the 6 weeks deployment commonly used medications and medical supplies required replenishment. Obtaining additional oxygen required daily negotiations with local authorities.

4. *Pay attention to your own health and that of your team members.*

Prior to deployment it is important to be aware of the potential threats to your personal health that should be addressed. This includes ensuring you have the appropriate vaccines for the region and prophylaxis against common infectious diseases such as malaria. In addition, personal protective equipment should be considered as appropriate for the region. In this case due to the high burden of

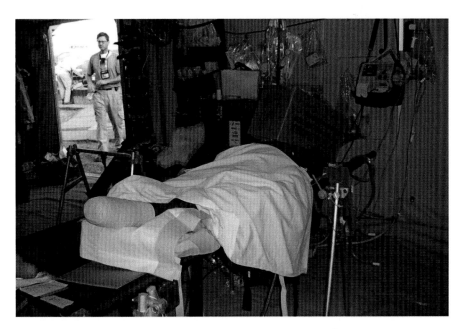

Fig. 11.4 Patient with severe tetanus following amputation of infected ankle wound. A box is placed over patients head to minimize sensory stimulation

mosquitoes and potential infectious disease exposure, insect repellant and mosquito netting for sleeping were important items. In addition, due to the heat and humidity of the environment, sunscreen and a source of safe drinking water to prevent heat illnesses, waterborne diseases and dehydration were vital.

A safety officer should be appointed to ensure the safety of team providers. Following an earthquake, aftershocks are common and may further threaten the structural integrity of remaining buildings. For each aftershock, an alert system was developed to ensure accountability of the team and to reassess the buildings in use.

Healthcare providers are anxious to help and will often sacrifice their own health to continue to provide care in a post-disaster scenario. Thus it is important to establish a shift schedule that gives providers mandatory time to rest. For this deployment all care providers were designated to 12 h shifts and "on-call" schedules were created to manage emergencies at night. Emotional support should be provided for team members during and after the event as well. IMSuRT teams also deploy with mental health personnel who are part of the team, both in training and deployments.

5. *Understand the chain of command and your role in it.*

Most surgeons are used to being the leader of the clinical team and do not routinely work under a strict command structure. In a disaster situation, establishing an incident command structure is critical to the success of the team [12]. Through an incident commander, the team can have consistent communication with local authorities and other supporting agencies. Thus it is critical that the surgeon understand this command structure and who to appeal to when additional resources are needed. There is online training available in incident command terminology available through FEMA (http://training.fema.gov/is/crslist.aspx)

6. *Look for creative solutions to make do with limited resources.*

As a clinician in an austere environment you must be willing to be flexible and adapt to the resources available. Diagnostic tools are frequently limited and decisions must frequently be made based solely on the clinical presentation of the patient and the findings on physical examination. For example, Fig. 11.5 shows how anemia can be diagnosed based on the color of the palm.

During this deployment several creative solutions were developed to adapt to limited equipment. Figure 11.6 shows how earthquake rubble can be used as a traction weight and how water bottles can be used to create an abduction splint for a patient with a pelvic fracture. We had no incubators but a large number of neonates to manage. Incubators were therefore fashioned from cardboard boxes lined with foil blankets and IV bags, which were warmed by placing them on the surface of the generator (Fig. 11.7).

7. *Know your limitations and have a patient evacuation plan if possible.*

Understanding the principles of triage and the fact that there are some patients that cannot be saved in a setting of limited resources is very important. It is important to know what your options are for evacuation to more definitive care as that will also factor into this decision making.

8. *Be sensitive to cultural differences.*

It is important to understand and respect the local culture of those affected by the disaster. Interpreters are vital to deal with the language barrier and help explain these cultural issues. Our team was fortunate to employ local Haitian personnel, including local medical students and teachers, as interpreters during this deployment. One example of an important issue to understand in Haiti is that living with a colostomy is not a viable option. There are no resources for ostomy supplies and creating an ostomy may commit the individual to life on the street. Thus every effort must be taken to avoid a colostomy.

In summary, responding to major international disasters, such as earthquakes, can be a very rewarding experience, but to have an effective response the surgeon should consider registering

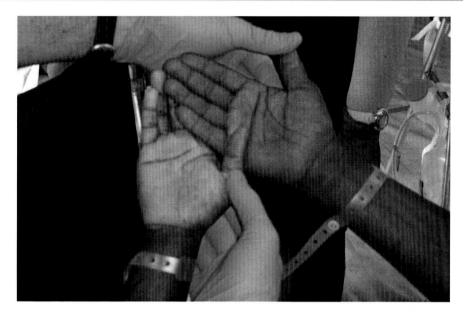

Fig. 11.5 Diagnosing anemia. Clinical diagnosis of anemia may be made by comparing the patient's palm color to that of her sister. Many patients with prior amputations presented with severe anemia requiring transfusion

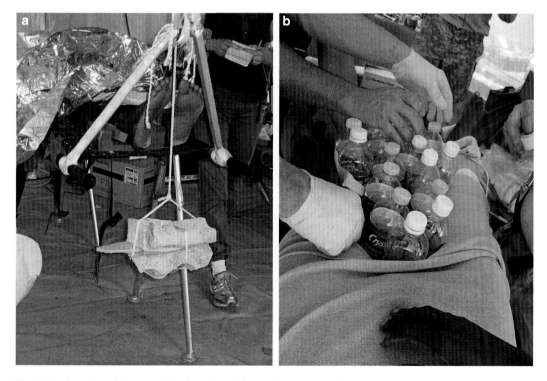

Fig. 11.6 Creative solutions. (**a**) Earthquake rubble used as a weight for femoral traction. (**b**) Water bottles taped together to create an abduction splint for a patient with a pelvic fracture

Fig. 11.7 (**a**) Neonatal incubators were created by lining boxes with foil warming blankets and heater with IV fluid bags which were warmed by placing them on the generator. (**b**) A neonate being prepared for transport to the USS Comfort

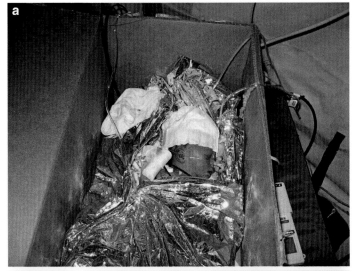

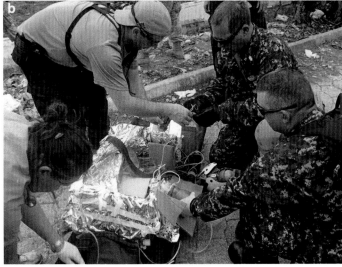

in advance with organizations such as IMSuRT or an established disaster relief agency. Such organizations have the resources to support a sustainable and safe response. The surgeon should consider training in advance in the principles of incident command and disaster triage and become familiar with the equipment to be used during the deployment. Prior to deployment the surgeon should consider the personal protective measures needed, develop an understanding of endemic diseases, and be prepared to treat a wide spectrum of surgical and medical diseases in all age groups.

This also from Dr. Briggs: During my 6 weeks deployment to Port-au-Prince, Haiti as Team Commander of the US Field Hospital, I encountered many amazing situations reflecting the resilience and compassion of the Haiti population. One of the most memorable was an 8-year-old Haitian girl who not only sustained a devastating crush injury to her head but also lost 12 members of her family. Despite her injuries, while awaiting evacuation to the US for definitive surgical care, she wanted to do something to help us in the field hospital. We taught her to play the harmonica and she went through the various tents, including the pediatric tent, playing for the other patients. Music in an integral part of the Haitian culture and this was better therapy than pain medication. The smiles she brought to the faces of the other victims of the disaster were incredible.

Editor's Note: Dr. Eileen Bulger is a professor of surgery at the University of Washington and the Chief of Trauma at Harborview Medical Center, Seattle, WA. She has been active with the West Coast International Medical Surgical Response Team (IMSuRT) since its inception in 2003 and has served as the acting Chief Medical Officer for the past 4 years. She was deployed to the Haiti earthquake in 2010.

Dr. Briggs has been deployed to six other natural disasters around the world aside from Haiti to include: Armenia, China, El Salvador, Iran, Russia, and the Virgin Islands. In the United States, she led surgical teams during Hurricanes Andrew and Katrina and during the bombings of 9/11 in New York and marathon in Boston. Dr. Briggs also spent 6 years in the U.S. Army Reserves and was deployed as a surgeon in Desert Storm I.

References

1. Doocy S, Daniels A, Packer C, Dick A, Kirsch TD. The human impact of earthquakes: a historical review of events 1980-2009 and systematic literature review. PLoS Curr. 2013;5. doi: 10.1371/currents.dis.67bd14fe457f1db0b5433a8ee20fb833.
2. Doocy S, Cherewick M, Kirsch T. Mortality following the Haitian earthquake of 2010: a stratified cluster survey. Popul Health Metr. 2013;11(1):5. doi:10.1186/1478-7954-11-5.
3. Doocy S, Jacquet G, Cherewick M, Kirsch TD. The injury burden of the 2010 Haiti earthquake: a stratified cluster survey. Injury. 2013;44(6):842–7. doi:10.1016/j.injury.2013.01.035.
4. Earthquake Overview. www.usaid.gov. www.usaid.gov/haiti/earthquake-overview. Accessed 1 Jan 2015.
5. CNN Library. Haiti earthquake fast facts. www.cnn.com. www.cnn.com/2013/12/12/world/haiti-earthquake-fast-facts. Accessed 1 Jan 2015.
6. Briggs SM. The role of civilian surgical teams in response to international disasters. Bull Am Coll Surg. 2010;95(1):13–7.
7. Owens PJ, Forgione A, Briggs S. Challenges of international disaster relief: use of a deployable rapid assembly shelter and surgical hospital. Disaster Manag Response. 2005;3(1):11–6. doi:10.1016/j.dmr.2004.10.004.
8. Reis ND, Better OS. Mechanical muscle-crush injury and acute muscle-crush compartment syndrome: with special reference to earthquake casualties. J Bone Joint Surg Br. 2005;87(4):450–3. doi:10.1302/0301-620X.87B4.15334.
9. Briggs SM, Bulger EM. Crush InjuriesIn: Briggs SM, editor. Advanced disaster medical response manual for providers. 2nd ed. Woodbury, CT: Cine-Med Publishing, Inc; pp. 148–154.
10. Goodman A, Black L, Briggs S. Obstetrical care and women's health in the aftermath of disasters: the first 14 days after the 2010 Haitian earthquake. Am J Disaster Med. 2014;9(1):59–65. doi:10.5055/ajdm.2014.0142.
11. Afshar M, Raju M, Ansell D, Bleck TP. Narrative review: tetanus-a health threat after natural disasters in developing countries. Ann Intern Med. 2011;154(5):329–35. doi:10.1059/0003-4819-154-5-201103010-00007.
12. Briggs SM. Regional interoperability: making systems connect in complex disasters. J Trauma. 2009;67 Suppl 2:S88–90. doi:10.1097/TA.0b013e3181adbcc0.

Surgery on Public Enemy #1

12

Alec C. Beekley

12.1 Introduction

Surgeons, particularly those involved in the care of trauma patients, may frequently find themselves required to treat individuals who have committed crimes. The most common "crimes" committed leading to an individual requiring surgical care likely involve traffic infractions, most of which are accidental or unintentional. These infractions range from relatively minor (e.g. failure to maintain close following distance, speeding) to major infractions with significant legal implications for the patient (e.g. driving while intoxicated, vehicular homicide). Unfortunately, a disproportionate amount of these injuries occur in young people. The CDC reported in 2012 that 7656 young people (aged 5–24) were killed in motor vehicle or traffic-related events and just over 804,000 were treated in an emergency department related to an unintentional motor vehicle-related event [1]. Legally minor traffic infractions may nevertheless result in serious injury and death. Because patients injured as a result of their traffic infraction rarely have crimi-

A.C. Beekley, M.D. (✉)
Divisions of Trauma/Acute Care Surgery and
Bariatric Surgery, Department of Surgery, Thomas
Jefferson University Hospitals, 1100 Walnut Street,
7th Floor Medical Office Building, Philadelphia,
PA 19107, USA
e-mail: alec.beekley@jefferson.edu

nal intent, they are generally not considered a flight risk nor pose a threat of physical harm to hospital personnel. They do not require special considerations beyond the routine delivery of standard care.

The second most common source of criminal behavior leading to a requirement of surgical care involves assault, which in 2012 was the 6th most common cause of non-fatal injury overall in the 24–35 years old age group [2]. A recent review of firearm-related hospital admissions from a population-based database demonstrated that 61 % of these admissions were related to assault with a firearm. The review found that almost 50 % of these patients were black, close to 90 % were male, and 34 % were uninsured [3]. Because these patients were sometimes engaged in criminal behavior at the time of their injury, they are more frequently a flight risk and more frequently of legal interest to authorities than those patients injured in the course of committing traffic infractions. Nonetheless, most of these patients' injuries arose due to conflicts with other, often criminal, elements outside the hospital. Many of these patients may often be the victims of criminals. These patients, therefore, are usually not opposed to those caring medically for them and hence usually do not pose a threat to themselves or hospital personnel.

Rarely, civilian surgeons will be called upon to provide care to patients serving prison sentences, patients with public notoriety for a history

© Springer International Publishing Switzerland 2016
C.R.B. Lim (ed.), *Surgery During Natural Disasters, Combat,*
Terrorist Attacks, and Crisis Situations, DOI 10.1007/978-3-319-23718-3_12

of known or suspected relationships with organized criminal elements, or patients with a recent history of criminal acts or violence. Recent examples of such patients that required surgical care include Nidal Malik Hasan (the Fort Hood shooter) and Dzhokhar Tsarnaev, the Boston Marathon bombing suspect. Such individuals provide unique challenges to surgeons, in that they may pose a direct threat to themselves and others while still in the hospital. In addition, legal authorities may exert pressure to have access to the patient to question or interrogate him or her during the recovery phase. Such patients often require around-the-clock armed guards, both to prevent their elopement and for their personal safety from threats to their well-being from outside the hospital. Finally, treating providers themselves may feel conflicted about caring for a patient they know may have committed terrible crimes against others or have an ideology completely at odds with their own.

In many respects, this last group of patients has many parallels with prisoners of war and detained personnel that military surgeons treated during Operations Enduring and Iraqi Freedom as well as earlier conflicts. U.S. Government and U.S. Military doctrine for care of casualties on the battlefield mandates triage and prioritization of treatment based solely on medical and surgical need, not on patient's gender, race, religion, nationality, ideology, politics, or any other such criteria. This doctrine is derived directly from the 1949 Geneva Convention(s) for the Amelioration of the Condition of the Wounded and Sick, Wounded, and Shipwrecked in Armed Forces in the Field and at Sea (Geneva Conventions I and II, August 12, 1949) [4]. Hence, military surgeons deployed in the wars of the last 13 years have frequently been called upon to save the lives of enemies of the United States (Fig. 12.1). Because U.S. military directives restrict research (eventually even retrospective data-gathering and analysis) on detained personnel, relatively sparse public data exist. In addition, research involving detained personnel or prisoners has, since wide adoption of the 1949 Geneva Conventions, been carefully reviewed to ensure the research has no punitive or retributive nature [5, 6]. Nevertheless, some published retrospective, observational reports provide some perspective and guidance on providing surgical care to this unique set of patients.

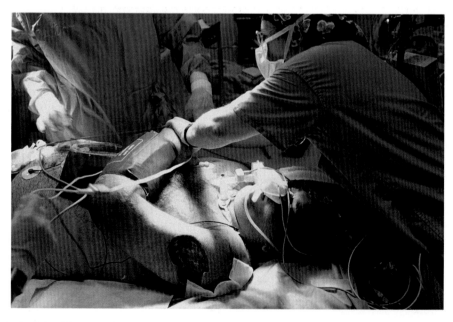

Fig. 12.1 An injured insurgent is treated by US Army (USA) Lieutenant Colonel (LTC) Kim Fedele, at the 31st Combat Support Hospital for gunshot wounds in Baghdad, Iraq, during Operation Iraqi Freedom, 06/26/2004 [23]

12.2 Security

The first non-medical priority when a "public enemy" is brought for surgical care is establishing security, both *from* the patient and *for* the patient. Security procedures should be established in hospitals' standard operating protocols, and health care personnel should insist that such security routines always be maintained. Such security routines are effective only when they are adhered to 100 % of the time. Depending on the patient's mental state and ideology, the patient himself may pose a threat to hospital personnel. Security from the patient includes ensuring he or she has no weapons, ensuring the patient cannot strike at personnel or gain control of items that could be used as weapons, and keeping the patient from escaping the hospital. Although law enforcement personnel may be in attendance when such a patient is brought to the hospital in an emergent setting, hospital personnel (and the surgeon as the team leader) should not automatically assume that the patient has been searched and cleared of all weapons. Rapid coordination with law enforcement personnel, if present, can establish if the patient has been searched and secured.

If law enforcement is not immediately present, hospital security personnel should be immediately contacted to assist in searching and securing the patient. If the patient is indeed under legal arrest or otherwise appears to pose a direct threat to hospital personnel, non-medical restraints should be used to ensure the patient cannot harm hospital personnel, attempt to find other weapons, or attempt to escape. If removal of these restraints is required for the patient's medical or surgical care, such removal should occur only with security or law-enforcement supervision. Security personnel should accompany the patient at all times and for all transports to other areas of the hospital, whether that transport is for diagnostic tests or procedures. Security personnel should also ensure that the patient does not have access to medical equipment or supplies that could be used to harm others or harm himself. Armed security personnel may need to accompany dangerous patients into the operating room, at least until sedation or anesthesia is induced. In some instances, calm and cooperative patients who are nevertheless considered a threat to

personnel may have mechanical restraints placed prior to movement to the operating room. Uncooperative or violent patients may require both mechanical and medical restraints (e.g. sedatives or general anesthesia) to allow for continuation of the therapeutic milieu, although providers should be aware that intubation for combativeness alone results in increased lengths of stay, increased incidence of pneumonia, increased cost, and affects discharge status [7, 8]. Hence, judicious use of narcotic, anxiolytic, and antipsychotic medications (e.g. morphine, midazolam, or haloperidol) may be able to calm agitated or combative patients without intubation. In instances where the patient is paralyzed and intubated, armed security can likely be on standby just outside the operating room.

Security *for* the patient may be even more important. This includes security from threats to the patient originating outside the hospital. One can imagine patients and settings—high profile, organized crime figures, for example—where the patient may be in the hospital secondary to a missed attempt on his life. The elements responsible may be desperate enough to try to murder the patient in the hospital. Although this type of circumstance may seem to be a gangster movie trope (e.g. the attempt on the hospitalized Vito Corleone's life in "The Godfather"), there are real-life accounts of similar events, which for various reasons may not be publicly reported [9, 10]. The Joint Commission reported 201 violent criminal events occurring in accredited hospitals between January 2010 and August 2014 [11]. Although a significant number of these reported events were patient on staff violence, the belief that hospitals are a safe and sacrosanct haven has unfortunately been proven incorrect [12, 13]. Finally, depending on the setting, the patient may also pose a threat to himself. For these reasons, patients should have around-the-clock direct supervision and may benefit from psychiatric evaluation.

12.3 Physical Location of Public Enemy Patients

Once a public enemy patient is stabilized, some consideration should be given for the physical location of the patient in the hospital. This location should also be codified into hospital security procedures. The patient's logistical needs (e.g. requirement for mechanical ventilation and other intensive care) may mandate that the patient be placed in an ICU. However, such patients can be located in lower traffic areas or isolation rooms where the patient's interaction with other patients and staff is limited and security presence is less obtrusive. In the event of multiple public enemy patients, a separate ward or floor should be used to keep these patients isolated; this may also concentrate the security presence. Such patients should nevertheless be isolated from each other as much as possible. The 31st Combat Support Hospital kept security detainee patients on a different area of the ICU and a different floor than Coalition patients. Other forward surgical units have documented such separation of patients based on detainee status [14].

Although physical separation of security detainees, public enemies, or criminals from the other patients can raise concerns that a different standard of care may be delivered, this concern does not appear to be borne out with the few studies that evaluated detainee care. For example, one Combat Support Hospital in Operation Iraqi Freedom demonstrated that fresh whole blood donated by U.S. Military personnel was transfused in equal amounts and proportions to U.S., Iraqi civilians, and enemy combatant patients, indicating a policy of administering a precious resource based solely on medical need [15]. Ingari and Powell demonstrated that casualties at an Air Force Theater Hospital in Balad, Iraq, received the highest level of care available in theater regardless of whether they were U.S. Military, local national civilians, or enemy combatants [16].

12.4 Surgical Treatment of Known or Suspected Criminals

12.4.1 Documentation and Informed Consent

The patient's legal status should not sway or influence the surgeon's clinical decisions; the standards of surgical and medical care remain the same. Preventing death, alleviating suffering, and restoring anatomy and function are the primary goals, regardless of the patient's ultimate legal fate. To that end, clinical documentation and informed consent should be meticulously documented, with the realization that such records may be exhaustively reviewed in legal and media settings in the future. Signed consent should be obtained for any surgical or invasive procedures, if possible. If the patient is unable to give informed consent because of medication effects or clinical status (e.g. intoxicated, brain injured, or in clinical shock), reasonable attempts should be made to gain informed consent from next of kin or power of attorney. Surgeons should keep in mind that a detained person's next of kin may be ashamed or angry with their detained family member for actions they may have done or been accused of doing. Whether these individuals are truly the best people to give informed consent is debatable. At any rate, controversy around the consent process or the reasons for the inability to get informed consent should be clearly documented. If the patient is unable to give informed consent because of the presence of medications or shock states, and no other surrogate, next of kin, or power of attorney is available, two physicians should document that the surgical procedure being proposed is the community standard of care and in the patient's best interest. Detained persons have the right to refuse surgical or invasive procedures. If such a refusal may lead to harm or death for the patient, their refusal should be clearly recorded. Preferably, this would be done with a document signed by the patient acknowledging their refusal or therapy and the physician's counseling of the potential outcomes that could befall them for such refusal.

Depending on the setting, surgeons may want to consider using high resolution photography to document patient's wounds and operative findings, particularly if an injury is likely to require amputation. Such documentation should become a part of the patient's private medical record. Standard medical photography techniques should be used that, if possible (and unlike most medical photography), clearly allow identification of the patient. This serves the dual purpose of establishing a photographic record of the patient's wounds on admission and can protect treating providers against claims of unnecessary operations or amputations [6, 17]. For example, in the wake of the Abu Ghraib scandal, Army urologists at the 31st Combat Support Hospital would routinely photograph the wounds of foreign national patients with external genitalia injuries, particularly if those injuries would likely result in permanent tissue and/or functional loss.

12.4.2 Surgical Care

The community standard of care should be applied to all injuries or surgical diagnoses. Surgeons should treat public enemy patients in the same fashion as every other patient. Where the typical course for a recovering trauma or surgical patient may vary with public enemies is in their disposition after the acute phase of their care. Patients who may derive benefit from inpatient rehabilitation may be difficult or inappropriate to place in private rehabilitation hospitals. Furthermore, since most of these patients are going from a hospital setting to custody in a detention facility or prison, treating providers must ensure that all residual medical and surgical needs (e.g. wound dressing changes, special medications, enteral feeds) can be handled by the receiving facility. These factors may lead to public enemy patients staying longer than expected at the acute care hospital.

12.4.3 The Surgeon's Ethical Responsibility

Perhaps one of the most difficult tasks that the surgeon faces when caring for a public or wartime enemy is to keep his own personal emotions and moral judgments about the patient from affecting his role as the patient's primary advocate and caregiver. Some providers may find it difficult to hold compassion for an individual who has committed horrific acts against other humans, although many surgeons report that they are easily able to place the surgical needs of their

patient paramount regardless of their race, sex, politics, ideology, or previous actions [18]. He or she may nevertheless face criticism from other hospital personnel for displaying such compassion, and strong advocacy on the patient's behalf may be viewed negatively by other hospital and non-hospital personnel.

A study of the ethical challenges involved in caring for detained personnel in Desert Storm by Major Brian S. Carter indicated that views of standard medical ethics regarding care of the wounded in war may not have uniform acceptance and application, even in a structured organization like the U.S. Military. Carter performed a survey study of over 350 physicians who had been deployed and cared for detained personnel during Operation Desert Storm. A majority (84 %) of these physicians reported familiarity with the Geneva Conventions of 1949 on care of the sick and wounded, and 60 % reported actually having read the document. When given a hypothetical scenario of a multiple patient treatment event made up of both friendly and enemy combatants and refugees, "most" (a percentage is not given) responders stated that they would treat each patient individually based solely on medical need. However, in a separate survey question, 33.5 % of respondents disagreed with the statement that "the only criteria used for triage should be medical status (need)." In addition, 27 % of respondents indicated that the Geneva Conventions did not necessary apply to their mission, and 22 % respondents indicated that "EPWs, no matter how severe their injuries, should only be treated after all Allied forces were treated [19]."

Perhaps one of the most difficult ethical challenges to arise for physicians during Operations Enduring and Iraqi Freedom was for them to remain the patient's staunch advocate in the face of Coalition personnel wishing to interrogate detained personnel before they had completely recovered from traumatic injury. This author personally experienced an interrogator requesting that pain medications be withheld from a post-surgical patient so that he could interrogate him. In this instance, the interrogator's request was refused, and nothing more came of the matter. There are now several well-researched articles and editorials in respected medical journals [20, 21], however, that in the setting of Abu Ghraib, "even without participating in the abuse, doctors may have become socialized to an environment of torture and by virtue of their medical authority helped sustain it" [15]. The physician's first duty, based on the Hippocratic Oath, is to do no harm. Treating physicians should be completely separate from any interrogation process. Furthermore, as the primary (and sometimes only) advocate for the patient, the physician should carefully document and report any signs of injury or abuse that may have arisen in an interrogation process. Due to entrenched institutional safeguards and widespread respect for the law in our country, surgeons in U.S. hospitals are unlikely to encounter a situation where a patient's rights to counsel or due process are compromised or where their right to dignity and freedom from coercion, abuse, harsh treatment, or torture is threatened. Such safeguards were likely eroded in the command climate and environment in Abu Ghraib.

Jones and colleagues from the Massachusetts Work Group on Law Enforcement Access to Hospital Patients provide a set of 5 principles to provide guidance regarding physicians' response to law enforcement's request to interview a patient [22]. The first principle is respect for patient autonomy. Surgeons should know that as the treating physician, they and the hospital facility have control of law enforcement access to the patient for the purpose of interview or interrogation, except in the event that law enforcement has a court order (search or arrest warrant) or if law enforcement is directly intervening in a crime or emergency on the hospital premises. However, if the treating surgeon determines that the patient is fit to make his or her own medical decisions, they are likely fit to decide whether or not to talk to law enforcement in a formal interview. The surgeon can inform the patient of law enforcement's interest in conducting an interview; the surgeon can also advise the patient (and law enforcement) regarding the patient's current medical and physical status and provide the surgeon's own medical opinion regarding the patient's fitness to undergo an interview.

The second principle is non-interference with medical care. In short, law enforcement interviews should not interfere with patient care or risk harm to the patient. Law enforcement interviews can only delay diagnostic or therapeutic interventions with valid informed consent from the patient. Hospitals should also consider adding physician observers to interviews to monitor the patient's medical status.

The third principle is protection of the patient's privacy. Information that the patient discloses to the physician, even if legally incriminating to the patient, may not be disclosed to the police unless the patient gives consent to do so (or unless the information may disclose risk of harm to another person). Surgeons should be aware that the Health Insurance Portability and Accountability Act (HIPAA) does not regulate police access to patients. HIPAA allows disclosures to law enforcement personnel if the patient is a suspected victim of abuse, neglect, or domestic violence; if law enforcement needs to locate or identify a person; if the patient is a crime victim; if the patient is receiving emergency care and reporting crime to alert police to the nature, location or commission of crime and the identity, description, and location of the perpetrator (even if it is the patient); if the surgeon believes in good faith that disclosure of protected health information is necessary to prevent serious or imminent threat to the health and safety of others; or if the disclosure is necessary for the police to identify or catch a suspect.

The fourth principle is the maintenance of professional boundaries. Providers observing a law enforcement interview of the patient should be sure the patient understands that they are NOT part of the interview team and are present only to protect the patient's medical condition. Lastly, "proactive interdisciplinary collaboration," with the creation of guidelines, means for conflict resolution, and liaisons between hospital personnel and law enforcement, and training of hospital personnel in this topic are critical to protect both the patient's well-being and the integrity of law enforcement interview process [22].

12.5 Conclusions

The surgeon's role in the care of the public enemy patient remains the same as for all other patients: the surgeon is the patient's primary caregiver and advocate. As such, the surgeon's job begins before such a patient ever comes to the hospital. Like the protocols and plans hospitals create for mass casualty events, the care of the high-profile criminal or public enemy should also be dictated by well-considered, multi-disciplinary protocols and plans. The surgeon should be involved in the hospital planning for such a patient.

If such a public enemy patient presents to the hospital for surgical care, the surgeon sets the tone and environment of care for the entire team. Security from and for the patient should be established based on previously established hospital standards. The standard of care should always be provided to the patient, including well-documented informed consent and right of refusal for all surgical or invasive procedures. Surgeons should consider taking extra steps to clearly document any physical findings, particularly if such findings may lead to permanent disfigurement, amputation, or functional loss.

Finally, the surgeon has an ethical responsibility to protect the patient from further harm, whether that harm arises from threats outside the hospital, threats within the hospital, or from the patient's threat to himself. This includes determining when the patient is medically fit for both interrogations by law enforcement and transfer to a prison or legal detainment facility.

Editor's Note: Dr. Alec Beekley served in the United States Army for 17 years and achieved the rank of Lieutenant Colonel. During that time he was deployed four times in support of Operations Iraqi and Enduring Freedom. He provided high-quality and timely care to several enemies of the United States.

References

1. Centers for Disease Control. http://www.cdc.gov/injury/wisqars/pdf/leading_causes_of_injury_deaths_highlighting_unintentional_injury_2012-a.pdf and http://www.cdc.gov/injury/wisqars/pdf/eading_cause_of_nonfatal_injury_2012-a.pdf. Accessed 5 Jan 2015.
2. National Center for Injury Prevention and Control. http://webappa.cdc.gov/sasweb/ncipc/nfilead2001.html and http://webappa.cdc.gov/cgi-bin/broker.exe, 10 Leading causes of nonfatal injury, United States, 2012, all races, both sexes. Accessed 5 Jan 2015.
3. Lee MK, Allareddy V, Rampa S, Nalliah R, Allareddy V. Longitudinal trends in firearm related hospitalizations in the United States: profile and outcomes in 2000 to 2008. http://www.thecrimereport.org/news/inside-criminal-justice/2013-11-the-public-health-cost-of-gun-violence and http://thecrimereport.s3.amazonaws.com/2/2d/4/2205/allareddy1_gun_victims_costs_more_than__16_billion_in_hospital_treatment_over_9_years.pdf. Accessed 5 Jan 2015.
4. Summary of the Geneva Conventions of 12 August 1949 and their Additional Protocols. https://www.icrc.org/eng/assets/files/publications/icrc-002-0368.pdf. Accessed 5 Jan 2015.
5. Stone TH. Discussing minimal risk in research involving prisoners as human subjects. J Law Med Ethics. 2004;32:535–7.
6. Place RP. Caring for non-combatants, refugees, and detainees. Surg Clin N Am. 2006;86:765–77.
7. Kuchinski J, Tinkoff G, Rhodes M, Becher Jr JW. Emergency intubation for paralysis of the uncooperative trauma patient. J Emerg Med. 1991;9:9–12.
8. Muakkassa FF, Marley RA, Workman MC, Salvator AE. Hospital outcomes and disposition of trauma patients who are intubated because of combativeness. J Trauma. 2010;68(6):1305–9.
9. Personal Communication. Gary Lindenbaum, M.D., Accessed 6 Jan 2015.
10. Special report: violence in hospitals: what are the causes? Why is it increasing? How is it being confronted? Hosp Secur Saf Manage. 1993;13:5–10.
11. Joint Commission. Preventing violent and criminal events. http://www.jointcommission.org/assets/1/23/Quick_Safety_Issue_Five_Aug_2014_FINAL.pdf. Accessed 6 Jan 2015.
12. Man detained for killing patient by stamping on head. 2011.http://www.bbc.co.uk/news/uk-england-london-13366062. Accessed 8 Jan 2015.
13. Teproff C. Lawsuit filed against Aventura Hospital after a patient was killed by another patient. 2014. http://www.miamiherald.com/news/local/community/miami-dade/aventura/article1975045.html. Accessed 8 Jan 2015.
14. Rush RM, Stockmaster NR, Stinger HK, et al. Supporting the Global War on Terror: a tale of two campaigns featuring the 250th Forward Surgical Team (Airborne). Am Journ of Surg. 2005;189:564–70.
15. Spinella PC, Perkins JG, Grathwohl KW, et al. Fresh whole blood transfusions in coalition military, foreign national, and enemy combatant patients during Operation Iraqi Freedom at a US combat support hospital. World J Surg. 2008;32:2–6.

16. Ingari JV, Powell E. Civilian and detainee orthopaedic surgical care at an Air Force theater hospital. Tech Hand Up Extrem Surg. 2007;11(2):130–4.

17. Westreich M, Waron M. Guidelines for a prisoner of war medical treatment center in a civilian hospital. Mil Med. 1988;153:549–54.

18. Ghert-Zand R. Once Inside Israel's Hospitals, the "terrorist" becomes the "patient." The Times of Israel. 12 Nov 2014. http://www.timesofisrael.com/once-inside-israels-hospitals-the-terrorist-becomes-the-patient/. Accessed 5 Jan 2015.

19. Carter BS. Ethical concerns for physicians deployed to Operation Desert Storm. Mil Med. 1994;159:55–9.

20. Miles SH. Abu Ghraib: its legacy for military medicine. Lancet. 2004;364:725–9.

21. Lifton RJ. Doctors torture. N Engl J Med. 2004;351(5): 415–6.

22. Jones PM, Appelbaum PS, Siegel DM. Law enforcement interviews of hospital patients: a conundrum for clinicians. JAMA. 2008;295(7):822–5.

23. National Archives. Online Public Access. http://research.archives.gov/description/6644091. Accessed 10 Jan 2015.

Lessons Learned in Combat Burn Care

13

Booker T. King

Being one of the few burn surgeons in the military, I have deployed to Iraq and Afghanistan as the theater burn consultant. In this role I was tasked to provide local (theater) expertise in the management of thermally injured coalition casualties and host nationals as well. The management of burn injury is complex in the tactical and operational environment. The patients often have severe traumatic injuries in addition to their burns. The traumatic injuries often take precedence for treatment as many of those injuries are immediately life-threatening. Once stabilized these patients should be evacuated out of theater expeditiously as their management and resuscitation will strain the resources of a field hospital.

Any Combat Support Hospital operating during a combat or humanitarian mission should be prepared to care for local nationals. But in the case of burn care, many patients will have injuries that were not sustained as a result of active combat. U.S. and coalition medical assets will often be diverted for the care of these patients as host nation medical assets will likely be unable to care for these patients acutely. It is imperative

B.T. King, M.D. (✉)
US Army Burn Center, San Antonio Military Medical Center, 3551 Roger Brooke Dr., JBSA Fort Sam Houston, San Antonio, TX 78234, USA

US Army Insititue of Surgical Research,
129 Blue Sage Lane, Cibolo, TX 78108, USA
e-mail: Bookerking@me.com

that a relationship is developed with host nation medical facilities in your area of operation in order to facilitate transfer once treatment at your facility is completed. Large burns in local nationals (over 50 % in Iraq and 40 % in Afghanistan) were often treated expectantly given the lack of resources available even at military theater hospitals.[1]

13.1 Case 1: Two Burned Soldiers from Early Operation Iraqi Freedom

I was assigned to a mobile surgical hospital that deployed in support of the initial phase of Operation Iraqi Freedom (OIF). We had two teams that convoyed from Kuwait and set-up a fully mobile hospital in an area just outside of An Najaf, Iraq. The initial days were very busy with 20–30 casualties treated per day. We were 10 days into OIF when we received a call in the Emergency Room (ER) that a rocket-propelled grenade (RPG) had struck a vehicle in a convoy and casualties from that incident were being evacuated to our hospital. Then we received a call from the medical evacuation (MEDEVAC) team that they were transporting these patients by ground ambulance and several critically ill patients were en route.

The patient I was assigned to had severe facial, neck, upper chest and bilateral hand burns, but

© Springer International Publishing Switzerland 2016
C.R.B. Lim (ed.), *Surgery During Natural Disasters, Combat, Terrorist Attacks, and Crisis Situations*, DOI 10.1007/978-3-319-23718-3_13

was awake and conversive. The plan was to evacuate this patient urgently to a Combat Support Hospital (CSH) in Kuwait as this severely burned patient would require prolonged fluid resuscitation and nearly deplete the resources of our mobile hospital. I was just a general surgeon at this point in my career and had not taken care of any trauma or burn patients since my general surgery residency some 3 years prior. I was initially concerned that my patient could develop airway compromise during transport. I wanted to electively intubate the patient. I was reassured that the patient would be travelling by rotary wing and their flight time would be about an hour unless delayed by hostile enemy action. Also the patient pleaded not to be intubated and he appeared to be oxygenating adequately, not exhibiting signs of airway compromise at the moment.

The MEDEVAC was delayed several hours due to weather. The patient began to have noticeable facial edema and mild hoarseness when he spoke. I consulted my anesthesia colleague to evaluate him and we both agreed that the patient should be intubated given these new, although subtle signs of airway compromise. A standard rapid sequence intubation was attempted but the nurse anesthetist could not visualize the vocal cords due to pharyngeal edema. The patient began to rapidly desaturate. I knew at this moment that I had to obtain a surgical airway but the patient had swelling of the face and neck and deep burns on the neck. I was able to do a tracheostomy but the procedure was very difficult due to marked tissue edema and bleeding from numerous branches of the anterior jugular veins. Just after completing the tracheostomy, we were alerted that the "skies were clear" and that the patients needed to be prepped for MEDEVAC. The first patient was evacuated to Kuwait without incident. When this case was reviewed we identified several areas for improvement. We came to the conclusion that his airway should have been secured upon arrival to our hospital. Even though he presented with a patent airway, the nature of his injuries made intubation the safest option for transport. If the MEDEVAC had not been delayed, he may possibly had died during transport due to the loss of this airway and the difficult tracheostomy.[2]

13.2 Case 2: Trauma and Burns in a Soldier in OIF

It is November of 2007 and I am deployed to Baghdad, Iraq with another CSH. I have just completed a trauma and surgical critical care fellowship and now assigned to US Army Burn Center. I am deployed as the theater burn consultant. The emergency room has just received a soldier who was traveling in a convoy and an RPG struck the gas tank of his vehicle causing a large explosion. Several soldiers were ejected from the vehicle and all the soldiers had severe burns and several had extremity and torso injuries as well. When the combat medics evaluated the injured, they found that only one of five soldiers was alive. This soldier was severely burned, unconscious but had no obvious signs of additional trauma. He was intubated at the scene and then transported to our CSH in Baghdad by rotary wing.

The transport took only 30 min as the incident occurred just outside of the city. When he arrived he was still unconscious and about 80 % of his body was burned and most of the burns were full thickness. Standard Adult Trauma Life Support measures were instituted in the ER. When his vital signs were obtained his mean arterial pressure (MAP) was 55 mmHg (normal is above 50) and his heart rate 140. He was given several liters of crystalloid but his MAP did not improve. On examination his abdomen was firm but difficult to completely assess due to the full thickness burns that covered his torso. Chest film was done but it was unremarkable.

Now his MAP was noted to be 45 mmHg so he was given a transfusion of PRBCs. I was summoned to the ER at that time which was the usual protocol to notify me of all burn patients. When I arrived I noted that his MAP was now 40 mmHg and heart rate was 145. When I inquired about the hypotension I was told that the chest films were unremarkable and that they suspected it was related to the patient's extensive burn injury. Several more units of blood and plasma was now being transfused. A patient with only a thermal injury should not require any blood so early after injury. These patients can become hypotensive but it occurs several hours into their resuscitation usually due to severe hypovolemia of "burn shock." Burn shock is the result of a severe systemic inflammatory response in burn patients that results in a marked increase in capillary permeability leading to the escape of fluid from the vascular space into the interstitial space in tissues and into the environment via the burn wound. This can result in profound hypovolemia and even death in larger burn injuries if not corrected. Burn resuscitation therefore usually involves the replacement of fluid by a continuous intravenous infusion of a crystalloid, most often lactated ringer's solution. All burn resuscitation formulas make adjustment in the rate of fluid replacement initially by using patient's weight (in kilograms) and the burn surface area (example: 2 cc/kg/%TBSA—Modified Brooke formula). This rate is then adjusted to achieve a target urinary output. Some patients become so hypovolemic that they become hypotensive and these patients may require vasoactive medications in addition to fluid resuscitation with crystalloid and colloid. But even in this situation a patient should not need blood transfusion unless there is occult bleeding.

I was concerned that there was occult blood loss most likely in his abdomen given the fact that he had no sign of extremity trauma and the chest films were normal. I performed a FAST examination but it was very difficult to visualize anything through the burned skin on his torso. It appeared that there was some fluid in the hepatorenal space and in the pelvis but the study was not definitive and my colleagues were not convinced. The patient was still "unstable" (MAP of 40 mmHg and heart rate of 148 now). I decided to go to the operating room. My operative plan was to perform a diagnostic peritoneal lavage (DPL) and proceed to an exploratory laparotomy if the DPL yielded gross blood. I would continue the resuscitation and superficially debride the wounds and dress them in the operating room if the DPL was negative. The DPL was positive right away with 10 cc of gross blood aspirated from the abdomen. My surgical assistant and I proceeded to emergent laparotomy. Upon entering the abdomen a large hemoperitoneum was noted. Significant bleeding was noted in the left upper quadrant. When we attempted to inspect the spleen we could not locate it in its normal anatomical location. After further inspection, several portions of the spleen were located in the left lower quadrant and pelvis. We immediately obtained control of the massive bleeding in multiple areas of the left upper quadrant. The distal pancreas appeared to be undamaged. The patient suddenly became profoundly hypotensive and remained so despite more transfusions of blood and plasma. The patient went into cardiac arrest and despite continued resuscitative efforts, the patient expired. After reflecting on all the events of the case I was reminded of what one of my mentors told me several years prior: "a burn patient is a trauma patient with burns first and foremost."

13.3   Case 3: Severe Inhalation Injury and Cyanide Toxicity

In May of 2010, we received word of a soldier who had sustained severe burns and inhalation injury from a gas explosion in a dining facility in Iraq. The patient was initially treated at CSH in Baghdad and then transferred to Balad air base. The patient had sustained 40 % total body surface area burns and had external signs and symptoms of inhalation injury. Upon arrival to the CSH the patient was immediately intubated and femoral venous central line placed. He has noted to be moderately hypotensive (BP—90/50 and HR—125). This was initially attributed to induction agents but hypotension persisted and oxygen saturation was 90 % despite the patient being mechanically ventilated with 100 % FiO_2. Arterial blood gas was significant for pH of 7.25, pO_2—75 mmHg, HCO_3—12 and lactate—10 mmol/L. Bronchoscopy was performed in the ER which showed moderate edema, carbon deposition down to the tertiary bronchioles and copious carboneous sputum all confirming inhalation injury. Hypotension persisted despite two intravenous fluid boluses. Cyanide toxicity was suspected at this time. Cyanide is a component of smoke inhaled from fire and this toxic gas is released upon the combustion of certain plastics and other polymers. Cyanide is a highly lethal substance that disrupts cellular respiration by irreversibly binding to cytochrome c oxidase in the mitochondria. Cyanide poisoning presents as seizures, obtundation, coma, hemodynamic instability, and cardiac arrest in patients with suspected smoke inhalation. This condition can be rapidly fatal if an antidote is not administered in a timely manner. Some antidotes include: amyl nitrate, sodium thiosulfate, and hydroxycobalamin. Hydroxycobalamin is a derivative of vitamin B12 and in the presence of cyanide is converted to the harmless chemical—cyanocobalamin that is excreted by the kidneys. Hydroxycobalamin was recently approved by Food and Drug Administration for treatment of cyanide poisoning and is marketed as Cyanokit®. Cyanokit® is now available in many of the ER's around the world.[3]

The patient was given hydroxycobalamin and within an hour symptoms and vital signs improved (BP—120/85, HR—115, oxygen saturation—97 %, and lactate—7 mmol/L). Wound care was performed in the ER in Baghdad and the patient was evacuated to Balad air base by rotary wing Air Ambulance. He was accompanied by ICU nurse and physician. At Balad his vitals remained stable and CCATT team was activated for transport to Germany. Unfortunately, the volcano at Mount Eyjafjallajokull in Iceland had erupted and many flights to and from Europe were canceled due to volcanic ash over the Atlantic Ocean. The patient could be evacuated to Germany but will likely be stranded in Germany for several days which would delay definitive treatment of his burn wounds. The decision was made to evacuate him directly to military Burn Center in San Antonio, Texas. He was evacuated without incident and after several months was discharged and recovered well from inhalation injury and burns.

13.4 Case 4: Comfort Measures for a Severely Burned Local National

It was February 2008, the later part of my second OIF deployment. I was called to the ER to evaluate a young woman who had sustained a burn injury after her clothes caught on fire while she was cooking. She was accompanied by her husband and she was in her late twenties. After assessing her injuries, her total burn size was estimated to be about 70 % with the vast majority full thickness burns on the lower three-quarters of her body. The husband was pleading for us to care for her and inquiring when she would be stable enough to go home. The reality was that this was essentially a non-survivable injury for a host national in Iraq. In the U.S. this would be a significant injury requiring great resources, several operations, and a hospital stay of several months. Even with all our resources in the U.S. her mortality would be greater than 40 %. The "Ibn Sina Rule" was an anecdote devised by my predecessors at the Army Burn Center that rotated through the Ibn Sina hospital (CSH) in Baghdad, Iraq. The rule simply stated that: "any burn greater than 50 % strongly consider comfort measures." This rule arose after several attempts (including myself) to treat patients with greater than 50 % burn. These patients universally died several weeks after injury of burn wound sepsis and multiorgan system failure. The resources are not available in Iraq to save these patients primarily due to lack of viable options for temporary wound coverage. This rule is mentioned in the Clinical Practice Guidelines for treatment of burn patients in combat.[4]

Given this bleak prognosis I admitted the patient and ordered Morphine and Lorazepam intravenous drips to be titrated for comfort in anticipation that she would expire within 24 h without burn resuscitation. She would be admitted to the ward instead of the Intensive Care Unit as this area was designated to treat expectant patients and the nurses had a protocol for this situation. I explained this all to the husband who was understandably distraught. As mentioned above, the protocol omitted any burn resuscitation and the patient was given only enough fluid to maintain the intravenous drips. The patient would usually become delirious in about 6 h. Some patients with greater than 50 % burn and severe facial burns would expire earlier due to airway compromise as we would keep them comfortable but only use supplemental nasal cannula oxygen per protocol. This patient had no facial burns but could possibly develop airway compromise but less likely in this situation. Several hours into her hospitalization the nurse summoned me and said that the patient wanted to speak to me. I was surprised that she was not completely delirious at this point. I was trying to think of what I could say to her as I know she would be pleading for me to attempt to save her. I walked in her room and she was surrounded by her family to include three young children. They had been brought to the hospital by a one of the combat units in the area. This was going to be tough and the interpreter and I were dreading the task. The women spoke to the interpreter and after they conversed, they both began to cry. I knew I was not ready to hear what the women had to say but asked the interpreter anyway. After she got her composure she told me that the woman said: "I know that you cannot save me. Thank you for making me comfortable and allowing me to have this time with my family. May Allah bless you and give you the strength to possibly save the next person. May Allah bless you and your family." When I heard this I had to hold back my tears, I was not expecting this but realized even though I could not save this young woman I was able to aide her in a comfortable and dignified death. She died a few hours later and I learned an important lesson that day, one I will never forget.[5,6]

13.5 Conclusions

The care of thermally injured patients can be difficult and its complexity multiplied when rendering care in tactical and operational environments. Initial reports can be misleading so careful evaluation of patients and constant suspicion of possible traumatic injuries in addition to burn injury is imperative. Life-threatening traumatic injuries must be addressed first but even with proper treatment of these patients, the mortality is high when severe burn injury is seen in conjunction with significant trauma. The airway should be definitively controlled if the patient exhibits signs of inhalation injury, have severe facial burns or have extensive burn surface area (>40 %). The potential of airway compromise during transport must be anticipated and definitive airway should be considered even in patients who are alert and verbal.

The resuscitation of casualties with burn and traumatic injuries is extremely complex. Burn resuscitation should not commence until all bleeding is controlled and blood volume replenished with blood products as needed. A search for occult sources of bleeding should be sought if a burn patient becomes unstable as even severe burn injury will not manifest as instability acutely in the absence of trauma or a severe medical condition (such as a myocardial infraction). Once the patient has all life-threatening traumatic injuries addressed burn resuscitation can begin. Cyanide toxicity should be considered in all patients that experience burns in a closed area or near plastics. It is important to monitor and document the entire burn resuscitation as this information will be useful once the patient arrives at the burn center. Equally important not to over-resuscitate these patients as this will greatly increase morbidity and mortality.

It is important to realize and prepare to treat host nationals. Often their care is hindered by lack of resources and experienced personnel. It is important to be mindful of local cultural norms and to respect them whenever possible. A good knowledge of the capabilities of the local host nation medical facilities is also essential as this medical community will need to assume follow-on care for these patients. Unfortunately in many situations the appropriate host national medical care is simply non-existent. Be prepared to render expectant care to local nationals with severe burn injury. Prepare your staff for this eventuality and have protocols and standard operating procedures for care of the expectant patient.[7]

Editor's Note: COL Booker King, MD is currently serving on Active Duty in the United States Army. He has been deployed four times in support of Operations Iraqi and Enduring Freedom. Dr. King is currently the director of US Institute of Surgical Research Burn Center at Joint Base San Antonio, Fort Sam Houston, TX.

References

1. Cancio LC, Horvath EE, Barillo DJ, Kopchinski BJ, et al. Burn support for operation Iraq Freedom and related operations, 2003 to 2004. J Burn Care Rehabil. 2005;26(2):151–61.
2. Cho J, Jatoi I, Morton T, Alacron A, King B. Operation Iraqi Freedom: surgical experience of the 212th Mobile Army Surgical Hospital. Mil Med. 2005;170(4):268–72.
3. Huzar TF, George T, Cross JM. Carbon monoxide and cyanide toxicity: etiology, pathophysiology and treatment in inhalation injury. Expert Rev Respir Med. 2013;7(2):159–70.
4. Lairet KF, Lairet JR, King BT, Renz EM, Blackbourne LH. Pre-hospital burn management in a combat zone. Prehosp Emerg Care. 2012;16(2):273–6.
5. Qader AR. Burn mortality in Iraq. Burns. 2012; 38(5): 772–775.
6. Renz EM, King BT, Chung KK, et al. The US Army burn center: professional service during 10 years of war. J Trauma Acute Care Surg. 2012;73 Suppl 6:S409–16.
7. Stout LR, Jezior JR, Melton LP, et al. Wartime burn care in Iraq: 28th Combat Support Hospital, 2003. Mil Med. 2007;172(11):1148–53.

Operating in a Tent

14

COL Robert B. Lim

14.1 Background

On the evening of March 19, 2003 I, along with the 19 other members of the 126th Forward Surgical Team (FST), stood on the boarder of Kuwait and Iraq as we watched the beginning of the Shock and Awe campaign. As we heard and watched the warplanes fly overhead and the munitions explode in front of us, we made the final preparations to our vehicles and equipment. Hours later we would enter into Iraq following the path laid out by the air support and cleared by the initial ground troops of the storied 3rd Infantry Division. Our surgical team followed some 3–5 km behind the ground troops but often times the fighting seemed to occur much closer than that. Our mission was to provide emergency surgical support to the United States led coalition forces. As an FST, we were a highly mobile surgical team with the ability to do 30 operations or continuous operations for 48 h. Our mission was dependent upon the ability to evacuate patients quickly to a tertiary-care facility and to get resupplied readily when the need arose. We also had to have the ability to set up and pack up quickly in

C.R.B. Lim, M.D., F.A.C.S. (✉)
Department of Surgery, Advanced Laparoscopic and
Metabolic Surgery, Tripler Army Medical Center,
1 Jarrett White Road, Honolulu, HI 96859, USA
e-mail: rob_lim@hotmail.com

order to keep up with the ground troops could as the invasion of Iraq led us up to Baghdad.

Over the next 18 days, we traveled slowly from Kuwait into Baghdad and during that time we formally set up our surgical suite five times. We did two operations and performed over 20 resuscitations. When we set up our surgical suite in a hangar bay of Baghdad International Airport on the 9th of April, we began to see patients more steadily. Until then we spent our days keeping our equipment as clean as possible and packing our vehicles so that we could set up a fully functional operating room within an hour even in the middle of the desert. For those 18 days we traveled in our chemical protective gear which made the almost 100° dry heat of the Iraqi desert even more oppressive. Bathing consisted of baby wipes only.

Our operative experience ran a gamut of combat and environmental extremes. In one example, we drove our vehicles almost 18 straight hours stopping only to hunker down for an impending sandstorm. Such storms are so bad, that one cannot see more than a few inches in front of one's face. Before the full effects of one such sandstorm hit, we set up to care for four casualties (Figs. 14.1 and 14.2). The first was a U.S. soldier with a penetrating injury to zone II of his neck. As he had no hard signs of bleeding and an intact airway, there was no indication for an operation. But we could not evacuate him out because air travel was limited due to the upcoming storm. The next three patients were Iraqi nationals. Two

© Springer International Publishing Switzerland 2016
C.R.B. Lim (ed.), *Surgery During Natural Disasters, Combat,*
Terrorist Attacks, and Crisis Situations, DOI 10.1007/978-3-319-23718-3_14

Fig. 14.1 One of the 126th FST General Surgeons traveling on a convoy during the Invasion of Iraq in 2003. His face is caked with sand

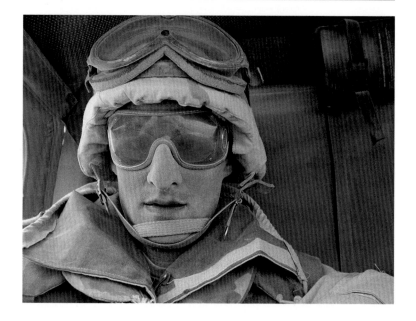

Fig. 14.2 The *orange sky* before the worst of a sandstorm or *shamal*. Any picture of an actual sandstorm would be completely *black*

were injured with penetrating wounds to their extremities but one had a large penetrating injury to his abdomen with clear penetration into his peritoneal cavity. The first two could be managed with local wound care and clean dressings. The third one, though, would require an operation.

With our entire team working together, we were able to set our surgical suite complete with an enclosed operating tent, an operating table, overhead lights, scrub table, and an anesthesia machine in an hour. An enclosed space was paramount because of the amount of sand flying around and so that there would not be a big light source for which the enemy could aim. In the time it took us to set up our suite, the visibility had gone from twenty or so feet to just a few inches. Two of our teammates actually got caught outside and because they could not see where to go, they just remained in place covering themselves up with a poncho until the storm subsided. When it did, they realized they were only about 25 yards from the operating room.

To make matters worse as the storm started to subside, our area started to take indirect fire from the enemy. Our forces returned fire causing the ground and our tent to shake. By this time, we had started our operation and opened the patient's abdomen to look for injuries. If that was not surreal enough, the first patient had a condition known as malrotation of his intestines. Here, the intestinal anatomy does not follow its usual pattern; and such a condition is estimated to occur in only about 0.2–0.5 % of all adults [1]. It did not make our operation any more difficult, but it did cause us to shake our heads in disbelief. The patient had a gunshot wound to his cecum, which we treated with resection of the injured intestine and a primary anastomosis. We also treated the malrotation anatomy with a formal Ladd's procedure.

The next such unique experience occurred a few days later after we had just packed our surgical suite onto our vehicles and trailers. We received a report the Iraqi National Army had intentionally blown up a weapons factory a few kilometers nearby that housed chemical weapons of mass destruction. Consequently, we were instructed to put on our full chemical protective gear to include our gas masks. About 30 min later, we received a call about an Iraqi National with penetrating trauma

to his chest and difficulty breathing; the patient has obvious chest injuries from shrapnel. He also had subcutaneous air, was dyspneic and with a low oxygen saturation. Moving while in such gear was extremely difficult and exhausting. Still because we knew where our equipment was, we were able to quickly find what we needed to attend to this patient. While in full chemical protection gear, I placed a chest tube and the nurse anesthetist was able to intubate the patient. A tension pneumothorax and hemothorax was relieved and the patient was stabilized for eventual transfer.

The next dramatic event was a MASCAL that occurred while we were located in the Baghdad airport. Our two-table operating room suite was set up and we were ready to take casualties when we received a report that an Infantry company received 22 injuries that would be evacuated to us within an hour. Our team of four surgeons (three general surgeons and one orthopedic surgeon) quickly began to assemble and establish other resources to assist with the anticipated casualties. Traveling with us was a Medical Company whose main function is to care for the non-trauma-related medical diseases like dehydration, infections, wound care, gastroenteritis, dental care, and musculoskeletal injuries to name a few. Their team had one internist, two physician assistants, a dentist, and a mental health provider, who was a social worker. We set up a triage area, then a resuscitation area with six trauma beds, and finally a holding area. I was the triage officer while my fellow surgeons, the internist, and the 2 PAs would run the resuscitations. The dentist along with the CRNAs were available for intubation. The remaining members of our team and the medical company would assist with IV placement, blood draws, wound care, and transport. Fortunately, none of the injured required surgery suffering mostly extremity wounds and musculoskeletal back and neck injuries. But within an hour we were able to triage and care for all 22 patients. Over the next two hours, we were able to evacuate all of them to a safer environment.

The surgical care in all these events took place in a tent. A mobile tent that was easy to set up with proper training and practice but a tent nonetheless. To do this effectively, there are some principles that providers should adhere to in order to deliver the health care in the most expeditious and safe manner possible. In an austere environment, though, "safe" care is a relative term. Early outcomes like a surgical site infection or the need for reoperation may be a neccessary evil when one is doing the best they can with what they have been dealt..

14.2 Situation

While it is unlikely that most non-military surgeons will find themselves in a situation where they would have to operate in a tent, like with other events detailed in this book, it is within the realm of possibility if one volunteers for a humanitarian mission, one responds to a natural disaster, or one's area is the victim of a terrorist attack where the infrastructure is severely damaged. The two overriding principles of this type of surgery are that (1) only damage control surgery to save a life, a limb, or eyesight should be employed. A gunshot wound to a leg causing a fracture in a hemodynamically stable patient will undoubtedly need at least a washout and a surgical repair of the fracture. But as the victim of such an injury is not likely to die, such a repair can be delayed until the patient can be transferred to a cleaner and more stable facility. (2) The surgical team has to be able and ready to move quickly to be closer to where the injuries are taking place. As such, the team should be able to pack as light as possible but at the same time carry as much as they can to care for as many patients as they can. (Figs. 14.3, 14.4, 14.5) If patient transfer is limited or hindered then the concept of the mobile operating team would bring the health care to the victim. The published data on the FST focus mostly on the teams that are in a static environment, often in buildings and under protection. The concepts of this chapter focus on the missions and events that require a mobile team, on the battlefield, and with minimal protection.

14.3 Knowing the Assets

This idea has been and will continue to be enforced throughout this book but preparation is extremely important for success. As terrorist acts and natural disasters are not scheduled events, one may not

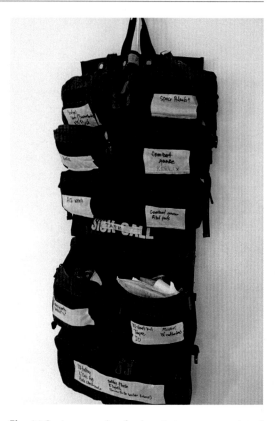

Fig. 14.3 An example of a bag that can carry a lot of equipment and medical supplies. Once opened, it can easily be hung for quick access to the supplies during a trauma resuscitation

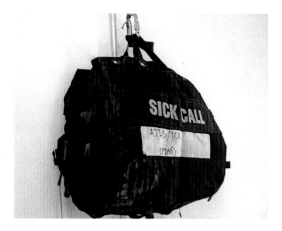

Fig. 14.4 Same bag in its easier to carry form

have the luxury of being prepared. But if one finds themselves in such an event, the first thing to do would be to determine what his or her assets are. Not just how many providers, but what type, and what kind of experience they have. One should at

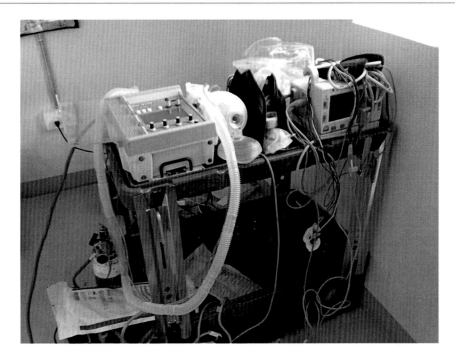

Fig. 14.5 This anesthesia table holds a ventilator, a monitor, intubation supplies, suction, and an electricity converter. The table can be converted into a single container to carry all of this equipment

least take the time to perform formal introductions of their personnel if only to learn the names of the people with whom they will be working.

The next step would be to determine what equipment they have and how they will be transporting such equipment. The latter will help determine how much they can take. The former should give the surgeon an idea of what his surgical capabilities are. For instance, if one is going to use surgical staplers for bowel surgery, they should be sure they are familiar with the type of stapler that they will be taking. It may indeed be different from the one they use in their regular practice. Orthopedic surgeons would need to be familiar with the different type of external fixation systems that are available.

The capabilities of the team would also include equipment to help with resuscitation. Rapid intravenous infusion devices may be available, its use would prevent someone from having to squeeze intravenous fluid into a patient. Fast reading lab analyzers are also available (Fig. 14.6) and these devices can quickly provide arterial blood gas, chemistry panel, complete blood count, and coagulation panel readings. Packed red blood cells

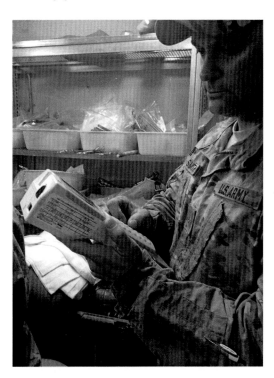

Fig. 14.6 This is a handheld blood-analyzing device that is commonly used in civilian hospitals in the United States. Its portable size makes it ideal for use in a mobile OR or FST

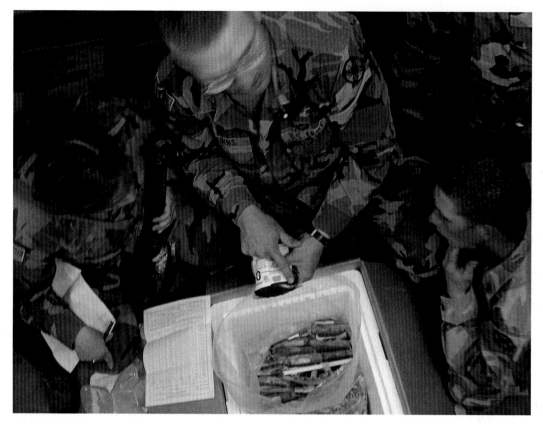

Fig. 14.7 Here the team is checking the expiration date of the packed red blood cells that it will transports during its mission. The blood is carried in coolers here but there are also portable refrigerators that can be utilized

and fresh frozen plasma can also be transported with the aid of refrigerators and/or ice chests (Fig. 14.7). It would be important, then to know their expiration dates and how long the refrigerators can last on battery power. Radiology equipment will not likely be available to the mobile team but an ultrasound device is portable. Physicians should be familiar with being able to do a focused abdominal sonography for trauma scan or FAST scan which may dictate their care especially in blunt trauma patients.

In addition to the surgical equipment or medical supplies, then a mobile team would ideally have a generator to produce power for its operating room. The power would be needed for lighting, the anesthesia machines, the refrigerators, the surgical electricity, and even the warming devices. The military uses fuel-based generators.

Inherent to knowing what the assets are is that everyone on the team should know how most if not all the equipment works, especially if it is a small 20-person team. If two surgeons are busy with a difficult operation that requires a massive transfusion, this would likely occupy two anesthesia providers, two operating room nurses, and probably two surgical technicians then 40 % of the team is engaged and unable to assist with any other casualties. As such the two other surgeons can help by getting other equipment, getting more blood, assisting with blood transfusion, and doing lab analysis. They can even help with the refueling of the generator or restocking for the next casualty.

When preparing for a mission and especially when there is down time, the team should be engaged with rehearsals, training, and teaching. Those with experience, in particular, should use the time to do everything they can to prepare younger and less experienced team members.

Our team practiced putting up our OR tent and surgical suite so many times, we could do it in an hour, in the dark, and during the middle of a sandstorm. I was so familiar where everything was packed, I knew which truck held the chest tubes and which container they were in.

14.4   Evacuation and Re-supply

The next important concept of operating in the field is to understand where and how far away the next hospital is. The military has a concept called the echelons of care so that an FST, at level II, would evacuate its patients to a Combat Support Hospital (CSH) or level III where there is more personnel, patient holding capability, and equipment like a computed tomography scanner (CT scan). Surgeons and surgical teams in the civilian world would have to know what hospital they could bring their patients and how long it would take to get there.

A mobile OR team, like an FST, is not designed to hold patients for a long period of time. Consequently, they must have a plan or assist in the planning of evacuation of the patients. Weather can prevent evacuation in a timely manner. The inability to evacuate a patient in a timely fashion may require the surgeon to operate on someone whom they fear has an injury that cannot wait for several hours. A gunshot wound to the kidney, for instance that destroys 50 % of the tissue may be something that can be salvaged at a high-volume civilian accredited trauma center with more blood, dialysis capability, and an urologist. But in the forward setting, this may consume all of the blood products and surgical supplies such that no other patients can be cared for. Additionally, it would likely keep the patient on the operating table for a longer period of time in an unsterile setting. If the patient cannot be evacuated to tertiary level trauma center in this situation, then, it may be more prudent to remove the kidney to stop the bleeding.

The mobile operating team would also need to know where its re-supply of equipment is coming from and how often. Since the mobile team can-not carry an endless supply of items, resuscitation of just a few patients may exhaust all of its assets. Subsequently, in order to be functional, the team would have to get re-supplied at regular intervals or when the need arose. Along these lines, good communication with the evacuation teams and the re-supply chain is very important. Without it, the team would not be able to treat patients.

14.5   Special Aspects of Patient Care

Triage: Because the supplies of a mobile operating team are limited, the philosophy of the team is to only perform surgery on those that would otherwise die or suffer greatly if surgery is not performed right then and there. About 22 % of battlefield deaths occur due to exsanguinations [2]. It is these patients that an FST will potentially have the greatest impact upon. Some believe this exanguination occurs within the first 60 min after injury and thus the term "golden hour" was coined. While it is hard to prove if 60 min is indeed the key, from a more practical perspective, if one includes the time needed to secure the combat area where the casualty occurred, the time it takes to remove the injured person from the hostile zone, and the actual time of transport, then it is very likely that an injured patient would not make it to the FST or 2nd echelon of care setting for a few hours much less to the 3rd level of care or the CSH [3]. Subsequently three categories of possible surgical patients make it to the FST: those that withstand the test of time and prove that they do not need emergent surgical care, those that are in extremis or near dead due to their injuries, and finally those that need emergent surgical care. Because the middle group can consume a lot of supplies, it is important to triage them appropriately and consider managing expectantly because of the futility of their injuries. On the other hand, those in the first category may need surgery eventually, but they can be safely transported back to a higher echelon of care. Proper triage then is vitally important to the success of the FST and mobile OR.

Language Barriers: As was true in the war in Iraq and continues to be true in the war in Afghanistan, many of the casualties are not English speaking. Since the mobile teams do not bring a CT scanner with them, providers in the austere environment rely heavily on their physical examination to make a diagnosis. In order to perform a good physical examination, the provider must be able to communicate with the patient. This is impossible if the provider does not speak the language of the patient. Thus a provider should try to learn at least a few phrases or words that would help him or her communicate with the injured patient. If there were interpreters available, this would also be an important adjunct to the mobile OR team.

Cultural sensitivity: Along those lines, it is important for the mobile OR team to be familiar with some of the local customs. In the Middle East, for instance, men might be very weary of female providers seeing them naked. They might view it as some kind of abuse. Additionally, waving hello with one's left hand is considered an insult and a patient may not answer questions in response to the slight. While this may not negatively affect the outcomes in patients with severe trauma, it may make a thorough examination difficult causing a missed injury.

Operations and Surgical Procedures: (Fig. 14.8) When it comes down to actually doing an operation, the technical aspects of the surgery are likely to be the easiest part of the mission for the surgeon because that is the part that he or she is most familiar with. Still there are some aspects of operating in a tent that make it different from operating in a hospital. The "OR" will be dirty. There will be sand and mud on the floors and dust and dirt in the air. Mobile ORs and open-air tents will not have a positive pressure system or a ventilator system to blow or suck dust particles away. The first time I asked for saline to irrigate an abdomen, the surgical technician poured saline into a basin to hand to me. But because of the dirt and dust in the air, when the saline was poured into the basin all it did was produce mud. After that we decided to pour the sterile saline directly from the bottle into the patient. Insects are likely to be in the OR as well. Because of the dirty environment, we rarely attempted an abdominal closure

and all wounds were extensively washed out and dressed meticulously to keep the wounds as clean as possible. The overwhelming majority of patients who receive an operation in the FST will need another operation within 24–48 h after their first surgery.

Temperature control is impossible in a tent also. When it gets cold, then it is imperative to keep the patient as warm as possible to prevent hypothermia and the lethal triad of trauma (academia, hypothermia, and coagulopathy). Multiple blankets should be used and so should "space blankets" or "casualty blankets" to help insulate the patient. If the team has a Bair Hugger™ or a forced air-warming blanket, this should also be utilized. The use of warm IV fluid should also be employed and keeping the instruments warm may help with the surgeon's comfort.

Heat, on the other hand, may affect the surgical team more than the patient. When it is too hot, this can cause sweat to hinder vision or fall into the surgical field. The use of cloth scrub caps with an absorptive headband or simply adding a headband can help to absorb the perspiration. The surgical gowns are designed to be water impermeable to keep fluids off the body of the team but this also causes heat to be retained inside the gown. If it gets very hot, it may cause the team to get dehydrated and even pass out. Before an operation in a hot environment, the providers should drink plenty of water. During the operation, the circulating nurses may have to provide water to the team that is scrubbed in. Some surgeons have also operated in shorts and light shirts underneath their gowns to help stay cool during an operation.

Aside from the environment, the surgical equipment will not be of the same caliber as a typical OR. The surgical table will most likely not be able to be rotated, raised, or lowered which would make some areas of the body easier to expose and visualize. Additionally, the surgical lights are likely to be inadequate. Headlamps are standard issue for the FST but like any light, they will be dependent on electricity or battery power so they must be maintained or supplied with power. Oxygen for anesthesia is very cumbersome and heavy to travel with. In addition to transporting the oxygen, it is important to know

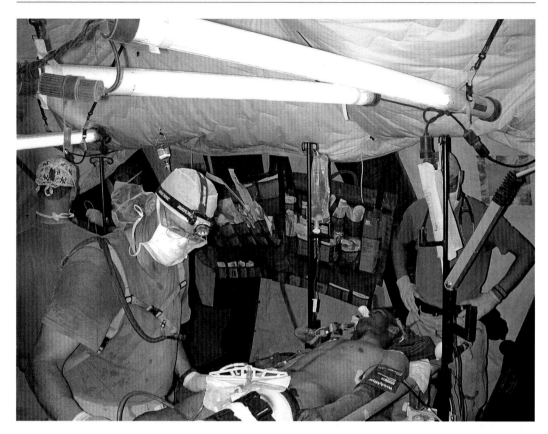

Fig. 14.8 Inside the operating room tent. Note the surgeon is using a headlamp because overhead lighting is limited and carrying water on his back because of the hot conditions

how much oxygen each tank takes. There are multiple sizes and how long a tank last also depends on how much one dispenses to the patient. So it may be wise to use the least amount of oxygen needed to treat a patient.

Another unique aspect of operating in the field or in a tent is security. In combat the mobile OR will be directly on the battlefield and some teams have operated while wearing their Kevlar body protection gear. The team members not directly involved in the operation may be called upon to provide security. On more than one occasion, I along with my fellow surgeons have pulled perimeter security. In a natural disaster, the team members may be needed to assist with other patients or just to help provide order to those who are seeking medical aid.

The final important task of the operation is communicating with the next level of care. An electronic record may not be readily available until a more permanent medical facility can be established, so the surgical team may have to rely on paper work. Paperwork, of course, can get lost especially during transport in a combat zone or in a disaster area. One tactic utilized in war is writing a brief operation report on the patient's bandages. Here, surgeons will write down details like how many units of transfusion the patient has received, the injuries and the repairs that were done, and in the case of open abdomens, they will write down how many packs were left inside the patient. This way the receiving team will have a good idea of what happened with the patient and there will not be confusion as to which patient it was because the report will have been written on the patients themselves. Aside from the written communication, every effort should be made to speak directly with a physician on the receiving end of the patient's evacuation.

14.6   Preparing for the Next Mission

Once the operations are over and the patients are evacuated to a higher level of care, substantial work must be done before the team can rest. The team must prepare for the next casualties, because, of course, he or she may arrive at any time. The operating room and the resuscitation areas must be cleaned and restocked. If supplies are low then this must be reported to the re-supply chain so that the team can continue to be functional. Surgical instruments need to be cleaned and sterilized. A short team meeting should occur when there is a time to discuss how things could be done better and what things went wrong.

The next thing the team should do is take care of itself. Team leaders should be responsible for making sure the team has plenty of food and water. Members should take the time for personal hygiene. Our team carried two outdoor shower bags that could each hold 5 gal of water. We would lay the bags outside in the hot sun so we could take showers at night with warm water. A 5-gal bag used appropriately would be enough to bathe 4–5 people. With appropriate rationing of the shower bags, people could take a shower every 2–3 days. Sleep should also be a priority for the team, even if surgeons are used to functioning well without it. Lastly, a good team will find time to bond and unwind together. This could be by playing a game, praying, playing music, sharing stories about their lives, watching movies, or any number of group activities. Of course, not everyone will react to stress in the same way and not everyone will want to participate in team activities. Leaders should seek out these team members and do their best to make sure their needs are met. This may include help from a chaplain or a mental health provider.

14.7   Conclusions

The recommendations in this chapter are meant to help surgeons and the surgical teams succeed in the most austere conditions and with the least amount of resources. While it is highly unlikely that the average surgeon will find him or herself in this situation, it may happen if there is a natural disaster like the earthquake in Haiti of 2010. As you have read in the chapter about that disaster, 300 surgeries were performed in tent conditions. Military health care providers may be deployed to a FST and if that particular team is not in a static environment, then the team will face the described challenges of being mobile. The United States Army has also recently deployed the idea of a GHOSTT team, which stands for Golden Hour Off-Set Trauma Team. The GHOSTT team is similar in concept to the mobile FST team. Here the team goes out on missions and locates itself closer to the war-fighters, so that they can be as close as possible to intervene with combat-related injuries. The GHOSTT teams travel with even less equipment than does a mobile FST team.

Integral to success is good teamwork, thorough knowledge of all the equipment, and preparation. All members of the team should help with packing and movement. All members of the team should have a basic idea of how the equipment works. All of the members of the team should be looking out for one another. These concepts allowed us to provide successful surgery during a sandstorm, under indirect fire, and in a massive casualty situation all inside of a tent. During the invasion of Iraq, the 126th FST saw roughly 84 patients and performed 27 surgeries with no deaths, during the first 5 months of the conflict.

References

1. Low S, Ngiu CS, Sridharan R, Lee YL. Midgut rotation with congenital peritoneal band: a rare cause of small bowel obstruction. BMJ Case Rep. 2014.
2. Eastridge B, Mabry RL, Seguin P, Cantrell J, Tops T, Uribe P, et al. Death on the battlefield (2001-2011): implications for the future of combat casualty care. J Trauma Acute Care Surg. 2012;73(6 Suppl 5): S431–7.
3. Apodaca A, Olson CM, Bailey J, Butler F, Eastridge BJ, Kuncir E. Performance improvement evaluation of forward aeromedical evacuation platforms in Operation Enduring Freedom. J Trauma Acute Care Surg. 2013;75(2):S157–63.

Dismounted Complex Blast Injuries

15

Joseph M. Galante and Carlos J. Rodriguez

15.1 Introduction

The authors were deployed together during the summer of 2010 in Southern Helmand Province, Afghanistan. That was the summer of the US troop surge into Afghanistan, and with it, combat casualty frequency dramatically increased. In fact, during a 6 month period, our hospital cared for over 1,700 combat trauma cases where approximately 43% of the injuries were from blast and over 25% had Injury Severity Scores greater than 15.

Of the many different patients we cared for that summer, one patient's story will forever live in our minds. It was early morning, the sun had just risen and our medical team was out for a morning run before the desert temperature rose too high while, unbeknownst to us, a young medic was on foot patrol in Sangin, Afghanistan when his foot triggered a pressure plate IED resulting in an above

J.M. Galante, M.D. (✉)
Division of Trauma, Acute Care Surgery and Surgical Critical Care, Department of Surgery, Davis Medical Center, University of California, 2315 Stockton Blvd., North Wing, Rm. 4206, Sacramento, CA 95817, USA
e-mail: joseph.galante@ucdmc.ucdavis.edu

C.J. Rodriguez, D.O., M.B.A.
Department of General Surgery, Walter Reed National Military Medical Center, 8901 Wisconsin Avenue, Bethesda, MD 20889, USA
e-mail: carlos.j.rodriguez4.mil@mail.mil

knee amputation so proximal, that it involved his external iliac vessels. His bleeding needed to be stopped quickly…his unit sprung to action by fashion an improvised tourniquet composed of a machine gun barrel used as a windlass and web belt.

He arrived to our trauma bay cold, clammy, and hypotensive. We took him directly to the operating room with barely enough time to transfer him from combat litter to a regular gurney. While securing his airway and initiating a massive blood resuscitation, we obtained proximal surgical control and took down his improvised tourniquet. The bleeding had stopped. It turns out, just the day prior, this medic had discussed and practiced making improvised tourniquets with his unit. That 20 minute training period, undoubtedly saved his life.

Unfortunately devastating blast injuries are no longer limited to the battlefields of Iraq and Afghanistan, as they are occurring on the streets of America. On April 15, 2013, an improvised explosive device (IED) packed with "ball bearings" and nails exploded at the finish line of the Boston marathon. Three were killed and 281 were injured. Many of the injuries involved lower extremities, including 16 amputations [1].

The traditional teaching of "land mine" pattern of injury as illustrated in the Emergency War Surgery (EWS) textbook (Fig. 15.1) is a gross underrepresentation of the modern-day battle injury pattern [2]. Dismounted complex blast injury (DCBI) from IEDs has become the signature injury of our nation's most recent war (Fig. 15.2).

© Springer International Publishing Switzerland 2016
C.R.B. Lim (ed.), *Surgery During Natural Disasters, Combat, Terrorist Attacks, and Crisis Situations*, DOI 10.1007/978-3-319-23718-3_15

Fig. 15.1 Traditional pattern injuries caused by antipersonnel mines. (Modified from Borden Institute, Emergency War Surgery, 4th edition, Fort Sam Houston, TX, 2013)

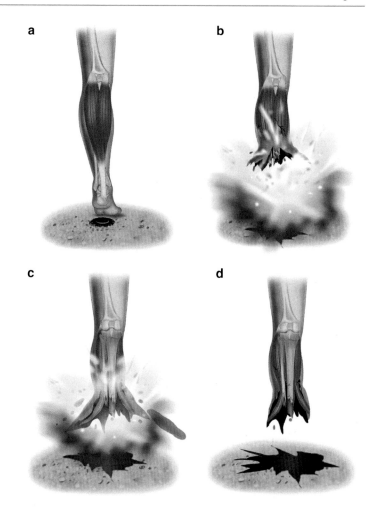

Fig. 15.2 Typical pattern of injuries caused by modern improvised explosive devices (Afghanistan 2010)

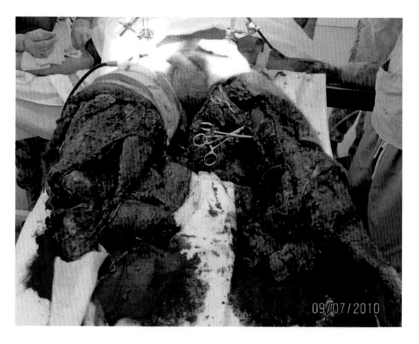

DCBI is a blast injury sustained while on foot patrol and carries a specific injury pattern that includes amputation of at least 1 lower extremity, a minimum of "severe" injury to another extremity, and pelvic, abdominal, or urogenital wounding [3]. Treating victims of DCBI requires a very specific systematic approach, beginning at the moment of the detonation.

15.2   Physics of a Blast

An understanding of blast physics is critical because it directs patterns of injuries. Blast physics can be explained via a diagram of concentric rings (Fig. 15.3a). The central point of blast is comprised of ignition and subsequent detonation of a fuel source. The burning fuel generates a thermal reaction where over-pressurized gas expands in a cir-

cumferential fashion from the point of detonation. Objects (ball bearings, rocks, etc.) within these two zones are propelled outward at very high velocities. The wave of over-pressurized gas is quickly followed by a negative pressure wave. The Friedlander curve illustrates the change in pressure during the period immediately after a blast (Fig. 15.3b). The over-pressurized wave causes direct impact on biological tissues, lung, and brain. The subsequent negative pressure wave then causes tissue cavitation.

Blasts can be classified as high energy and low energy [4]. The level of energy is determined by the type and amount of explosive material used and it also directly relates to injury patterns. For example, high-energy blasts, typical of DCBI, often result in complete mid-thigh or higher amputations, pelvic disruptions, extensive GU/perineal injuries, and intra-abdominal injuries. Low-energy blasts, which are common in traditional mines, cause a range of

Fig. 15.3 (**a**) Blast radius. (**b**) Pmax = maximum pressure. (From Mediavilla Varas J, Philippens M, Meijer SR, van den Berg AC, Sibma PC, van Bree JL, de Vries DV. Physics of IED blast shock tube simulations for mTBI research. Front Neurol. 2011 Sep 19;2:58)

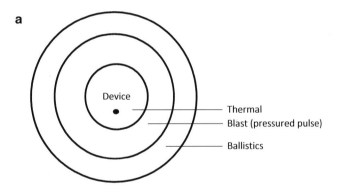

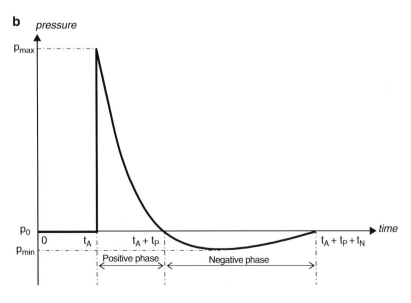

injuries from open long bone fractures to mangled extremities with possible amputations and are only occasionally associated with urogenital trauma (Fig. 15.1). The Boston Marathon bombing can be classified as a low-energy blast [5].

15.3   Patterns of Injury

Projectiles from IED fragmentation and surrounding debris, coupled with the positive and negative pressure waves and the physics and heat of a high energy explosion, result in blunt, penetrating, and burn trauma (Table 15.1.) Simultaneous injury to multiple body cavities adds to the complexity of blast injuries (Fig. 15.4).

DCBI-associated traumatic amputations can be a combination of mangled extremity and true amputations typically mid-thigh or more proximal with the blast force often causing pelvic fractures. The fracture pattern most commonly seen is a Tile Type C (Fig. 15.5). Given the frequent penetrating fragmentation injuries, pelvic fractures are typically open in nature and, as such, are often a source of massive hemorrhage.

Fragmentation or small projectiles, either as part of the explosive device or related to the surrounding debris create insidious and potentially life-threatening injuries. Since the 1940s, it has been known that blast injuries, particularly grenade and mine in origin, can cause an individual to sustain up to of 50 or more fragmentation wounds.

Table 15.1 Spectrum of blast-generated trauma

Trauma type	Phase explosions	Injury
Over-pressurized wave/blunt	Primary	Barotrauma ears, lungs TBI
Penetrating	Secondary ballistics/projectiles	Ballistic projectile-type injury
Blunt	Tertiary	Fractures, crush
Burns	Primary or quaternary	Inhalation

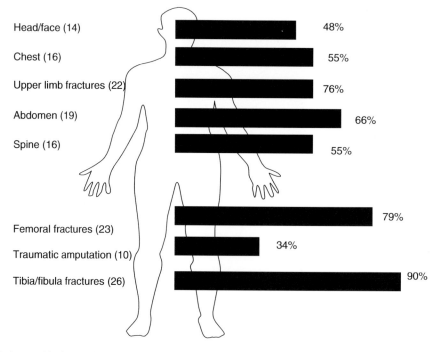

Fig. 15.4 Areas of body associated with blast injury

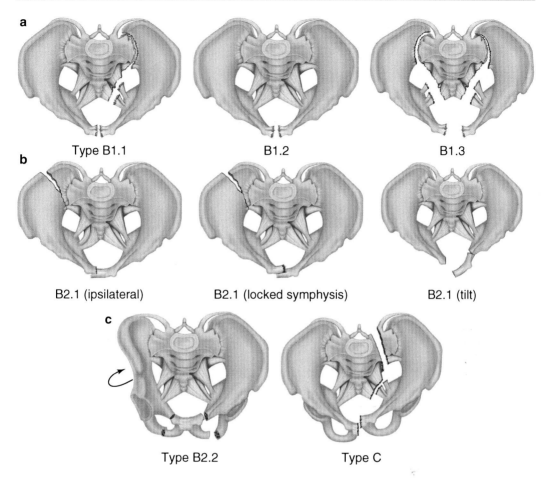

Fig. 15.5 Classification of pelvic fracture. (Modified from http://www.orthoassociates.com/SP11B26, accessed Dec 16, 2014)

Moreover, these injuries may not be immediately life threatening yet still have the potential to kill days or weeks later through complications associated with infection, traumatic arteriovenous fistulas, and arterial pseudoaneurysms [6]. Though fragmentation wounds might appear unimpressive and superficial, the wounds are caused by fragments which can travel at more than 5000 ft/s. This should prompt one to fully evaluate the patient radiographically with AP/lateral plain films and in those patients with fragments within the soft tissue of the extremity, a CT angiogram (Fig. 15.6).

Genital trauma occurs frequently. Almost 90 % patients who have sustained bilateral LE amputations also have testicular trauma from penetrating or over-pressurized compression [7].

Fragments can easily injure the penile shaft, urethra, prostate, or bladder.

Burns occur with DCBI but are frequently limited to the area immediately surrounding the initial combustion of material. Blasts occurring in Operation Enduring Freedom (OEF) typically occurred out in the open, not in enclosed spaces, so inhalation injuries were less frequent. Blast injuries in closed spaces can be much more damaging. In Operation Iraqi Freedom (OIF), troops encountered shaped charges which could penetrate armored vehicles and subsequently, cause fire and inhalation injuries within the vehicles. The presence of 2nd or 3rd degree burns has a significant impact on initial resuscitation, debridement, and reconstruction.

Traumatic brain injury (TBI) is frequently caused by the over-pressurized wave impacting

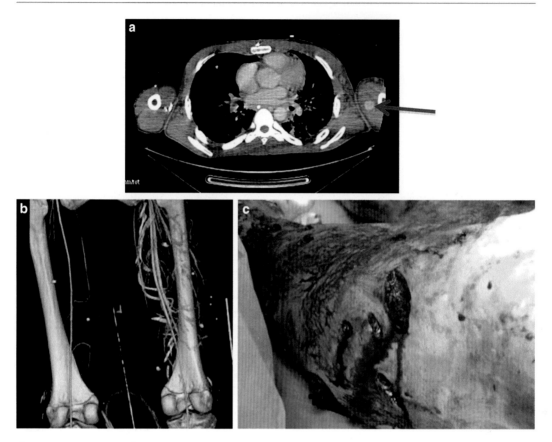

Fig. 15.6 (**a**) Brachial artery pseudoaneurysm caused by fragmentation of explosive device (Afghanistan 2010); (**b**) CTA of "superficial" wounds showing traumatic AV fistula, and (**c**) with patient prone (Afghanistan 2010)

the skull. This is very similar to the concussion mechanism encountered in professional sports such as football. The majority of victims from dismounted complex blast (DCB) have mild TBI and manifest through memory or visual disturbances [8]. There is a relative paucity of major TBI related to DCBIs. This may be due to the fact that blasts typically occur outside of a confined space.

A well-described injury related to blasts is tympanic membrane (TM) rupture. While this is frequently discussed, the incidence varies. Data from OIF suggest that only 16 % of patients involved in explosions had TM rupture but these perforations were large and the majority required surgical repair. Patients with perforation were noted to be symptomatic (77 % diminished hearing and 50 % tinnitus) but long-term hearing loss was uncommon [9]. This is in contrast to

findings from the Boston Marathon bombing where 90 % of the victims had TM rupture. Similar to patients from OIF, many required tympanoplasty. Long-term sequelae included hyperacusis and difficulty hearing in noisy surroundings [10].

The differences in TM injuries may or may not be related to the protective equipment used in OIF/OEF, but one area in which protective equipment does have a significant impact is ocular injuries. In combat, proper wearing of eye protection limited ocular blast injury to 0.5 % [11]. In the Boston Marathon bombing, 13.4 % of patients had ocular injuries [12]. The incidence is similar in other civilian blast events. In survivors from Oklahoma City, the most common ocular injuries were lid lacerations, globe rupture, orbital fracture, detached retina, and retained foreign bodies—mostly glass shards [13].

Dental and other maxillofacial injuries are common in DCBI, likely related to the lack of protective equipment around the jaw. The most common facial injury is mandible fracture [14]. Tooth injury is often related to these complicated, frequently open, mandible fractures.

Spine fractures may seem to be a likely injury after DCBI, but our experience and the literature does not support this belief. Spine fractures were more often seen in mounted blasts. Kinetic blast wave energy is distributed in such a way with dismounted blasts that there is little axial compression on the spine.

15.4 Treatment

15.4.1 Prehospital

Similar to American College of Surgeons, Advance Trauma Life Support (ATLS) philosophy, a systematic approach saves lives. But unlike the ABCs of ATLS, care for DCBI follows a different set of priorities, XABC (exsanguinating hemorrhage, airway, breathing, circulation) focusing first on hemorrhage control at the scene immediately after the blast, for without organized prehospital care, there is no need to discuss surgical priorities (Fig. 15.7).

Hemorrhage is the most common cause of immediate death. Total or near-total extremity amputation is a source of massive blood loss. Improvement in survival on the battlefield can be attributed to the increased use of tourniquets [15]. Tourniquets come in many forms from those that are commercially available to those that can be improvised. Whichever type is used, proper application will achieve the same goal—to stop exsanguinating hemorrhage [16]. Tourniquets are most effective in areas of compressible hemorrhage, where direct pressure can be applied to an artery proximal to the injury.

A review of all battlefield deaths by Eastridge in 2012 showed almost 25 % of prehospital deaths were preventable. Of these preventable deaths, 90 % were from hemorrhage. Junctional hemorrhage (bleeding from an artery not compressible by tourniquet) accounted for 19 % of preventable prehospital deaths [17]. As of this writing, several commercially available tourniquets, the CRoC TM clamp, the SAM Junctional Tourniquet, or the JETT (Junctional Emergency Treatment Tool) have been developed to stop junctional hemor-

Fig. 15.7 Immediate treatment after blast

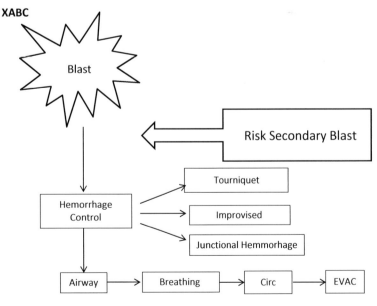

*Immediate priorities after blast

rhage, but none have been widely adopted in either military or civilian settings.

Blast injuries causing junctional hemorrhage in the groin are often associated with proximal femur amputations and pelvic fractures both of which are additional sources of major hemorrhage. Prehospital strategies for pelvic hemorrhage control include utilization of commercially available pelvic binders or wrapping a sheet tightly around the pelvis. These forces close the volume of the pelvis and theoretically decrease the space in which bleeding can occur. One of the commercially available junctional tourniquets is actually imbedded into a pelvic binder allowing for the ability to compress junctional hemorrhage and decrease pelvic volume with a single device.

Once hemorrhage is controlled Airway, Breathing, and Circulation (ABCs) become the priorities. Airway obstruction and tension pneumothorax are the second and third leading cause of preventable death on the battlefield and need to be specifically addressed.

Cardiopulmonary resuscitation in the field should be treated similarly to cardiac arrest from blunt trauma. Measures such as resuscitative thoracotomy have been debated, but we believe this should be avoided since rates of survival are extremely low, and the cause of arrest is typically blood loss, for which restoration of blood volume is the appropriate therapy vice a correctable cause of arrest in the thorax such as tamponade. Civilian literature in less complex trauma has dismal outcomes with resuscitative thoracotomy [18, 19].

Evacuation from the site of the blast is extremely important but can be dangerous. A common enemy tactic has been to have secondary or delayed explosions targeting medical personnel. In the civilian sector, structural damage to a building from a explosion may cause the building to be unsafe such that removing rubble to access injured patients may cause other injuries to the victim or to the rescuer. Individuals, such as law enforcement, should deem the area safe before medical teams enter.

Upon entering a blast scene, the systematic process of triage begins. Individual prehospital providers should have a basic understanding of resources available at system and hospital levels. Hospital team leaders receiving casualties should have an understanding of available hospital resources—i.e. blood bank, surgical capacity (OR, surgical teams, etc.). Hospitals receiving patients should perform a tertiary triage and conduct patient sanitation to ensure firearms or explosives do not make their way into the ED. The receiving hospital may not know if an arriving patient was a victim or participant in the blast with ulterior motives. Tertiary triage and sanitation should be conducted in a safe location outside and away from the hospital—i.e. not at the ED entrance.

15.4.2 Resuscitation

After hemorrhage control is established, resuscitation should begin. With a focus on hemostatic resuscitation, efforts in Afghanistan led to limiting infusion of crystalloid. Through the development of prehospital blood transfusion protocols, this effort was pushed as close to the point of injury as possible [20, 21]. Tactical Combat Casualty Care (TCCC) guidelines and the US Military's Joint Trauma System clinical practice guidelines suggest that for patients in shock (altered mental status without evidence of TBI and absent or weak radial pulse), whole blood should be transfused in order to achieve a palpable radial pulse (estimated SBP of 80–90 mmHg) [22]. If whole blood is not available, the preferred order of fluid administration is plasma, packed red blood cells, Hextend, and then crystalloid.

The early use of blood and blood products is the key element of hemostatic resuscitation. This is part of a broader concept called "Damage Control Resuscitation" (DCR). DCR is centered on disrupting the "trauma lethal triad" of acidosis, coagulopathy, and hypothermia with the target of reversing (or halting) acute traumatic coagulopathy (ATC). ATC is a result of the endogenous response to injury with the activation of both pro- and anticoagulation mechanisms. ATC is complicated by exogenous sources of coagulopathy such as infusion of large volumes of crystalloid or packed red blood cells without subsequent plasma infusion.

Many of these patients require large volume resuscitation due to the nature of their injuries

Table 15.2 Blood products

Blood product	Mean per patient (range)
Packed red cells	28.6 (2–98)
Fresh frozen plasma	25.5 (0–97)
Cryoprecipitate	2.41 (0–11)
Platelets	3.8 (0–18)

Reproduced with permission and copyright © of the British Editorial Society of Bone and Joint Surgery. Ramasamy A, Evans S, Kendrew JM, et al. The open blast pelvis. *J Bone Joint Surg Br.* 2012 June;94(6)829–35

Table 15.3 Physiological derangement associated with DCBI and hemostatic

Time	1545	1730
pH	6.6	7.4
HCO_3^-	<10	21
Base excess	−30	−4
Temp (°C)	35.6	37
INR	1.9	1.3

Between 1545 and 1730, patient received 40 units of packed red blood cells, 40 units of fresh frozen plasma, five packs of platelets, activated factor 7×2, and 2 g of TXA. No crystalloid was administered during this resuscitation

and immediate blood loss (Table 15.2). A 1:1:1 ratio of PRBCs to fresh plasma to platelets can achieve resolution of acidosis and coagulopathy within hours of initiating resuscitation. A DCR resuscitation example is presented of a DCBI patient over two hours in Afghanistan (Table 15.3). High volume crystalloid use does not achieve similar results [23].

15.4.3 Tranexamic Acid (TXA)

In 2010, the CRASH-2 study demonstrated decrease in mortality from bleeding with administration of TXA, an antifibrinolytic plasmin binding lysine analog, in civilian trauma. The study included >20,000 patients across the globe [24]. In 2011, the MATTERs study analyzed TXA use in Afghanistan with injured service members and identified a decrease in mortality from bleeding when given within 3 h of injury [25]. TXA administration has also been shown to provide a survival benefit to injured children in Afghanistan [26].

15.4.4 Vascular Access

If large bore peripheral or central venous catheterization is not available, intraossous (IO) lines are a viable alternative for administering large volume resuscitation [27]. The tibia is the preferred site, if available, with the humeral head, iliac crest, and sternum being suitable alternatives. Care must be taken when selecting the proper device for sternal IOs as this location calls for shorter needles. Using the longer humeral IO for the sternum may lead to the needle traversing the sternum, therefore, fluid may be directly administered to the sub-sternal space (or potentially injuring superficial structures of the mediastinum). Sternal IOs are commonly used in DCBI patients as it can be difficult to establish peripheral IVs or IO catheters in patients with multiple amputations. Peripheral or central IV access becomes more feasible as the intravascular volume expands with resuscitation.

15.5 Surgical Priorities

Complex trauma associated with DCBI requires a systematic approach to surgical care. Multidisciplinary surgical teams, sometimes operating in parallel, are critical to successful outcomes given the whole-body injury patterns seen in the DCBI patient.

There are two important principles governing surgical management of DCBI:

1. Distilling this complex trauma to simple principles.
2. Establishing the goals of index procedure—hemostatic resuscitation and debridement.

Priority of surgical management is based on the condition most likely to cause death from exsanguination. The algorithm (Fig. 15.8) is based on the principle of hemorrhage control. Survival rates from high-energy blasts is reliant upon by early hemorrhage control and reversal of acidosis and hypercoagulability [3]. Tourniquet reassessment and reapplication is critical (Fig. 15.9). As resuscitation begins and blood

Fig. 15.8 Basic algorithm for treatment plan for DCBI

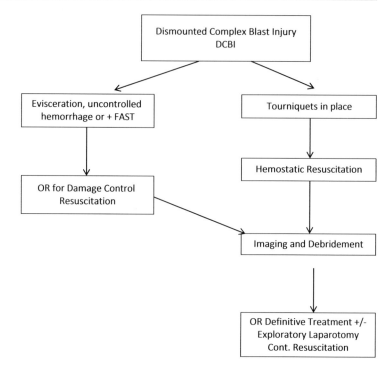

Fig. 15.9 Protocol for managing DCBI patients who arrive with tourniquets in place

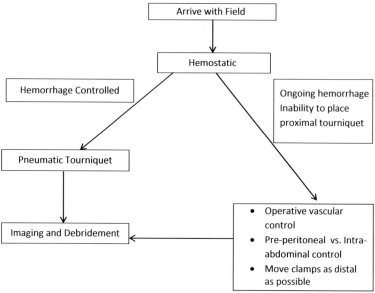

pressure rises, tourniquets, which once were hemostatic, may lose their effectiveness.

As long as hemorrhage is controlled in the ED, tourniquet reassessment should be done in an optimal setting for surgeons—the operating room. This is particularly true when dealing with junctional hemorrhage. Junctional hemorrhage may be temporized in the prehospital setting with specialized tourniquets but more definitive control should be sought in the OR setting.

Resuscitative endovascular balloon occlusion of the aorta (REBOA) devices have been advocated in certain settings but may not be available in all hospitals [28]. Angioembolization is an additional method of noncompressible hemorrhage control. While this resource may be available, given the potential for hemodynamic instability, it should be avoided initially [29]. Open vascular control is a most definitive method for vascular control and is the preferred method.

15.6 Open Vascular Control

There are several principles for open vascular control. The first is to proceed with most proximal control at first and then work to most distal point on the artery that can be safely clamped. The purpose is to preserve uninjured artery and to avoid further ischemia to blasted tissue. Some have advocated for cross-clamping the distal intra-abdominal aorta but this is dangerous due to the increased ischemic burden on the pelvic muscles, which have been exposed to the blast. Other than the obvious avoidance of further injury, the musculature needs to be preserved for future reconstruction (i.e. gluteal flaps).

Depending on the extent of the injuries, a trans-abdominal approach may need to be performed for proximal vascular control. However, an ex lap is always not warranted. In a case such as this, a unilateral extraperitoneal incision (similar to those used for renal transplants) may be used for control of the external iliac artery.

15.7 Pelvic Fractures

Pelvic fractures can be the most anxiety-provoking injury for the civilian general surgeon since exposure to these injuries in typical practice is quite limited. Preperitoneal pelvic packing coupled with external fixation has emerged as standard of care at trauma centers without ready access to angioembolization or for those patients who present in extremis [30].

To safely pack a pelvis, one requires firm structure to pack against, ideally an intact pelvis. If the injury is so unstable to not allow for firm packing, external fixation (ex-fix) may be required to achieve effective pelvic packing. If ex-fix is

required, it should be performed simultaneously with pelvic packing. While one team is placing the pelvic fixation pins, the second team is gaining access to the preperitoneal space through a Pfannensteil incision, removing the pelvic clot, and placing folded laparotomy pads as packs. The ex-fix crossbars should be tightened in place as soon as the last (sixth) preperitoneal pack is placed. If the pelvis is already wrapped in a sheet or binder, holes can be cut for the pins to be inserted with the temporary pelvic stabilization still place. This combined approach can be performed very rapidly, but relies on clear communication between the general surgeon and orthopedic surgeons.

Outside of austere environments, in modern trauma centers, angioembolization is potentially an option. This option is often negated in DCBI by the need to provide open vascular control for tourniquet removal. Ideally, resuscitation and other injuries can be addressed simultaneously hence vascular control is done in the operating room as opposed to the interventional suite.

15.7.1 Intra-abdominal Damage Control

Care for intra-abdominal injuries in DCBI patients follows the basic tenets of damage control surgery: stop hemorrhage, control contamination, and save definitive reconstruction for a second operation—definitive procedures should not be performed during the index operation.

Rectal injuries are common in DCBI given the mechanism of the blast. Historically, penetrating injuries to the rectum have been treated with diverting colostomy, washout of the affected area, and drainage. Since the early to mid 1900s, there have been multiple studies advocating both for and against diverting colostomies. Our algorithm was conservative given the high risk of infection these patients already have. An examination of the rectum was performed digitally followed by a rigid proctoscopy—findings of blood or other evidence of injury necessitated a diverting colostomy.

Bowel injury, in either small or large bowel, was cared for in a straightforward manner.

The segment or segments were resected and the patient was left in discontinuity. While this impacts the ability to deliver early enteral nutrition, it is outweighed by the leak risk encountered by performing bowel anastomosis in the setting of ongoing shock. Definitive repair with a stapled or hand-sewn anastomosis can be done at subsequent washout procedures.

Solid organ injuries were treated in a similar manner to typical civilian trauma. Liver injuries should be packed for hemostasis and if necessary a Pringle maneuver was performed to facilitate suturing of large hepatic arteries or hepatic veins.

Any splenic injury, regardless of ongoing hemorrhage, should be treated with splenectomy. The patient will have ongoing blood loss, and one does not want to worry about a delayed splenic rupture. Renal injuries are treated as in civilian trauma—based upon blunt or penetrating mechanisms of abdominal injury. Fragments or holes identified in Zone 2 of the retroperitoneum are considered penetrating injuries and should be explored. If the injury was from blunt trauma, a non-expanding hematoma need not be explored.

15.7.2 Genitourinary

As stated earlier, nearly 90 % of DBCI patients with lower extremity amputations have genitourinary injuries. The treatment algorithm is clear and relies upon a high index of suspicion (Fig. 15.10). Immediate care is wrapping an exposed testicle in a moist dressing [31]. However, exposed and ruptured testicles often have a large amount of contamination from debris.

Combat surgeons have observed that physical appearance of the scrotum was not a reliable predictor of testicular injury. Index of suspicion should be heightened in DCBI patients even in the presence of small scrotal lacerations as occult injuries could be present. Scrotal exploration should be considered in these patients [32].

When treating testicular rupture, preservation of seminiferous tubules is paramount; however, nonviable tubules should be debrided. The tunica albuginea should be closed with absorbable suture. The repaired testicle should be replaced into the scrotum in a tension-free manner, if possible. Stretch on the vas deferens can initiate contraction of the tubules

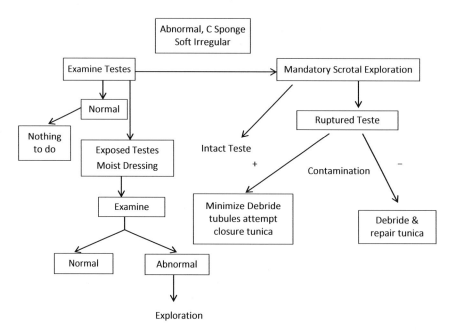

Fig. 15.10 Algorithm for testicular trauma

and loss of viable sperm. Finding a suitable tension-free location in which to replant the testicles is more difficult after a blast injury. In order to avoid stretching the vas deferens, placement of the testicle into the thigh is contraindicated. Early consultation with a fertility team is most important [31].

Bladder injuries occur and require immediate drainage. Drainage can be either transurethral or suprapubic depending on the ability to pass a Foley [31]. As in civilian trauma, intra-abdominal (and some extraperitoneal) bladder injuries require two-layer repairs with absorbable suture. If need to fully expose the injury, the bladder can be opened posteriorly, safely, in the midline.

Urethral injuries and penile shaft injuries do occur. If possible, a Foley should be passed into the bladder even with injuries. This requires an experienced surgeon or urologist, but placement will provide a long-term benefit to the patient rather than going straight to a suprapubic tube.

15.7.3   Amputations

Amputations are the defining injury in DCBI, with a significant percentage of patients losing three limbs (Table 15.4). Many amputations are incomplete upon arrival and surgeons need to make the decisions to complete the amputations. The decision can range from obvious, the mangled extremity hanging on with just a flap of skin, to the not so obvious. The UK Limb Trauma Working group examined the care of DCBI patients in Afghanistan [33]. The Working Group's recommendations for absolute indications for amputation are:

1. Avulsed extremity.
2. Unreconstructable boney damage.
3. Severe combined injury and warm ischemia time >6 h and soft tissue necrosis.
4. Potentially lethal reperfusion injury.

The applicability of scoring systems is useless in DBCIs. This is in part due to the insidious effects of blast to normal-appearing musculature. This blast-affected tissue has an increased risk of infection and therefore worse outcomes.

When an amputation appears to be indicated based either upon the absolute indications or clinical judgment of two surgeons, the UK Limb Working Group suggests the following:

1. Document the examination and indications for amputation.
2. Avoid reference to any limb salvage scores.
3. Photograph all wounds prior to amputation.
4. Do not base amputation on any neurological criteria—more than 50 % cases recover.
5. Radiographs should be obtained of the extremities unless the delay would negatively impact care [33].

With respect to other fractures, which do not require amputation, initial treatment should be external fixation as internal fixation is complicated by very high infection rates. Greater than 50 % patients with early internal fixation required subsequent implant removal secondary to infection [34].

Table 15.4 Injury patterns for patients with bilateral lower limb amputations

	N (%)
Lower limb (43)	
Bilateral trans-tibial	4 (9)
Trans-tibial/knee disarticulation	1 (2)
Trans-tibial and trans-femoral	9 (21)
Bilateral knee disarticulation	0
Knee disarticulation and trans-femoral	4 (9)
Bilateral trans-femoral	25 (58)
Concurrent upper limb loss (9) (triple amputation)	
Trans-radial	3 (33)
Elbow disarticulation	0
Trans-humeral	6 (66)

Reprinted from Injury, 45(7), Penn-Barwell JG, Bennett PM, Kay A, et al., Acute bilateral leg amputation following combat injury in UK servicemen, pp. 1105–10, Copyright 2014, with permission from Elsevier

15.8   Sepsis

After the initial hemorrhage is controlled, sepsis becomes the primary cause of long-term death. This can be countered to an extent, with the early use of antibiotics, which have been advocated for by the US and UK [31].

Aggressive initial debridement with frequent returns to the operating room for ongoing debridement is a critical element in DCBIs. Every effort to remove all debris and devitalized tissue should be made at the initial operation. This can take a few hours to accomplish. The only way this OR time is possible is to move all ICU resuscitative capacities to the operating room so the patient can continue an ongoing resuscitation while undergoing adequate debridement. Following debridement, all wounds should initially be left open to allow for drainage and demarcation. Negative pressure therapy works well in these wounds to control effluent, limit pain, and minimize bedside wound care.

The debridement does not end with the first operation, but it is a step-by-step process. The blasted tissue may initially appear viable. Then, at subsequent operations, the tissue may appear necrotic, necessitating further debridement. Reconstruction may be a major concern, but a mindset similar to debridement of necrotizing soft tissue infections is needed during the initial debridements. One must cut away all dead and devitalized tissue to save the patient's life. Tissue culture tissue may seem appropriate at the initial surgery but often identifies multiple organisms making differentiation between infection and colonization difficult [31]. One must then differentiate infectious agents vs. colonizers. As a general rule, we do not culture wounds unless there is concern for infection.

In OEF, invasive fungal infections were common in this patient population. This was likely due to multiple factors including severity of injury, soil contamination of tissue, and immunosuppression from transfusions [35].

15.9   Conclusion

Blast injuries are complex wounds. Success is rooted in a systematic but simple treatment algorithm. Providers need to first focus on hemorrhage control via proper tourniquet application. Control of hemorrhage in patients with very proximal amputations may require intraoperative vascular control. This type of control needs to be done as distally on the artery as possible. Once bleeding is

controlled, resuscitation should begin with blood and blood products. Further damage control surgery techniques are incorporated in the initial phase to prevent immediate death. Once the patient is stable, which is frequently during the first trip to the operating room, debridement and prevention of infection become the major focus. Long-term survival is dependent on the surgeons' abilities to remove all debris and devitalized tissue.

Seeing the wounds immediately after blast causes one to pause and ask how does anyone survive this? With a systematic approach, the chances of surviving skyrocket, one does not need to ask how they survive. Instead, we are left admiring our patients' strength and courage as they return to seemingly normal lives.

Editor's Note: CDR Joseph Galante, MD, FACS serves in the United States Navy Reserves. He was deployed to western Afghanistan in 2010. He is currently the Vice Chair of Education and the Chief of the Trauma and Acute Care Surgery Division of the University of California at Davis.

CDR Carlos J. Rodriguez, DO, MBA, FACS is currently serving on Active Duty in the United States Navy. He is Chief of the Trauma Surgery Division at Walter Reed National Military Medical Center. He has been deployed three times to Operations Iraqi and Enduring Freedom.

For the aforementioned patient, Drs. Rodriguez and Galante performed life-saving surgery. Despite his devastating injury and because of his ingenuity and the medical training he provided his unit, the patient is reported to be doing well and able to ambulate short distances with the use of crutches and prosthetics.

References

1. Gates JD, Arabian S, Biddinger P, et al. The initial response to the Boston marathon bombing: lessons learned to prepare for the next disaster. Ann Surg. 2014;260(6):960–6.
2. Emergency war surgery. 3rd ed. Weapons Effects and Parachute Injuries. Washington D.C.: Borden Institute, 2004; 1–14. Print.
3. Dismounted complex blast injury. DCBI Task Force Report. 2011.
4. Mamczak CN, Elster EA. Complex dismounted IED blast injures: the initial management of bilateral lower extremity amputations with and without pelvic and perineal involvement. J Surg Orthop Adv. 2012;21(1): 8–14.
5. http://www.ctvnews.ca/world/how-pressure-cooker-bombs-boost-the-deadliness-of-low-explosives-1.1241516. Accessed 8 Jan 15.

6. Elkin DC, Woodhall B. Combined vascular and nerve injuries of warfare. Ann Surg. 1944;119(3):411–31.

7. Paquette EL. Genitourinary trauma at a combat support hospital during operation Iraqi freedom: the impact of body armor. J Urol. 2007;177(6):2196–9.

8. Anderson RC, Fleming M, Forsberg JA, et al. Dismounted complex blast injury. J Surg Orthop Adv. 2012;21(1):1–7.

9. Ritenour AE, Wickley A, Ritenour JS, et al. Tympanic membrane perforation and hearing loss from blast overpressure in operation enduring freedom and operation Iraqi freedom wounded. J Trauma. 2008;64 Suppl 2:S174–8.

10. Remenschneider AK, Lookabaugh S, Aliphas A, et al. Otologic outcomes after blast injury: the Boston marathon experience. Otol Neurotol. 2014;35(10):1825–34.

11. Breeze J, Horsfall I, Hepper A, et al. Face, neck, and eye protection: adapting body armour to counter the changing pattern of injuries on the battlefield. Br J Oral Maxillofac Surg. 2011;49(8):602–6.

12. Yonekawa Y, Hacker HD, Lehman RE, et al. Ocular blast injuries in mass-casualty incidents: the marathon bombing in Boston, Massachusetts, and the fertilizer plant explosion in West Texas. Opthalmology. 2014;121(9):1670–6.

13. Mines M, Thach A, Mallonee S, et al. Ocular injuries sustained by survivors of the Oklahoma City Bombing. Opthalmology. 2000;107(5):837–43.

14. Tucker DI, Zachar MR, Chan RK, et al. Characterization and management of mandibular fractures: lessons learned from Iraq and Afghanistan. Atlas Oral Maxillofac Surg Clin North Am. 2013;21(1):61–8.

15. Kragh Jr JF, Walters TJ, Westmoreland T, et al. Tragedy into drama: an American history of tourniquet use in the current war. J Spec Oper Med. 2013;13(3):5–25.

16. Stewart SK, Duchesne JC, Kahn KA. Improvised tourniquets: obsolete or obligatory? J Trauma Acute Care Surg. 2015;78(1):178–83.

17. Eastridge BJ, Mabry RL, Seguin P, et al. Death on the battlefield (2001-2011): implications for the future of combat casualty care. J Trauma Acute Care Surg. 2012;74(6 Suppl 5):S431–7.

18. Duron V, Burke RV, Bliss D, et al. Survival of pediatric blunt trauma patients presenting with no signs of life in the field. J Trauma Acute Care Surg. 2014;77(3):422–6.

19. Battistella FD, Nugent W, Owings JT, et al. Field triage of pulseless trauma patient. Arch Surg. 1999;134(7):742–5.

20. Malsby 3rd RF, Quesada J, Powell-Dunford N, et al. Prehospital blood product transfusion by US Army MEDEVAC during combat operations in Afghanistan: a process improvement initiative. Mil Med. 2013;178(7):785–91.

21. O'Reilly DJ, Morrison JJ, Jansen JO, et al. Initial UK experience of prehospital blood transfusion in combat casualties. J Trauma Acute Care Surg. 2014;77(3 Suppl 2):S66–70.

22. Joint theater trauma system clinical practice guideline. http://www.usaisr.amedd.army.mil/assets/cpgs/High_Bilateral_Amputations_7_Mar_12.pdf. Accessed 12 Jan 2015.

23. Duchesne JC, Heaney J, Guidry C, et al. Diluting the benefits of hemostatic resuscitation: a multi-institutional analysis. J Trauma Acute Care Surg. 2013;75(1):76–82.

24. Crash-2 Trail Collaborators, Shakur H, Roberts I, et al. Effects of tranexamic acid on death, vascular occlusive events and blood transfusion in trauma patients with significant hemorrhage (CRASH-2): a randomized, placebo-controlled trial. Lancet. 2010;376(9734):23–32.

25. Morrison JJ, Dubose JJ, Rasmussen TE, et al. Military application of tranexamic acid in trauma emergency resuscitation (MATTERs) study. Arch Surg. 2012;147(2):113–9.

26. Eckert MJ, Wertin TM, Tyner SD, et al. Tranexamic acid administration to pediatric trauma patients in a combat setting: the pediatric trauma and tranexamic acid study(PED_TRAX). J Trauma Acute Care Surg. 2014;77(6):852–8.

27. Leidel BA, Kirchhoff C, Bogner V, et al. Comparison of intraossous versus central venous vascular access in adults under resuscitation in the emergency department with inaccessible peripheral veins. Resuscitation. 2012;83(1):40–5.

28. Brenner ML, Moore LJ, DuBose JJ, et al. A clinical series of resuscitative endovascular balloon occlusion of the aorta for hemorrhage control and resuscitation. J Trauma Acute Care Surg. 2013;75(3):506–11.

29. Holcomb JB, Fox EE, Scalea TM. Current opinion on catheter-based hemorrhage control in trauma patients. J Trauma Acute Care Surg. 2014;76(3):888–93.

30. Tosounidis TI, Giannoudis PV. Pelvic fractures presenting with haemodynamic instability: Treatment options and outcomes. Surgeon. 2013;11(6):344–51.

31. Mossadegh S, Midwinter M, Tai N, et al. Improvised explosive device-related pelviperneal trauma; UK military experience, literature review and lessons for civilian trauma teams. Ann R Coll Surg Engl. 2013;95:S24-31.

32. Hudak JS, Hakim S. Operative management of wartime genitourinary injuries at Balad Air Force Theater Hospital, 2005 to 2008. J Urol. 2009;182(1):180–3.

33. Brown KV, Guthrie HC, Ramasamy A, et al. Modern military surgery: lessons from Iraq and Afghanistan. J Bone Joint Surg Br. 2012;94(4):536–43.

34. Ramasamy A, Evans S, Kendrew JM, et al. The open blast pelvis. J Bone Joint Surg Br. 2012;94(6):829–35.

35. Rodriguez CJ, Weintrob AC, Shah J, et al. Risk factors associated with invasive fungal infections in combat trauma. Surg Infect. 2014;15(5):521–6.

Surgery Under Fire

16

George E. Black IV and Scott R. Steele

16.1 The Event

In the early morning hours on an otherwise routine day in the summer of 2008 and after weeks of an eerie quietness in the Southeastern Iraqi desert, our small medical team was awoken by shaking ground and deafening explosions. Our forward surgical team had been attached to a larger unit to provide medical support for their mission to secure the Iran-Iraq border and prevent the further influx of weapons. We were located on a small forward operating base (FOB), but had the surgical equipment necessary to handle any expected injury patterns and about 30 patients. We also had two medical evacuation (medevac) helicopters at our disposal.

As the first of several missiles landed in close proximity of our 4-tent hospital, what was likely only minutes felt like days. The initial priorities

G.E. Black IV, M.D. (✉)
Department of Surgery, Madigan Army Medical Center, 9040a Fitzsimmons Dr., Fort Lewis, WA 98431, USA
e-mail: george.e.black20.mil@mail.mil

S.R. Steele, M.D., F.A.C.S., F.A.S.C.R.S.
Department of Surgery, Division of Colorectal Surgery, University Hospitals Case Medical Center, Case Western Reserve University, 11100 Euclid Avenue Cleveland, OH 44106, USA
e-mail: scott.steele@UHhospitals.org; harkersteele@mac.com

of donning our protective gear, accounting for each member of the team, and preparing for incoming casualties—all under the "fog of war"—was the easy part, as we had prepared for that *ad nauseum*. With only two surgeons, a CRNA and an anesthesiologist as the "providers" on the team, performing triage while simultaneously providing care took on a whole new meaning. Interspersed with executing ATLS protocols and readying the operating room, thoughts of "these are our guys," "what can we handle here?" and "when is the next round of fire coming?" entered my mind. Anger, anxiety, and fear had to be quickly replaced with calmness, composure, and focused attention. The team was looking for a leader, and more importantly, the patients were looking for our help (Fig. 16.1).

I was the lead on the first major injury through the door, a shrapnel wound through the right chest combined with hypotension. As I instructed the anesthesia provider to intubate the patient and to start transfusing blood, I prepared to place a tube thoracostomy. The young man, going in and out of consciousness, gripped my left wrist, looked into my eyes, and whispered, *"Please, Doc.....I got kids...."* Chills went down my back in the 100+ degree heat; and I somehow managed to respond, "No worries, I got you." With only the aid of a small portable radiographic machine and a hand-held ultrasound, I placed the chest tube, continued resuscitation and began a secondary survey, identifying only concomitant

© Springer International Publishing Switzerland 2016
C.R.B. Lim (ed.), *Surgery During Natural Disasters, Combat, Terrorist Attacks, and Crisis Situations*, DOI 10.1007/978-3-319-23718-3_16

Fig. 16.1 Typical triage area for a forward surgical team

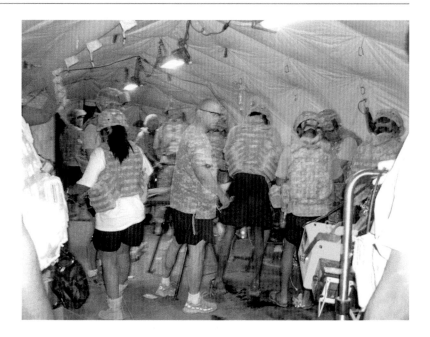

orthopedic injuries. With stabilization, he would be ready for a flight to larger US facility for continued and more definitive care.

Shortly thereafter, I was called by my fellow surgeon to help with another soldier who had been struck and was hemorrhaging severely from his right lower extremity, despite the presence of tourniquets. Blood was pouring through the gurney onto the floor of our tent and I saw several "Swiss cheese-like" wounds in both legs, his right upper thigh, and groin. He was intubated and was undergoing our massive resuscitation protocol, utilizing the limited blood products that were intrinsic to our team. We brought him urgently to the operating room, completed a guillotine amputation and began to explore the right leg. The principles of attaining adequate exposure, gaining proximal control in the groin, and stopping the hemorrhage echoed over and over in my head. Ultimately we were able to identify several injuries, and had to make a decision between ligation/shunting, or repair, opting for the former in many situations, and understanding this was no place for the latter. Time was of the essence, not only for this patient, but also because additional casualties awaited, resources were scarce, and the threat of further imminent attacks loomed.

We treated several other patients that day, some more injured than others. I was thankful for the skilled care of each member of our team, as well as for the unit's partial "Charlie-med" holding company. All provided valuable expertise and resources to help with the care of those not requiring emergent interventions as well as those less injured—if there ever is such a thing in war. Looking back, I had heard that caring for battlefield injuries is different, no matter how minor—physiologically and psychologically—for the patient and the provider alike.

16.2 Introduction

The narrative above outlined a real situation encountered while deployed in a combat zone. To account for all that happened that day in a few paragraphs and capture what truly took place is nearly impossible. Sights, sounds and even smells are only a simple "closing of the eyes" away from reliving the event in full detail. While an episode such as this one would be extremely uncommon in the USA today, it is not too far-fetched to imagine similar situations, especially in light of the events of the Boston Marathon and Oklahoma City bombings, the Sandy Hook Elementary school shootings, and other domestic terrorist activities. In these situations there are many other factors influencing the care that is rendered to an injured person. The ideas and tenets of damage control resuscitation (DCR) and damage control surgery (DCS) play a large role in determining the best approach and treating someone when faced with a situation where time, resources, and personnel are at a premium and your life and the lives of those helping you are also at stake. While many injuries were cared for over the course of four deployments, these concepts and their practical application in the treatment of peripheral vascular injuries will be the focus of this chapter.

Injury patterns witnessed during these events are different, especially when high-energy explosive weapons are used to cause damage and incite terror. In the combat environment, explosive injuries predominate, with the majority of injuries occurring in the exposed extremities [1]. Body armor and helmets, in large part, help protect against truncal and head injuries. On the other hand, the extremities have little protective gear at the present time, especially when confronted with this type of mechanism. This injury distribution differs both from prior military conflicts as well as from the typical injury patterns seen in the typical civilian trauma [2]. The differences witnessed in the current battlefield environment are thought to be mostly due to enhancements and advances in body and vehicle armor. But these improvements don't prevent all injuries. Overall, over 50 % of battlefield injuries are of the extremities and peripheral vascular injuries occur at a rate of between 9 and 15 % [3]. Being familiar with the tools and techniques to potentially save an injured person's life and limb are important for any surgeon who may be faced with treating these injuries.

In addition to taking care of an injured person with wounds not often encountered in one's daily practice, multiple other challenges exist in the austere and possibly dangerous environment. These include the need for a safe and secure area to assess and treat the injured person, and a potential lack of necessary supplies and equipment [4]. In the scenario presented, a secure area was not an option, as tents provide no overhead cover, and bunkers or other protective structures were unavailable. Supplies were also a constant concern, both for the patients at hand and the ever-present possibility of additional casualties, especially in a remote environment with limited re-stocking ability. Combine these trepidations with the stress of the overall situation, and one can imagine how this may potentially influence a surgeon's ability to function at his or her optimal level. As such, we will also discuss the impact that operating under extreme pressure can have and offer some tips on ways to prepare for and mitigate that stress.

16.3 Damage Control Surgery

Over the last decade plus, advances in military medicine in combat and austere environments have led to the increased usage of tourniquets, (Fig. 16.2) [5], hemostatic dressings [6, 7] and changes in fluid resuscitation strategy [8, 9]. These changes have led to improvements in the care of multiply-injured trauma patients and tie into the concept of damage control surgery [10]. Damage control surgery (DCS) is utilized in order to try and prevent the development or halt the downward spiraling of the "lethal triad" of hypothermia, coagulopathy, and acidosis in the severely injured trauma patient. DCS is undertaken in three phases. These phases are (1) initial surgery to stop hemorrhage and control contamination, (2) resuscitation and correction of coagulopathy and other physiologic abnormalities, and (3) a return to the operating room after the patient is physiologically better able to tolerate definitive procedures to repair the injuries sustained [11, 12].

The concept of damage control has its origins in the Navy's response to a damaged ship [13] and has its surgical roots in the management of severe liver injuries [14]. These concepts can be used in the treatment of injuries sustained in any area of the body to include peripheral vascular injury. Utilization of DCS techniques for peripheral vascular injury in the combat setting has returned good outcomes with high rates of limb salvage and low rates of amputation in some studies [15].

The decision to utilize the damage control route is usually based on the extent of injury the

Fig. 16.2 Bilateral
lower extremity injuries
with tourniquets in
place. Courtesy of James
Sebesta, MD

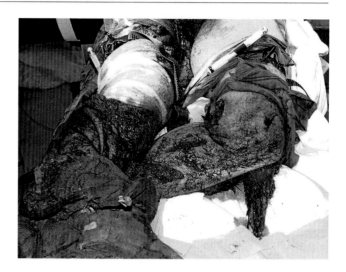

patient has suffered as well as their physiology at the time of presentation. In an austere environment, the equipment that measures many of the parameters commonly used in most intensive care units to determine the current physiologic state of a patient is not available. Depending on location, blood pressure monitoring devices, pulse oximetry, or laboratory services to include blood gas analysis may not be available for use in extreme situations. It is under these circumstances that reliance on observation and physical examination skills become of the utmost importance. When caring for injured patients in these environments, only basic first aid supplies may be available. If not located close to a unit with surgical capabilities, only basic surgical instruments (or none) may be available. Understanding the pre-hospital interventions that will stop bleeding, help ward of hypothermia, and in turn stave off worsening coagulopathy is also extremely important. More detailed information on these topics, especially as they relate to care for the injured patient in combat, can be found in the Combat Casualty Care manual, available through the Borden Institute (http://www.cs. amedd.army.mil/borden/) [16]. Some of these topics will also be discussed in more detail below.

16.4 Peripheral Vascular Injury

16.4.1 Epidemiology of Battlefield Peripheral Vascular Injury

Extremity injuries are common the modern battlefield. In recent series looking at the distribution of combat wounds in the wars in Iraq and Afghanistan, the rate of extremity injury is over 50 %. Most of these injuries occur secondary to explosive mechanisms; however, around 20 % of extremity injuries are due to gunshot wounds [17]. Battlefield vascular trauma occurs at a rate of around 12 % [3]. In addition to tension pneumothorax and airway compromise, uncontrolled bleeding from peripheral vascular trauma remains a top cause of preventable battlefield or pre-hospital death [18]. The causes of trauma in the civilian sector have rather different mechanisms of injury, with blunt trauma such as motor vehicle crashes and injury from falls predominating [2, 19]. Recent events such as the Boston Marathon Bombing, however, have reminded us of the fact that battlefield-like injuries can occur even in the domestic Western world and having the tools to properly treat and manage these injuries is vitally important [20].

16.4.2 Pre-hospital Intervention

Practices to decrease the number of preventable deaths during our most recent and current conflicts have often focused on the pre-hospital setting. Within that realm there are usually three groups of injured individuals: those who sustain instantly or near instantly fatal injuries, those who sustain nonfatal injuries, and those who sustain injuries which could be fatal if not treated within a short period of time. Peripheral vascular injuries most often fall under the last category, especially if the injury is isolated to the extremities without concomitant wounds.

One of the most successful changes in pre-hospital or pre-surgical intervention in the wars in Iraq and Afghanistan has been the early and frequent use of a properly applied tourniquet for controlling extremity bleeding. This intervention alone has led to an 85 % decrease in mortality from peripheral-extremity hemorrhage in combat over the course of the last decade [18]. Of note, tourniquets (including hastily assembled improvised versions) were also used successfully in injured patients in the Boston Marathon Bombings [20]. This intervention, coupled with swift evacuation to a facility with the capacity for definitive treatment, as well as early implementation of damage control principles has played as big of a role as any in improving outcomes in this patient population.

Another important adjunct in the pre-hospital setting is the hemostatic dressing. These dressings have been used in the current combat environment to help control hemorrhage especially in the case of junctional hemorrhage not amenable to tourniquet use. Becoming familiar with the different types and application of these products is also useful in the pre-hospital care of bleeding trauma patients [6].

The two most commonly utilized, commercially available agents are QuikClot® (Z-medica, Wallinford, CT) and HemCon® (HemCon Medical Technologies, Portland, OR). QuikClot® is available in a granular form made from zeolite and as various gauze forms which are impregnated with kaolin. The zeolite forms are from earlier generations of the product and work by

absorbing water from the site of injury. The main problem with this form of QuikClot® is the exothermic reaction that occurs upon its application that raises the risk of thermal injury to the tissues on which it is applied. For the most part, this form of QuikClot® is no longer in use. There are various surgical dressing forms of QuikClot® that are impregnated with kaolin. Kaolin is an inert mineral which acts by inducing the coagulation cascade. These dressing forms do not lead to the same exothermic reaction as the zeolite form and have the added benefit of being easily removed from a wound when no longer needed [21]. Multiple animal studies have demonstrated the effectiveness of QuikClot®, mainly the Combat Gauze form, in decreasing bleeding from artery and vein injuries and improving survival. There is a relative paucity of human data to support the use of QuikClot Combat Gauze® (Fig. 16.3). One Israeli case series of 14 patients showed a success rate at controlling hemorrhage of 79 % with a 93 % survival rate and advocated for its use in the pre-hospital trauma setting [22].

HemCon® is a chitosan-based product produced by deacetylation of the structural element chitin found in crustacean exoskeletons. It is also available predominately as a dressing [21]. The data for the use of HemCon® is similar to that of QuikClot® in that there are no randomized controlled human trials that show the effectiveness of either. Most of the data is in the form of animal trials and case series from various trauma centers

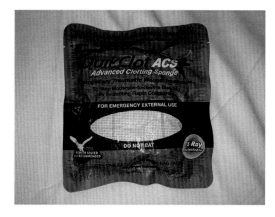

Fig. 16.3 QuikClot Advanced Clotting Sponge®, one of the various QuikClot® products

and the recent conflicts in the Middle East. HemCon® has similarly been shown to be effective at decreasing or controlling bleeding in a wide variety of situations [6].

16.4.3   Initial Assessment

It is important to remember that with any trauma patient the mechanism of injury and the possibility of multiple injuries in one patient is very real. Each patient should be evaluated and treated using standard trauma algorithms. The ability to rule out and treat airway and breathing compromise, control bleeding, and help keep the patient from becoming hypothermic secondary to environmental exposure are also as critical today as ever before. Especially with blast injuries, do not be blinded by the mangled extremity or external bleeding initially encountered and forget to search for other life-threatening injuries. Be cognizant of potential concomitant bony injuries, and splint fractures as needed to stabilize the bone, and help decrease the risk of worsening whatever vascular injury is already present.

16.4.4   Damage Control Principles for Peripheral Vascular Injury

Remember that when dealing with extremity injuries, once you have control of the major external bleeding you have given the patient and yourself more time. If a tourniquet was placed to control bleeding it should be monitored for effectiveness, especially once any resuscitation has begun [23]. There are times when a tourniquet will control bleeding in a hypotensive patient, but will need to be tightened once their blood pressure has been restored from fluid or blood product administration.

The main tenets of damage control for peripheral vascular injuries are control of hemorrhage, reperfusion of a threatened limb, and prevention of compartment syndrome [23]. One of the major decisions that must be made in peripheral vascular injury is the decision to place a vascular shunt, ligate the vessel or to attempt a definitive repair.

If the patient is hypotensive, cold, and coagulopathic, this is not the time to try and harvest vein or sew in a synthetic graft. Placing a temporary vascular shunt will assist with reperfusion of the patient's limb and will help buy more time to transport the patient to an ICU for resuscitation or to a definitive care facility [24].

16.4.5   Diagnosis of Peripheral Vascular Injury

As with the diagnosis of any trauma, the mechanism of injury will give great insight for predicting the injury sustained. Try to find out as many details as possible about how the patient was injured. Was the mechanism blunt or penetrating? What caused the penetrating injury? How far was the patient from the blast? These are examples of some of the questions that should be asked. After finding out as much as you can about how the patient was injured, perform your physical examination. Always keep in mind that most trauma patients, unless they have a single penetrating injury, will likely have multiple injuries, and more than one could be life threatening. Stick with your ATLS principles for your initial assessment and management, then move on to a more specific examination of the peripheral injury once other life threatening injuries have been ruled out or managed.

Table 16.1 Hard and soft signs of vascular injury [24]

Hard signs	Soft signs
Nearly 100 % predictive of significant vascular injury [41]	Significant vascular injury in up to 27 % [41]
– Active hemorrhage – Expanding hematoma – Palpable thrill – Continuous murmur – Signs of ischemia (pain, pallor, pulselessness, paralysis, poikilothermia)	– Proximity of wound to a major vascular structure – Stable hematoma – Ipsilateral neurologic defect – Unequal pulses – Shock – Report of pre-hospital hemorrhage

Palpation of pulses is very important in peripheral vascular injury, though depending on the overall clinical condition of the patient, they may or may not be present. In addition, a pulse may still be present, even in the setting of a vascular injury. When dealing with lower extremity trauma, the femoral, popliteal, and pedal pulses should be characterized. Remember the hard and soft signs of vascular injury. The hard signs include pulsatile or active bleeding, an expanding hematoma, palpable thrill or audible bruit and evidence of distal ischemia. A patient with any of these signs will almost always require an intervention to manage their injury. Soft signs that suggest a vascular injury, but may not need immediate intervention and include a history of hemorrhage prior to your evaluation, proximity of an injury to a major vascular structure, unequal pulses in the injured vs. non-injured side, a non-expanding hematoma, or an ipsilateral neurologic deficit (Table 16.1) [25].

The ankle-brachial index (ABI) can also be useful when it is unclear if a vascular injury has been sustained. This is measured by using a manual blood pressure cuff at the ankle and a 9-MHz continuous wave Doppler probe over both the dorsalis pedis and posterior tibial pulses to determine the pressure at which those pulses disappear. This pressure is then divided by the patient's highest brachial artery pressure. An ABI of less than 0.9 in a patient with no evidence of peripheral vascular disease is an indication for more definitive testing, usually in the form of angiography or duplex ultrasonography [23]. As is the theme of this chapter, the definitive tests will often not be available in the austere setting and will require transfer in order to obtain them. However, an ABI is easily calculated and provides valuable information. Additionally, contrast dye, a 30 or 60 cc syringe, butterfly needle and plain film radiology capabilities are all that is required to perform an on-table angiogram. While not "optimal," they are available in most settings and becoming facile with the technique will reap rewards.

16.4.6 Vascular Exposure

Once a vascular injury that requires operative intervention has been identified, the patient must be prepped accordingly. In the case of lower extremity trauma, the patient's abdomen should be prepped as there will be times when an abdominal or pre-peritoneal approach will be necessary to gain proximal control of the bleeding. This is especially the case in high femoral injuries. Both legs should also be circumferentially prepped, as vein from the opposite leg may be needed to perform a reconstruction if the patient can tolerate it.

With lower extremity injuries control of the proximal common femoral artery is necessary. As a general rule, performing a longitudinal incision over the common femoral artery will give the best exposure for control (Fig. 16.4) [23]. Identifying the inguinal ligament will help in guiding dissection into the femoral canal so ensure the incision extends far enough superiorly. When the injury is higher the inguinal ligament may need to be divided in a lazy-S fashion or control of the distal external iliac vessel may be

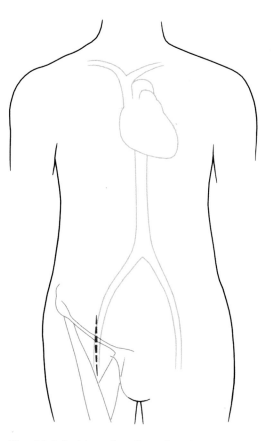

Fig. 16.4 Incision for femoral artery exposure. Illustration by Thomas R. Pierce

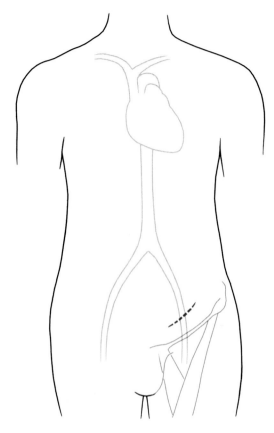

Fig. 16.5 Lower abdominal incision for pre-peritoneal exposure of the external iliac artery. Illustration by Thomas R. Pierce

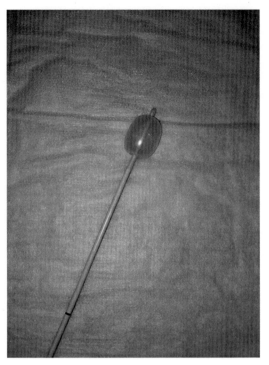

Fig. 16.6 Example of a Fogarty balloon catheter

necessary through a lower abdominal incision, with dissection through the pre-peritoneal space (Fig. 16.5) [26]. Control of the vessels can then be maintained with manual pressure, silastic vessel loops, or atraumatic clamps, if these tools are available.

16.4.7 Shunt vs. Graft

Once control of bleeding and exposure has been obtained and the injured vessel or vessels identified, then debridement of the injured vessel should be performed to healthy and viable appearing tissue. All contamination should be removed from the wound. In an austere environment or after a blast injuries, the wounds should be considered at an extremely high risk for infection effectively ruling out the possibility of using

synthetic graft. After this it is prudent to check both back bleeding and bleeding from the proximal vessel. If no flow is noted from either of these, then thrombectomy using a Fogarty catheter should be carefully performed (Fig. 16.6). If available, heparinized saline at a ratio of 10 units/mL of normal saline should be flushed proximally and distally to the injury prior to shunting or repair.

If there are combined venous and arterial injuries, the arterial injury should be completed first. If time and patient physiology permits, the venous injury can be repaired at this time as well; however, this is not as critical as restoring arterial flow [23]. Edema is the main potential complication of vein ligation and this is more common when the popliteal vein is ligated vs. the femoral vein. Despite rather high rates of edema regardless of if the choice to repair or ligate the vein is made, most patients will eventually have resolution of their edema [27]. The other dreaded complication of vein ligation is thromboembolism. This complication is more common following ligation vs. repair; however the risk of developing

Fig. 16.7 Exposed femoral artery with temporary shunt in place. Courtesy of Eric K. Johnson, MD

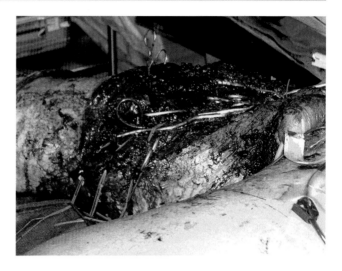

a pulmonary embolism is no different between the two techniques [28]. In most cases, the vein can simply be ligated, and the extremity wrapped to provide compression and decrease edema. Care should be taken to avoid too much compression that may result in cutting off arterial flow.

The decision to place a shunt or to perform a more formal repair will depend on many factors. If the patient will not tolerate a longer procedure due to their physiology, placement of a temporary shunt while the patient is resuscitated and transported may be prudent (Fig. 16.7). Individual skill and ability to perform a technically proficient vascular repair will also play a role. Placement of a shunt may be the safest option if you are not comfortable with the necessary techniques to harvest vein and perform a repair of the vessel. Shunts have been used successfully during the recent conflicts in the Middle East and have become a viable option for returning blood flow to an ischemic limb prior to definitive repair [24, 29]. In one series 57 % of patients treated at a forward surgical facility were managed with a temporary shunt with a patency rate after transfer of 86 % for proximal shunts. The patency rate for more distal shunts was much lower at 12 %; however, the placement of a distal shunt allowed for more time to transfer the patients to higher levels of care for definitive repair. Overall the early viability of limbs which underwent temporary shunting was 92 % in this series [24]. It is impor-

tant that when the shunt is placed, it is adequately secured at both ends, and the extremity is protected from excess movement, which may require splinting, or physical contact that could result in dislodgment of the device.

16.4.8 Fasciotomy

The old adage of "the main indication for fasciotomy is thinking about performing a fasciotomy" holds true today, especially in peripheral vascular injuries in the austere or combat environments. The risk for reperfusion injury and development of compartment syndrome is high in patients who have sustained peripheral vascular injury in a remote setting. The tools to measure compartment pressures may not be available, the time for evacuation may be long, and the extent of injury may be such that without fasciotomy the patient will develop compartment syndrome. Indications for fasciotomy in a combat or austere setting can be found in Table 16.2 [23]. Fasciotomy was shown in a recent review of the National Trauma Data Bank to be associated with improved outcomes. In this series patients were divided into early (i.e., performed within 8 h of vascular repair) and late (i.e., performed greater than 8 h after vascular repair) groups. The authors found that patients in the early fasciotomy group had a statistically significant lower amputation rate of 8.5 % vs. 24.6 %,

Table 16.2 Indications for fasciotomy in the austere environment [22]

- Greater than 4–6-h delay to revascularization
- Combined arterial and venous injuries
- Severe crush injuries or high-energy mechanism of injury
- Vascular repair
- Arterial or venous ligation
- Altered mental status or decreased sensation to the extremity (epidural anesthesia, spine injury, etc.)
- Concern for compartment syndrome

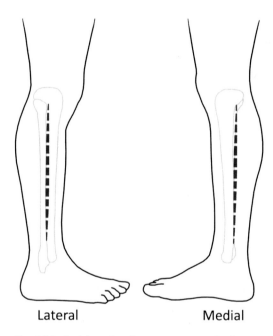

Lateral   Medial

Fig. 16.8 Incisions for four-compartment fasciotomy. Illustration by Thomas R. Pierce

lower infection rate, 6.6 % vs. 14.5 %, and shorter total hospital stay, 18.5 days vs. 24.2 days [30].

The technique for performing fasciotomy of the lower extremity includes both medial and lateral incisions to open the four compartments of the lower leg (Fig. 16.8). The lateral incision is placed lateral to the tibia along the predicted course of the intramuscular septum between the anterior and lateral compartments. Once the intramuscular septum is identified, two separate parallel incisions on either side of the septum are made in the fascia and extended approximately 15 cm to allow these compartments to decompress. Be careful with the proximal extent of these incisions

as the common superficial and deep peroneal nerves run near the fibular head and are at risk of injury in this region. The medial incision is placed 1 or 2 cm posterior to the tibia to decompress the superficial and deep posterior compartments. Beware of the saphenous vein and nerve in the subcutaneous tissue. Open the gastrocnemius fascia to decompress the superficial compartment and take the soleus down off the tibia to expose the fascia of the deep compartment. Open this fascia as well but be careful as the posterior tibial artery runs through this compartment [27]. Finally, ensure that the lateral and deep posterior compartments are opened adequately to avoid inadvertently missing a compartment and leading to loss of the limb despite performing the procedure.

16.4.9 Amputation

One big question that remains when discussing lower extremity vascular injury is whether or not to amputate a limb. Amputations in the combat environment are often of the traumatic type and a surgeon will be called upon to perform a completion amputation. Other indications for amputation following trauma include an unrepairable vascular injury, a life-threatening infection of the limb, or a patient at the extremes of physiology who has severe soft-tissue or bony injuries to the limb that would not likely lead to a functional recovery. The considerations above must be weighed against the patient's other injuries and current physiologic reserve when deciding either to perform an amputation or proceed with a temporary or definitive revascularization procedure.

Table 16.3 Principles to consider with lower extremity amputation [31, 42]

- All devitalized muscle, skin, and bone should be removed as early as possible
- The greatest residual length without osseous prominences should be retained
- Function of the proximal joint should be present—this helps with future prosthetic functionality
- The greatest amount of viable and durable soft tissue should be retained in order to cushion areas of shear and high pressure

Additionally the surgeon must also be cognizant of his or her resources. If blood transfusion products are low or there are many more patients that need surgical care, an amputation may be more practical for the surgical team and the injured patients. As always, the main goals of caring for a traumatically-injured patient in an austere environment is to save their life, get the patient prepared for evacuation to a higher level of care and not burn any bridges for the surgeon(s) who will assume their care at that higher level [31].

Once the decision has been made to perform an amputation, the next question that must be answered is how to actually perform the amputation. In the combat or austere setting there are some guiding principles that can be utilized to help promote better long-term outcomes. The overarching principle is to preserve as much bony length and soft tissue as possible, while at the same time, debriding all nonviable tissue. These principles are outlined in Table 16.3 [32]. When performing the amputation it is also necessary to ligate all major arteries and veins in order to prevent hemorrhage during transport. Nerves should also be identified and transected; however this should be performed at a point where there is sufficient muscular coverage to help mitigate patient pain. Finally, during transport ensure that a tourniquet is readily available (but not on) in case the patient begins to hemorrhage from their amputation site [31].

16.5 Operating Under Fire

Understanding all that goes into the care of traumatically injured patients in austere and dangerous environments has been highly impacted by the conflicts in Iraq and Afghanistan. The military has made great strides in this arena and has compiled the lessons learned from these conflicts into multiple texts such as the Combat Casualty Care manual [16] and Emergency War Surgery [31]. Training in these concepts has also become more standardized and emphasizes the interventions that will help a patient in a combat zone reach a level of care where their injuries can be appropriately treated [33]. Caring for patients in austere and potentially dangerous environments brings about another set of stressors and considerations as well. For health-care providers, and specifically surgeons, these stressors may also affect your performance and long-term mental health.

16.5.1 Caring for Patients in Dangerous Environments

It may seem overly obvious to say that practicing in a remote combat environment is different than caring for patients at an established hospital with a modern support structure—but it is still worth noting. At times, the downtime in either situation can lull one into complacency. Yet, one must always be aware of and use all the resources available, which frankly may not be much. Another facet that must be considered is the safety of the situation in which you find yourself caring for these patients. As our vignette at the beginning of the chapter relates, the environment may not be safe. It is not a stretch to imagine that the terrorists in the Boston Marathon bombing may have placed bombs at hospital Emergency Rooms to reduce the ability of providers to care for the injured. If this is the case one may be forced to provide only absolutely life-saving care initially in order to move the patient to an area that is safer. If those situations the most important medical tenants remain the same: stop any ongoing blood loss and making sure that the patient has an adequate airway and breathing capacity. If the supplies are available one may need to intubate a patient to include performing a surgical airway or decompress a tension pneumothorax quickly in order to get them to safety. During an event where both the provider's life and the patient's life are in danger, the concept of situational awareness becomes very important. This concept is not foreign to surgeons. We use it often in the operating room when we listen to the sounds of the anesthesia machine coming from the head of the table. It is evident when we are planning our next move of a surgery and the circulating nurse or operating room technicians are preparing the needed instruments or supplies.

When in a dangerous environment, situational awareness is even more important. Focusing solely on the patient's problems can very easily put one's own life at risk. One also has to seek safety for the patient, themselves, and whatever team they have available to them at the time. Although one still may not have many options, becoming an unnecessary casualty helps no one. Here one should strive to communicate with the people in charge of security. In the civilian environment, this may be the police or fire department.

16.5.2   Stress and Its Effect on Surgical Performance

The impact of stress on surgical performance is difficult to study as the literature on this topic is somewhat variable and difficult to interpret. While seemingly intuitive that performance under extreme duress may result in degradation in performance, measuring the impact and degree to which this happens is more difficult. A systematic review from 2010 concluded that proving a link between operative stress and performance is difficult at best. The authors did conclude that surgeons who were able to cope with stress effectively were technically more skilled than those who were unable to effectively cope with the stress encountered in the operating room [34]. An additional study taught a group of medical students a surgical skill (placing a chest tube), and then tested their ability to perform that skill under the stress of a simulated combat environment in both day and night time conditions. The authors found that while the skill was retained in the simulated combat or low-light settings, the procedures took longer and the quality of the tube placement was lower in the more stressful environment [35]. Another study assessed the ability of novice surgeons to perform laparoscopic tasks under different mentally stressful conditions. They showed that performance of the tasks was worse when the subjects were mentally stressed [36]. Other studies have attempted to assess the coping mechanisms of surgeons with different levels of experience and have found that more

experienced surgeons have developed coping mechanisms for stress throughout their careers. These coping mechanisms included reassessment of the situation or taking a step back to think, practicing or mentally rehearsing a surgery or situation ahead of time, and ensuring adequate communication with the surgical team. Unfortunately, for many surgeons these coping strategies are not often talked about or formally taught during surgical training and the impetus to acquire these skills falls upon the individual surgeon [37]. These studies suggest that while stress can affect one's surgical skill or ability to think clearly in very stressful situations, appropriate coping mechanisms and training both in stress management and simulation can help mitigate that stress.

Undoubtedly, combat and dangerous environments are stressful. Yet, treating a traumatically injured patient in any environment can be stressful, even when one has all the necessary resources available to care for that patient. These stressors are simply often multiplied several fold when in an austere or dangerous environment. Recognizing the triggers that increase individual stress levels and planning coping strategies ahead of time could make a difference in both surgeon's life and the patient's life he or she is trying to save.

16.5.3   Mental Effects of Caring for Trauma Patients in Dangerous Environments

A correlation has been shown between combat experience and new onset post-traumatic stress disorder (PTSD) and depression [38]. While it might be presumed that treating a large number of trauma patients could lead to PTSD, this correlation has not been validated. One interesting study from 2013 attempted to correlate PTSD symptoms with treatment of trauma patients. The authors did not find a direct correlation between the time treating trauma patients and PTSD, but did find that surgeons with lower resiliency were at a higher risk of developing PTSD than surgeons who were more resilient to stress. They concluded that learning coping skills and seeking psychological treatment, if necessary, were important in combating the stress of treating these patients [39].

Therefore, when dealing with the aftermath of a traumatic experience, whether one's own life was in danger or one was caring for those who underwent a significant traumatic event, it is important to take stock of how that event affected oneself mentally. Developing coping mechanisms and training prior to traumatic events is important and can help with decreasing the impact those events have. It is also crucial that one seeks whatever help they need to recover from a traumatic experience [40]. For some that means taking time off to rest or spend time with family and loved ones. For others, they may need to talk about the event and how it affected them either with friends or a professional counselor. One must do whatever it is they need to do to keep themselves mentally and physically healthy and ready to tackle the next stressful or unexpected situation.

16.6   Conclusion

Caring for the injured patient in a combat environment involves so much more than simply performing the operation. As it relates to peripheral extremity injuries, the age-old principles of exposure, identification, and control are as crucial as ever. The difficulties inherent in operating in an austere or dangerous environment add complexity and higher levels of stress to what are already stressful situations. How one deals with stress both in these situations and after can make a huge difference in the patient's life as well as one's own. Taking stock of their own skillset and ability to handle stressful situations is worthwhile and finding opportunities to enhance one's skills and resiliency will go far in helping them operate at a high level, even when faced with dire and life-threatening events. While no one wants to ever have to take care of a seriously injured patient in the type of environment described at the beginning of this chapter, one may never know when one will have to perform surgery under fire.

Editor's note: LTC Scott R. Steele, MD, is a graduate of the USMilitary Academy at West Point, NY. He served on active duty in the US Army from 1998 to 2015. He has been deployed to combat zones four times-twice each in Afghanistan and Iraq, being awarded the Combat Medical Badge and Bronze Star.

CPT George E. Black, IV, MD, is General Surgery Resident currently on Active Duty in the US Army. Prior to starting his medical education, he was deployed to Iraq from 2003 to 2004 where he earned the Combat Action Badge.

References

1. Schoenfeld AJ, Dunn JC, Bader JO, Belmont Jr PJ. The nature and extent of war injuries sustained by combat specialty personnel killed and wounded in Afghanistan and Iraq, 2003-2011. J Trauma Acute Care Surg. 2013;75(2):287–91.
2. Schreiber MA, Zink K, Underwood S, Sullenberger L, Kelly M, Holcomb JB. A comparison between patients treated at a combat support hospital in Iraq and a Level I trauma center in the United States. J Trauma. 2008;64 Suppl 2:S118–21. discussion S21–2.
3. White JM, Stannard A, Burkhardt GE, Eastridge BJ, Blackbourne LH, Rasmussen TE. The epidemiology of vascular injury in the wars in Iraq and Afghanistan. Ann Surg. 2011;253(6):1184–9.
4. Venticinque SG, Grathwohl KW. Critical care in the austere environment: providing exceptional care in unusual places. Crit Care Med. 2008;36(7 Suppl):S284–92.
5. Kragh Jr JF, Walters TJ, Baer DG, Fox CJ, Wade CE, Salinas J, et al. Survival with emergency tourniquet use to stop bleeding in major limb trauma. Ann Surg. 2009;249(1):1–7.
6. Granville-Chapman J, Jacobs N, Midwinter MJ. Prehospital haemostatic dressings: a systematic review. Injury. 2011;42(5):447–59.
7. Wedmore I, McManus JG, Pusateri AE, Holcomb JB. A special report on the chitosan-based hemostatic dressing: experience in current combat operations. J Trauma. 2006;60(3):655–8.
8. Duke MD, Guidry C, Guice J, Stuke L, Marr AB, Hunt JP, et al. Restrictive fluid resuscitation in combination with damage control resuscitation: time for adaptation. J Trauma Acute Care Surg. 2012;73(3):674–8.
9. Langan NR, Eckert M, Martin MJ. Changing patterns of in-hospital deaths following implementation of damage control resuscitation practices in US forward military treatment facilities. JAMA Surg. 2014;149(9):904–12.
10. Rotondo MF, Schwab CW, McGonigal MD, Phillips 3rd GR, Fruchterman TM, Kauder DR, et al. "Damage control": an approach for improved survival in exsanguinating penetrating abdominal injury. J Trauma. 1993;35(3):375–82. discussion 82–3.

11. Germanos S, Gourgiotis S, Villias C, Bertucci M, Dimopoulos N, Salemis N. Damage control surgery in the abdomen: an approach for the management of severe injured patients. Int J Surg. 2008;6(3):246–52.

12. Blackbourne LH. Combat damage control surgery. Crit Care Med. 2008;36(7 Suppl):S304–10.

13. Navy U. Surface ship survivability. Washington, DC: Department of Defense, Navy War Publications; 1996.

14. Walt AJ. The surgical management of hepatic trauma and its complications. Ann R Coll Surg Engl. 1969;45(6):319–39.

15. Fox CJ, Gillespie DL, Cox ED, Kragh Jr JF, Mehta SG, Salinas J, et al. Damage control resuscitation for vascular surgery in a combat support hospital. J Trauma. 2008;65(1):1–9.

16. Savitsky E, Eastridge B, editors. Combat casualty care: lessons learned from OEF and OIF. Fort Detrick, MD: Borden Institute by the Office of The Surgeon General; 2012. 719 p.

17. Belmont Jr PJ, McCriskin BJ, Sieg RN, Burks R, Schoenfeld AJ. Combat wounds in Iraq and Afghanistan from 2005 to 2009. J Trauma Acute Care Surg. 2012;73(1):3–12.

18. Eastridge BJ, Mabry RL, Seguin P, Cantrell J, Tops T, Uribe P, et al. Death on the battlefield (2001-2011): implications for the future of combat casualty care. J Trauma Acute Care Surg. 2012;73(6 Suppl 5):S431–7.

19. Sise RG, Calvo RY, Spain DA, Weiser TG, Staudenmayer KL. The epidemiology of trauma-related mortality in the United States from 2002 to 2010. J Trauma Acute Care Surg. 2014;76(4):913–9. discussion 20.

20. Caterson EJ, Carty MJ, Weaver MJ, Holt EF. Boston bombings: a surgical view of lessons learned from combat casualty care and the applicability to Boston's terrorist attack. J Craniofac Surg. 2013;24(4):1061–7.

21. Georgiou C, Neofytou K, Demetriades D. Local and systemic hemostatics as an adjunct to control bleeding in trauma. Am Surg. 2013;79(2):180–7.

22. Ran Y, Hadad E, Daher S, Ganor O, Kohn J, Yegorov Y, et al. QuikClot Combat Gauze use for hemorrhage control in military trauma: January 2009 Israel Defense Force experience in the Gaza Strip – a preliminary report of 14 cases. Prehosp Disaster Med. 2010;25(6):584–8.

23. Starnes BW, Beekley AC, Sebesta JA, Andersen CA, Rush Jr RM. Extremity vascular injuries on the battlefield: tips for surgeons deploying to war. J Trauma. 2006;60(2):432–42.

24. Rasmussen TE, Clouse WD, Jenkins DH, Peck MA, Eliason JL, Smith DL. The use of temporary vascular shunts as a damage control adjunct in the management of wartime vascular injury. J Trauma. 2006;61(1):8–12. discussion-5.

25. Moore WS. Vascular and endovascular surgery: a comprehensive review. Philadelphia: Saunders, 2013. pp. 721–53.

26. Hirshberg AMK. In: Allen MK, editor. Top knife: the art and craft of trauma surgery. Harley, UK: Tfm Publishing Ltd; 2005. p. 234.

27. Cronenwett JL, Johnston KW. Rutherford's vascular surgery. Philadelphia: Saunders, 2014. pp. 2485–500, 544–54.

28. Quan RW, Gillespie DL, Stuart RP, Chang AS, Whittaker DR, Fox CJ. The effect of vein repair on the risk of venous thromboembolic events: a review of more than 100 traumatic military venous injuries. J Vasc Surg. 2008;47(3):571–7.

29. Chambers LW, Green DJ, Sample K, Gillingham BL, Rhee P, Brown C, et al. Tactical surgical intervention with temporary shunting of peripheral vascular trauma sustained during Operation Iraqi Freedom: one unit's experience. J Trauma. 2006;61(4):824–30.

30. Farber A, Tan TW, Hamburg NM, Kalish JA, Joglar F, Onigman T, et al. Early fasciotomy in patients with extremity vascular injury is associated with decreased risk of adverse limb outcomes: a review of the National Trauma Data Bank. Injury. 2012;43(9):1486–91.

31. Cubano MA. Emergency war surgery. Fort Sam Houston, TX: Borden Institute, Office of the Surgeon General; 2013. 565 p.

32. Pinzur MS, Gottschalk FA, Pinto MA, Smith DG. American Academy of Orthopaedic S. Controversies in lower-extremity amputation. J Bone Joint Surg Am. 2007;89(5):1118–27.

33. Butler Jr FK, Holcomb JB, Giebner SD, McSwain NE, Bagian J. Tactical combat casualty care 2007: evolving concepts and battlefield experience. Mil Med. 2007;172 Suppl 11:1–19.

34. Arora S, Sevdalis N, Nestel D, Woloshynowych M, Darzi A, Kneebone R. The impact of stress on surgical performance: a systematic review of the literature. Surgery. 2010;147(3):318–30. e1–6.

35. Schmidt EAS, Mark W, Bliss JP, Hanner-Baily Hope S, Garcia, Hector M, Weireter, LJ Jr, editors. Surgical skill performance under combat conditions in a virtual environment. Human Factors and Ergonomics Society 50th annual meeting; 2006.

36. Conrad C, Konuk Y, Werner PD, Cao CG, Warshaw AL, Rattner DW, et al. A quality improvement study on avoidable stressors and countermeasures affecting surgical motor performance and learning. Ann Surg. 2012;255(6):1190–4.

37. Arora S, Sevdalis N, Nestel D, Tierney T, Woloshynowych M, Kneebone R. Managing intraoperative stress: what do surgeons want from a crisis training program? Am J Surg. 2009;197(4):537–43.

38. Jacobson IG, Horton JL, Leardmann CA, Ryan MA, Boyko EJ, Wells TS, et al. Posttraumatic stress disorder and depression among U.S. military health care professionals deployed in support of operations in Iraq and Afghanistan. J Trauma Stress. 2012;25(6):616–23.

39. Warren AM, Jones AL, Shafi S, Roden-Foreman K, Bennett MM, Foreman ML. Does caring for trauma patients lead to psychological stress in surgeons? J Trauma Acute Care Surg. 2013;75(1):179–84.

40. Palm KM, Polusny MA, Follette VM. Vicarious traumatization: potential hazards and interventions for disaster and trauma workers. Prehosp Disaster Med. 2004;19(1):73–8.

41. Frykberg ER, Dennis JW, Bishop K, Laneve L, Alexander RH. The reliability of physical examination in the evaluation of penetrating extremity trauma for vascular injury: results at one year. J Trauma. 1991;31(4):502–11.

42. Tintle SM, Forsberg JA, Keeling JJ, Shawen SB, Potter BK. Lower extremity combat-related amputations. J Surg Orthop Adv. 2010;19(1):35–43.

Lessons Learned from the Boston Marathon Bombing

17

David R. King and Tomaz Mesar

17.1 Introduction

The practice of trauma surgery in the aftermath of the Boston Marathon bombing took place within the walls of the five Boston Level I trauma centers, as well as several adjacent community hospitals. The approach to these patients reflected the general philosophy of rapid damage control, abbreviated surgery, frequent returns to the operating room in a staged fashion, and high ratio blood transfusions. The real lesson for surgeons, however, is learned from careful examination of the prehospital treatment of the large number of extremity injuries resulting from the two improvised explosive devices detonated on Boylston Street during the running of the 117th Boston Marathon at 14:49 on April 15, 2013. The late Dr Norman McSwain often said that trauma is a surgical disease from start to finish, and that surgeons need to re-engage in the prehospital care of the bleeding trauma patient. He was right.

As a surgeon, soldier, Bostonian, 50+ time chronic marathoner, and participant of the 117th Boston Marathon (3:12 marathon, I crossed the finish line roughly an hour before the blasts), I will forever remember the events of that day and how they altered our city forever. I remember those who died (29-year-old Krystle Campbell, 23-year-old Lu Lingzi, 8-year-old Martin Richard, and 27-year-old Sean Collier) and celebrate those who lived: the survivors. This chapter is dedicated to the survivors of the Boston Marathon bombing.

17.2 History Repeats Itself

Described in antiquity, tourniquets have been used to control extremity bleeding during amputations. This evolved to encompass the use of tourniquets as a first aid maneuver for extremity bleeding. The merits of tourniquet use as a first aid hemorrhage control maneuver have been repeatedly debated, mostly based on historical battlefield experiences that traditionally condemned the practice for its dreaded limb-threatening complications [1, 2]. Data collected throughout the most recent decade of war in Iraq and Afghanistan [3, 4], however, have caused physicians, first responders, and policy-makers to reconsider previously held beliefs around tourniquet use in the prehospital management of

D.R. King, M.D., F.A.C.S. (✉) • T. Mesar, M.D.
Division of Trauma, Emergency Surgery, and Surgical Critical Care, Department of Surgery, Harvard Medical School, Massachusetts General Hospital, 165 Cambridge Street, Suite 810, Boston, MA 02114, USA
e-mail: dking3@mgh.harvard.edu

© Springer International Publishing Switzerland 2016
C.R.B. Lim (ed.), *Surgery During Natural Disasters, Combat, Terrorist Attacks, and Crisis Situations*, DOI 10.1007/978-3-319-23718-3_17

severely bleeding extremities [1]. This contemporary military wartime experience demonstrates that while improvised tourniquets are rarely effective, the ubiquitous availability and early use of commercial, purpose-designed tourniquets reduces death rates from extremity wound exsanguination [5–8]. The Boston Marathon bombing was the first major, modern terrorist event on US soil, with multiple, severe, wartime-like lower extremity injuries [9]. Mass casualty events with multiple, severe extremity injuries are common on the battlefield but uncommon in the homeland. In Boston, trained medical professionals, civilian first responders, and non-medical bystanders rushed to aid the injured, mostly attending to extremity wounds [10].

17.3 The Bombing

Two ground level improvised explosive devices were detonated on Boylston Street in downtown Boston during the running of the 117th Boston Marathon, at 14:49:43 and 14:49:57 on April 15, 2013. Two-hundred-forty-three injured patients presented with a myriad of injuries (Fig. 17.1). Of the total population of 243 injured casualties, 152 patients presented to the Emergency Department (ED) within 24 h of the explosions. Among the 152 patients presenting with 24 h, an extremity injury was present in 66 patients. Among these patients, most sustained concomitant injuries to other body regions, depicted and summarized in Fig. 17.2.

Of the 66 patients with extremity injury, 4 patients had only upper extremities affected, 56 patients had only lower extremities affected, and 6 patients sustained combined upper and lower extremity injuries. There were 17 lower extremity traumatic amputations (LETA) in 15 patients; of these patients, ten suffered a below knee traumatic amputation (BKA), three suffered an above knee traumatic amputation (AKA), one patient suffered bilateral BKAs, and one suffered a BKA and an AKA.

Among patients with a lower extremity injury but no traumatic amputation, 14 major vascular injuries (MVI) were present in 12 lower extremities in ten patients with severe soft tissue extremity injury. Seven of the latter were arterial (1 femoral, 2 popliteal, and 4 other named arteries) and seven were venous (1 femoral, 3 popliteal, and 3 other named veins). Two lower extremities had combined arterial–venous injuries (1 combined femoral arterio-venous and 1 combined popliteal arterio-venous injury). The burden of extremity injury is presented in Fig. 17.3.

Of all 66 patients with extremity injuries, 29 (44 %) were recognized and documented as having life-threatening extremity exsanguination at the point-of-injury, including all 15 (100 %) LETA patients, 7 of 10 (70 %) MVI patients, and 7 of 41 (11 %) non-LETA and non-MVI patients with other massive soft tissue and open long-bone fractures.

Among the 29 patients with recognized exsanguination, 27 tourniquets were applied at the point-of-injury: 94 % of the LETA extremities, 42 % of the lower extremities with major vascular injuries, and 6 of the 7 additional extremities with major soft tissue injury. No patient had more than one tourniquet per extremity and no junctional injuries with significant hemorrhage were identified. Of the 16 LETA patients with tourniquets, four had improvised tourniquets applied by EMS, seven had improvised tourniquets applied by non-EMS responders (some of whom had known medical training but were not acting as part of the official Boston EMS response, including physicians, off-duty soldiers, etc.), and five had improvised tourniquets of unknown origin. Of the five lower extremities with MVI, two had improvised tourniquets applied by EMS, two had improvised tourniquets applied by non-EMS responders, and one had an improvised tourniquet of unknown origin. Of the six additional extremities with major soft tissue injury and exsanguination, four had improvised tourniquets applied by EMS and two had improvised tourniquets of unknown origin. Figures 17.4 and 17.5 reflect the sources of the tourniquets recovered. In total, 37 % of tourniquets were applied by EMS. Eight limbs presented to the ED with life-threatening exsanguination and had no prehospital tourniquet in place on arrival.

All tourniquets were improvised, including those applied by EMS, and no commercially available and purpose-designed tourniquets were

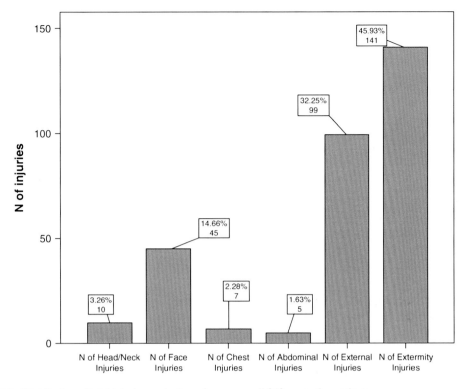

Fig. 17.1 Distribution of total injuries per body region among all 243 presenting patients

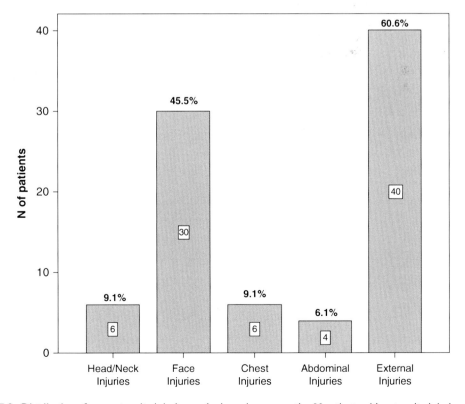

Fig. 17.2 Distribution of non-extremity injuries per body region among the 66 patients with extremity injuries

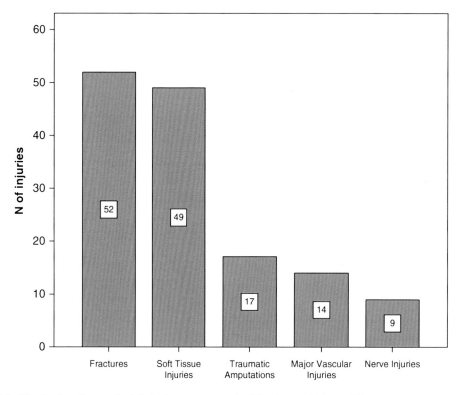

Fig. 17.3 Distribution of extremity injuries by type among the 66 patients with injured limbs

Fig. 17.4 Sources of
the 27 tourniquets

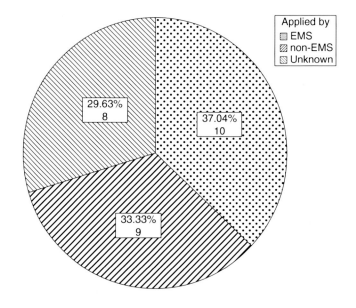

identified. A review of photography and video from the scene response demonstrates a single extremity with soft tissue injury (but not a LETA) identified with a Combat Application Tourniquet (CAT) in place. We have no knowledge of this patient's trauma burden or outcome. At the Massachusetts General Hospital, all six improvised tourniquets encountered were venous tourniquets and required replacement with a CAT tourniquet to prevent ongoing extremity exsanguination and effect hemostasis upon arrival in the ED. Similar reports exist from other Boston hospitals. The most commonly encountered EMS tourniquet was an improvised tourniquet consisting of rubber tubing and a Kelly clamp (Fig. 17.6). None of the 66 patients with extremity injuries died.

17.4 Analysis of the Unthinkable

Although the Boston Marathon bombing was not the first terrorist event in the United States, it was the first modern event to create mass casualties with a pattern of severe lower extremity blast injury commonly seen on the battlefield from improvised explosive devices. The Boston experience demonstrated the nearly universal use of improvised tourniquets as a primary prehospital and presurgical attempt at hemostatic intervention for life-threatening extremity hemorrhage. A recent study conducted in Boston describes the city's informal tourniquet protocol and use of the commonly seen improvised tourniquet after the bombing, however this manuscript conspicuously omits data regarding effectiveness of the improvised tourniquet or why this device was specifically selected over others [11]. Recent data derived from military experience do not support the use of improvised tourniquets as best practice, as multiple studies [3–8] have consistently reported superior hemostatic results with the use of commercial, purpose-designed tourniquets. Our collective military experience has also established the hemostatic superiority of the commercially available devices by directly comparing them to improvised devices [12–14]. As a result, US combat personnel are now trained in self and buddy application of these purpose-designed

tourniquets [1, 3–8], and each US military service-member carries at least one CAT tourniquet (often two). The translation of this military posture (general availability of tourniquets and widespread training on how to apply them correctly) to the homeland has not been realized, unlike other battlefield lessons such as early use of anti-fibrinolytics, high-ratio transfusion, and abbreviated surgery, which have gained far more translational traction in the homeland [15]. Had translation been more successful, one may have expected far more than a single commercial tourniquet identified after the bombing.

Additional evidence from the civilian community [14, 16] demonstrates an obvious deficiency in the translation of the military's extremity hemorrhage control posture. A retrospective study on trauma registries at two large Level 1 Trauma centers in Canada [14] revealed that of 190 patients who suffered isolated extremity injuries with arterial injury, only four patients had a tourniquet present upon arrival. Those were all improvised tourniquets (neck tie, belt, or handkerchief) applied by police or bystanders. In the non-tourniquet group, six deaths were recorded as a direct result of exsanguination. While statistically significant differences were difficult to observe given the small number of patients who received a prehospital tourniquet, this study highlights the profound absence of systematic use of tourniquets in the prehospital environment. Following this, the 2012 Adult Traumatic Hemorrhage Control Protocol was introduced to all EMS providers in the province of Alberta, Canada—a protocol that advises the use of a Combat Application Tourniquet for uncontrolled extremity bleeding and completes the translation of battlefield lessons to the homeland. Each state in the United States should consider adopting a similar protocol.

Although it is certainly possible to improvise an effective arterial tourniquet, the data suggest this is uncommonly done appropriately, especially under stress [4, 10–16]. An improvised tourniquet should be (1) wide enough to compress arterial and venous vasculature without creating pressure necrosis of the skin or neuropraxia (as may occur with narrow tourniquets, such as rubber tubing), and (2) have a device attached to

Fig. 17.5 Sources of the 27 tourniquets among 66 patients with extremity injury categorized by injury type

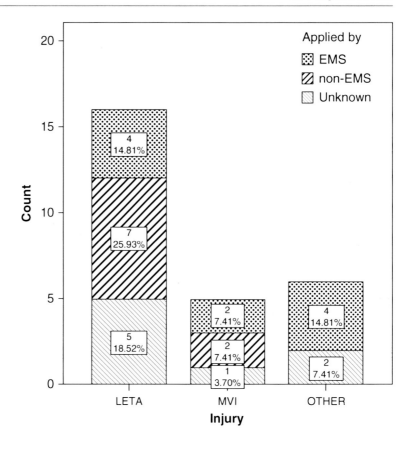

Fig. 17.6 Typical EMS improvised tourniquet

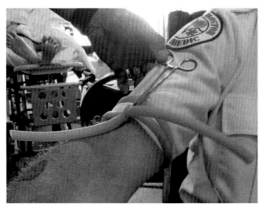

create a mechanical advantage in order to generate adequate circumferential pressure (such as a windlass). The improvised tourniquets used in Boston met only the second of these two fundamental criteria. It is important to note that as materials science and tourniquet technology advances, it may be possible to create an effective arterial tourniquet device without a windlass. This will likely translate to a simpler tourniquet application method and broader use by both first responders and bystanders [17, 18].

While full translation of the military posture regarding extremity hemorrhage control and tourniquet use may be ideal, one must accept that, in the setting of sudden disaster, tourniquets will continue to be improvised despite all efforts at translation by policy-makers. It is clear that improvised tourniquets, and the temporary hemorrhage control they offer, will always be used in mass casualty scenarios and their role should not be entirely discounted. An improvised venous tourniquet can provide temporary hemorrhage control [3, 5, 6], however a comprehensive review of emergency tourniquet use recently highlighted the significance of unintentional venous tourniquets as potentially deadly [2], particularly in the minutes following initial bleeding control. The experience in Boston, with apparent, initial hemostasis using improvised tourniquets at the point-of-injury, supports this notion and appears to echo that of known paradoxical bleeding after venous tourniquet application. Venous tourniquets can create initial adequate hemorrhage control that soon worsens as a time-dependent function, until hemorrhage control is lost and supplanted by paradoxical hemorrhage, with ensuing worsening of hemorrhage than if no tourniquet were used at all [3]. Perhaps an educational campaign to teach the correct way to apply a purpose-designed tourniquet, as well how to improvise an effective arterial tourniquet, may be appropriate since it is nearly certain that limbs will have improvised tourniquets applied after the next, unfortunate, bombing in the homeland. Several studies suggest that adequate training can be minimal (less than a minute) and still result in trainees who can apply effective tourniquets [17, 18].

Despite some possible limitations with respect to prehospital extremity hemorrhage control, there were no in-hospital deaths. The mean transport time from point-of-injury to ED was 24 min, substantially faster than the range of commonly reported evacuation times in the military and civilian literature, which could vary from well under 1 h to over 2 h after time of wounding, depending on the setting and circumstances [10, 12, 19–22]. The high number of Boston area metropolitan trauma centers all co-located in a very small geographic area in close proximity to the Boston Marathon finish line likely contributed to this rapid evacuation time, as well as the robust medical infrastructure already in place at the finish line for the expected event-related illnesses.

The Boston bombing experience suggests that (1) instances of multiple exsanguinating extremity injuries, similar to battlefield wounds, can occur in the homeland and (2) improvised tourniquets likely provided initial hemorrhage control, but the absence of purpose-designed devices in the bombing response probably created some cases of paradoxical bleeding. When contrasted to the wealth of evidence gathered from the last decade of military experience, these findings call for a reconsideration of our practices. We recommend that all EMS services translate a military posture with an extremity hemorrhage control protocol that emphasizes appropriate training with liberal availability of commercial,

purpose-designed tourniquets. Proper tourniquet application techniques should be presented in the Advanced Trauma Life Support and Prehospital Trauma Life Support training manuals, among others. Several notable organizations, including the Hartford Consensus and the American College of Surgeons, are recommending translation and adoption of military posture toward prehospital extremity hemorrhage control [23, 24]. Physician leaders and policy-makers should insist on translation of a prehospital extremity hemorrhage control posture similar to the ubiquitous adoption and presence of automated external defibrillators in nearly every ambulance, federal building, cafeteria, and other public gathering area in the United States.

17.5 By the Numbers

Although much attention has been given to the obvious absence of purpose-made tourniquets in the Boston bombing response, other lessons were also learned of significant importance. For sake of completeness, the entire list of Lessons Learned is presented here.

1. *No tourniquetsor advanced topical hemostatic agents were available.* Unfortunately, this is a posture that was poorly translated to the homeland from the battlefield.
2. *Improvised tourniquets do not work.* Although we must not discourage bystanders from responding to disaster to aid the injured, we must also be intellectually honest and recognize that (despite the lay press reporting) the improvised tourniquets applied on Boylston were likely not arterial tourniquets. Improvisation of an arterial tourniquet is a skill-set that can be taught and should be widely incorporated into general first aid classes.
3. *There was no formal tourniquet training or protocol.* If purpose-made tourniquets had been available, proper training to ensure correct application is necessary. The Committee on Tactical Combat Casualty Care publishes guidelines regarding tourniquet use, and formal

training and written protocols are widely available. These should be adopted as permanent part of every first responder educational curriculum.

4. *There was too much "stay and play" in the medical tent at the finish line.* While the finish line medical tent instantly became the *de facto* triage area after the bombing, the transport times recorded for many severely injured patients was over an hour. By either design or by a matter of mass-confusion, some patients remained in the medical tent for an extended period of time. In a city with five Level I trauma centers, and hundreds of patients with surgical injuries, patients should be moved to hospitals in a swifter fashion.

5. *Electronic medical record systems are slow.* For some patients, electronic registration in the ED became a bottleneck for fastest care. In most cases, patients cannot even receive a single unit of blood without an assigned medical record number. During a mass casualty event, this electronic registration system becomes bogged down and slow, possibly limiting expediency of care. Hospitals should create a contingency plan to have pre-assigned mass casualty medical record numbers, or implement a system capable of rapid registration of hundreds of patients.

6. *Sequential medical record numbers are dangerous.* Assigning patients sequential medical record numbers in simple escalating numerical fashion creates an unacceptable margin of error since there will be many simultaneous patients with medical record numbers differing by only a single digit (1234567, 1234568, 1234569, …). This creates an unacceptable environment for a potential clerical error, single key-stroke mistake, that would potentially result in a surgeon looking at the hemoglobin value of the wrong patient or (worse yet) ordering tests or procedures on the wrong patient. Medical record numbers during disasters should vary widely to prevent this error.

7. *The most visually stimulating injury is often not the most life threatening one.* The Boston bombing patients arrived with extremely devastating, and visually stimulating, limb injuries. These injuries, despite their appearance, were easily controlled with a proper tourniquet. Some patients also had co-existing intra-cavitary hemorrhage. This can often be overlooked when the clinician inappropriately focused on the limb injury and neglects a complete trauma evaluation, particularly of the peritoneal and thoracic cavities. Once an effective tourniquet is in place, the limb injury becomes (temporarily) forgettable.

8. *Don't Go Home Just Yet: The tertiary trauma survey is extremely important.* In disasters, it is a common urge to "take a break" once each patient's index operation is complete and all the bleeding and contamination is controlled. This approach and attitude, however, may result in adverse results in patient management. Once the initial surgery is done, the entire trauma team has to re-assemble to go over each patient again, in extreme detail. The purpose of this is twofold. First, the entire team needs to understand each patient's condition and status so appropriate planning for operative take-backs, additional imaging, and other interventions can be planned and prioritized. Second, small injuries are commonly missed and will only be identified by a careful tertiary survey. Although most of our patients had non-life-threatening ruptured tympanic membranes, for example, these were largely not identified until post trauma day two on a careful tertiary examination. This is, of course, an appropriate injury to miss on initial evaluation in a mass casualty situation, however failure to recognize and treat this injury (and others like it) could result in long-term disability.

17.6   In a Nutshell

After the Boston Marathon bombings, extremity exsanguination at the point-of-injury was either left un-treated or treated with an improvised tourniquet in the prehospital environment. An effective prehospital extremity hemorrhage control posture should be translated to all civilian first responders in the United States, and should mirror the military's posture toward extremity bleeding control. Physician leaders and policy-makers should support this initiative. The prehospital response to extremity exsanguination after the Boston Marathon bombing demonstrates that our current practice is an approach lost in translation from the battlefield to the homeland.

Editor's Note: LTC David King, MD US Army, has been deployed three times to the combat zone in support of Operation Iraqi Freedom and Operation Enduring Freedom. Within a few hours of finishing the Boston Marathon himself, he himself was amazingly treating and performing surgery on the victims of the blasts. Dr. King also testified about the injuries and wounds of the bombing victims at the trial of Dzhokhar Tsarnaev which ended in Tsarnaev's conviction.

References

1. Welling DR, McKay PL, Rasmussen TE, Rich NM. A brief history of the tourniquet. J Vasc Surg. 2012;55(1):286–90.
2. Kragh Jr JF, Swan KG, Smith DC, Mabry RL, Blackbourne LH. Historical review of emergency tourniquet use to stop bleeding. Am J Surg. 2012;203(2):242–52.
3. Kragh Jr JF, O'Neill ML, Walters TJ, Dubick MA, Baer DG, Wade CE, et al. Minor morbidity with emergency tourniquet use to stop bleeding in severe limb trauma: research, history, and reconciling advocates and abolitionists. Mil Med. 2011;176(7):817–23.
4. King DR, van der Wilden G, Kragh Jr JF, Blackbourne LH. Forward assessment of 79 prehospital battlefield tourniquets used in the current war. J Spec Oper Med. 2012;12(4):33–8.
5. Beekley AC, Sebesta JA, Blackbourne LH, Herbert GS, Kauvar DS, Baer DG, et al. Prehospital tourniquet use in Operation Iraqi Freedom: effect on hemorrhage control and outcomes. J Trauma. 2008;64 Suppl 2:S28–37.
6. Kragh Jr JF, Walters TJ, Baer DG, Fox CJ, Wade CE, Salinas J, et al. Survival with emergency tourniquet use to stop bleeding in major limb trauma. Ann Surg. 2009;249(1):1–7.
7. Kragh Jr JF, Littrel ML, Jones JA, Walters TJ, Baer DG, Wade CE, et al. Battle casualty survival with emergency tourniquet use to stop limb bleeding. J Emerg Med. 2011;41(6):590–7.
8. Lakstein D, Blumenfeld A, Sokolov T, Lin G, Bssorai R, Lynn M, et al. Tourniquets for hemorrhage control on the battlefield: a 4-year accumulated experience. J Trauma. 2003;54 Suppl 5:S221–5.
9. Kapur GB, Hutson HR, Davis MA, Rice PL. The United States twenty-year experience with bombing incidents: implications for terrorism preparedness and medical response. J Trauma. 2005;59(6):1436–44.
10. Gates JD, Arabian S, Biddinger P, Blansfield J, Burke P, Chung S, et al. The initial response to the Boston marathon bombing: lessons learned to prepare for the next disaster. Ann Surg. 2014;260(6):960–6.
11. Kalish J, Burke P, Feldman J, Agarwal S, Glantz A, Moyer P, et al. The return of tourniquets. Original research evaluates the effectiveness of prehospital tourniquets for civilian penetrating extremity injuries. JEMS. 2008;33(8):44–6. 49–50, 52, 54.
12. D'Alleyrand JCG, Dutton RP, Pollak AN. Extrapolation of battlefield resuscitative care to the civilian setting. J Surg Orthop Adv. 2010;19(1):62–9.
13. Evaluation of self-applied tourniquets for combat applications, second phase. 2013. http://archive.rubicon-foundation.org/xmlui/handle/123456789/6870?show=full. Accessed 19 Sept 2013.
14. Passos E, Dingley B, Smith A, Engels PT, Ball CG, Faidi S, et al. Tourniquet use for peripheral vascular injuries in the civilian setting. Injury. 2014;45(3):573–7.
15. Duchesne JC, Islam TM, Stuke L, Timmer JR, Barbeau JM, Marr AB, et al. Hemostatic resuscitation during surgery improves survival in patients with traumatic-induced coagulopathy. J Trauma. 2009;67(1):33–7. discussion 37–9.
16. Dorlac WC, DeBakey ME, Holcomb JB, Fagan SP, Kwong KL, Dorlac GR, et al. Mortality from isolated civilian penetrating extremity injury. J Trauma. 2005;59(1):217–22.
17. Wall PL, Duevel DC, Hassan MB, Welander JD, Sahr SM, Buising CM. Tourniquets and occlusion: the pressure of design. Mil Med. 2013;178(5):578–87.
18. Wall PL, Welander JD, Singh A, Sidwell RA, Buising CM. Stretch and wrap style tourniquet effectiveness with minimal training. Mil Med. 2012;177(11):1366–73.
19. Ingalls N, Zonies D, Bailey JA, Martin KD, Iddins BO, Carlton PK, et al. A review of the first 10 years of critical care aeromedical transport during Operation Iraqi Freedom and Operation Enduring Freedom: the importance of evacuation timing. JAMA Surg. 2014;149(8):807–13.
20. Ball CG, Williams BH, Tallah C, Salomone JP, Feliciano DV. The impact of shorter prehospital transport times on outcomes in patients with abdominal vascular injuries. J Trauma Manag Outcomes. 2013;7(1):11.

21. Crandall M, Sharp D, Unger E, Straus D, Brasel K, Hsia R, et al. Trauma deserts: distance from a trauma center, transport times, and mortality from gunshot wounds in Chicago. Am J Public Health. 2013;103(6):1103–9.

22. Bulger EM, Guffey D, Guyette FX, MacDonald RD, Brasel K, Kerby JD, et al. Impact of prehospital mode of transport after severe injury: a multicenter evaluation from the Resuscitation Outcomes Consortium. J Trauma Acute Care Surg. 2012;72(3):567–73. discussion 573-5.

23. Jacobs LM, McSwain Jr NE, Rotondo MF, Wade D, Fabbri W, Eastman AL, et al. Improving survival from active shooter events: the Hartford Consensus. J Trauma Acute Care Surg. 2013;74(6):1399–400.

24. Bulger EM, Snyder D, Schoelles K, Gotschall C, Dawson D, Lang E, et al. An evidence-based prehospital guideline for external hemorrhage control: American College of Surgeons Committee on Trauma. Prehosp Emerg Care. 2014;18(2):163–73.

Chemical Warfare: A Brief History and Summary of Current Threats and Initial Management

18

LCDR Jami L. Hickey and Sean M. Bryant

18.1 Introduction: Tokyo, 1995

On March 20, 1995 at 8:09 a.m. the Tokyo Metropolitan Fire Department (TMFD) received an emergency call from a Tokyo subway station. Within 1 h, there were calls from 15 different subway stations with similar reports, symptoms ranging from mild visual complaints to cardiopulmonary arrest. The incoming information rapidly overwhelmed the communication abilities of the ambulance control center. During the incident, 1364 EMTs and 131 ambulances were dispatched. A total of 688 patients were transported by TMFD in ambulances or minivans and more than 4000 additional patients arrived at hospitals in the area either on foot, in taxis, or in personal vehicles.

It took several hours to appreciate that incident was initiated by members of a religious cult who had deposited bags of liquid sarin in five

LCDR J.L. Hickey, M.D., M.C., U.S.N. (✉)
Emergency Department, Naval Medical Center
Portsmouth, 620 John Paul Jones Circle, Portsmouth,
VA 23708, USA
e-mail: jami.l.hickey@gmail.com

S.M. Bryant, M.D.
Emergency Medicine/Medical Toxicology,
Cook County Hospital (Stroger), 1900 West Polk,
10th Floor, Chicago, IL 60612, USA
e-mail: sbryant@cookcountyhhs.org

subway cars. Sarin is a potent nerve agent that acts by inhibiting the enzyme acetylcholinesterase, leading to a cholinergic toxidrome. Its effects are immediate and life threatening. The sarin began to vaporize once the bags were opened. This resulted in immediate symptoms in the passengers who then hurriedly exited the cars all the while allowing the gas to continue to disperse. Communications between the police department, EMS, and hospitals were overwhelmed. The police department confirmed 3 h after the incident that the substance was sarin, not acetonitrile as originally reported. The staff at the treating hospitals only became aware of the nature of the exposure after it was reported on the news [1].

The most severe cases were transported immediately, but due to laws in place in Tokyo EMS personnel were unable to perform rescue airway procedures or even place IVs without consent from a physician. As they had lost contact with the control center, no communication with the physician was available and no rescue airways were performed in the field. Only one IV was placed prior to a patient arriving at the hospital.

St. Luke's Hospital received a report at 8:16 a.m. that a gas explosion had occurred at a subway station. Hospital staff began preparation to care for expected burns and carbon monoxide poisonings. The first patient arrived on foot at 8:28 complaining of eye pain and visual disturbance. Within the first hour over 500 patients were received at the St. Luke's

© Springer International Publishing Switzerland 2016
C.R.B. Lim (ed.), *Surgery During Natural Disasters, Combat,*
Terrorist Attacks, and Crisis Situations, DOI 10.1007/978-3-319-23718-3_18

emergency department, including three patients in cardiopulmonary arrest.

Once the agent was known to be sarin, hospital staff began administering appropriate and focused antidotal therapy (i.e., atropine and pralidoxime (2-PAM)). Severe cases of organophosphate poisoning may require extremely high atropine dosing, on the order of several hundred milligrams. In storage, St. Lukes had 100 ampules of 2-PAM, each containing 500 mg, and 1030 ampules of atropine sulfate, each containing 0.5 mg. At early stages, orders were made for more medications. In total, 700 ampules of 2-PAM and 2800 ampules of atropine sulfate were used [2].

As a result of this attack, 12 were killed and over 5500 sought medical care. Of 1364 EMTs, 135 showed symptoms of secondary exposure. At St Luke's Hospital, 23 % of the staff surveyed after the incident reported symptoms of secondary exposure. Throughout the incident, only standard personal protective equipment, limited mostly to gloves, was worn by EMS and hospital staff.

Although this attack was a peacetime event, it illustrates how easily a chemical weapon attack can in any setting overwhelm any medical or disaster response system. There is much to be learned from such an uncommon, large-scale local event, both nationally in Japan and internationally [3]. A chemical weapons attack differs from usual warfare tactics or large-scale attacks in that decontamination and prophylaxis play a large role in limiting casualties [4]. It is vital for every physician or provider to be familiar with the possibilities of chemical warfare, the presentations of key agents, and the interventions necessary to save lives.

18.2 History of Chemical Warfare

Chemical weapons have been part of warfare for as long has history has been recorded. A chemical weapon can be defined as any chemical agent that is designed to seriously injure, kill, or incapacitate opposing forces. Throughout history this has taken many forms and the acceptance of such methods of warfare has undergone numerous and sophisticated evolutions.

Early chemical weapon use included poison darts and arrows that utilized the natural venom extracted from scorpions, snakes, and frogs. The Laws of Manu, a Hindu text circa 500BC, was against the use of poison arrows and darts as part of warfare, but advocated the use of poisons in the enemy's water and food. Ancient Chinese texts describe the use of arsenical smoke to incapacitate the enemy. In ancient Greece, various plants were used as weapons to poison the enemy. In the Siege of Kirrha, a battle that took place during the First Sacred War in 590BC, hellebore was used to poison the aqueducts of Kirrha, causing severe, incapacitating diarrhea in the city's inhabitants [5].

In the early modern era, use of chemical weapons continued to evolve. Leonardo da Vinci advised throwing chalk, arsenic, or powdered verdigris on enemy ships to cause asphyxiation. In 1675 the Strasburg agreement, the first international agreement to ban the use of poison projectiles, was signed by France and Germany in response to the use of belladonna alkaloids during the siege of Groningen, part of the Franco-Dutch War [5].

Moving forward, the use of chemical weapons continued to be controversial. In 1894, during the Siege of Sevastopol, a British chemist by the name of Lyon Playfair advised the use of cacodyl cyanide artillery shells against enemy ships to solve a stalemate. The Admiral of the Royal Navy backed the idea, but the British Ordinance Department rejected the proposal on ethical grounds. Lyon Playfair's response was that the use of chemical weapons is no different from other forms of warfare; and this defense was used well into the twentieth century to justify their use [5].

More modern forms of chemical warfare came into play in World War I, also called the Chemist's War. The first notable use was in Yper, Belgium. On April 22, 1915, the Germans released 160 tons of chlorine gas over the French and Algerian military, killing over 1000 soldiers and injuring over 4000 more. Yper became a testing ground for German chemical weapons. Mustard gas was introduced later in the war, often nick-named "yperite" and within 6 weeks of introduction was responsible for 20,000 casualties [6].

While the use of chemical weapons in WWI was limited to Germany, the development of these technologies was not. Within 1 year of the United States entering the war on April 16, 1917, Johns Hopkins, Harvard, and Yale all had programs dedicated to the development of chemical weapons as well as initiating preventive measures including more advanced gas masks and antidotal treatments. The French also had several medical schools and universities with chemical weapon programs [6].

World War II saw further development of chemical weapons from Germany, with the first nerve agents developed from chemicals previously intended to be pesticides. While several countries, Allied and Axis alike, had stockpiles of chemical weapons, there are no documented incidences of chemical weapons use in combat during WWII, although the constant threat of use in combat loomed over both sides for the duration of the war [6].

Since WWI, chemical weapons have remained a threat both during wartime and peacetime. In the Iran–Iraq war in the 1980s, 5 % of Iranian casualties were due to chemical weapons, again drawing attention to the threat [6]. During the Cold War, the stockpiles held by the US and the Soviet Union totaled tens of thousands of tons, enough to destroy most of life on earth.

International ongoing efforts to both identify and destroy stockpiles of chemical weapons have had some success, however, until there is 100 % cooperation internationally, the possibility of chemical attack remains a real one. The remainder of this chapter will cover the individual presentations, prophylaxis, decontamination, and treatment for individual chemical agents.

18.3 Agents: Presentation and Management

18.3.1 Asphyxiants

An asphyxiant is any substance that prevents the body from utilizing oxygen. Two categories include simple asphyxiants like carbon dioxide and nitrogen, and systemic asphyxiants such as cyanide. Cyanide is the most notorious asphyxiant relevant to chemical warfare. Although little research exists focusing on mass exposures to cyanide, there are some case reports and small series available on cyanide toxicity primarily through exposures in civilian settings from burning synthetic materials. These data, in addition to several animal studies, are our best resource for determining best treatment for cyanide if used as a chemical weapon.

In civilian settings, cyanide toxicity is usually diagnosed through a combination of historical and physical examination findings. Patients have generally been exposed to an explosion or fire in which synthetic materials were burned. They will often present with concomitant burns or even carbon monoxide poisoning, complicating the clinical picture. These confounding factors may or may not be present in an intentional chemical attack, so high clinical suspicion will be paramount to proper treatment [7, 8].

As cyanide exerts its effects through inhalation or GI tract absorption, superficial decontamination and secondary exposure do not play a large role. Effective prophylaxis may be limited to on-scene rescuers wearing proper protective clothing, however, given that the identity of the gas or toxin involved may not be known at the time, rescuers and those assisting in the area should be instructed to don full gas mask and protective Mission-Oriented Protective Posture (MOPP) gear. The potential for release of more than one toxin in any attack also warrants this precaution.

Patients exposed to cyanide will exhibit a host of vague symptoms including but not limited to anxiety, altered mental status, shortness of breath, tachycardia, bradycardia, hypotension, hypertension, nausea, vomiting, dizziness, headache, seizures, and coma [7, 8]. Classically it is described as having a bitter almond odor, but this may not always be present and a significant percentage of people are genetically unable to detect this odor. The variability of symptoms again makes the diagnosis difficult. Cyanide levels in the blood take too long to obtain to be useful in the initial evaluation and treatment. If cyanide is suspected, a lactate level is recommended to help determine likelihood of cyanide toxicity. Studies have shown a lactate level of >10 mmol/L is consistent with cyanide toxicity in patients with less than 15 % body surface area burns [8]. If not already started, this may prompt clinicians to initiate antidotal treatment for cyanide when the history and clinical picture fit the possibility.

At the cellular level, cyanide is a potent noncompetitive inhibitor of cytochrome c oxidase, leading to cellular hypoxia and tissue death. Cyanide is metabolized by the enzyme rhodanase to thiocyanate. Rhodanase requires thiosulfate as a substrate. Treatments for suspected cyanide toxicity work in one of three ways: (1) by binding cyanide, (2) by generating methemoglobin, which then binds cyanide, or (3) by increasing metabolism of cyanide via addition of substrate.

Today, there are several commercially available antidotes for cyanide. Hydroxycobalamin, if available, is the preferred method of treatment for cyanide toxicity [7, 8]. Hydroxycobalamin is a potent competitive binder of cyanide and binds both free and cytochrome bound cyanide, forming cyanocobalamin, which is then easily excreted by the kidneys. The efficacy of hydroxycobalamin in treating cyanide toxicity has been shown in multiple animal studies [7–10]. Studies in humans have been very limited. Several case series and case reports showed positive results. The usual dosing of hydroxycobalamin is 5 g IV over 15 min (see Table 18.1) [8].

The longest standing antidote for cyanide is the Lilly Cyanide Antidote Kit, or Lilly kit. The Lilly kit is comprised of amyl nitrite, which is inhaled, followed by IV sodium nitrite and IV sodium thiosulfate. The nitrites form methemoglobin, which then binds cyanide. The sodium thiosulfate provides substrate for rhodanase to then metabolize cyanide to thiocyanate. While the goal of using nitrites is the production of methemoglobin, this may compromise oxygen transport and become problematic in patients from fires with smoke inhalation and/or carbon monoxide poisoning which further exacerbate functional anemia and cellular shock (see Table 18.1) [11].

Other available treatments include 4-DMAP, available commercially in Germany. 4-DMAP also induces methemoglobinemia at unpredictable levels. In France and Great Britain, dicobalt edetate is approved for use. It forms a complex with cyanide that can be excreted in the urine, but has potential for cardiac toxicity, seizures, and anaphylaxis (see Table 18.1) [7, 8].

Hydroxycobalamin remains likely the safest treatment for cyanide toxicity and has shown efficacy in animal trials. Potential side effects are limited to transient hypertension, bradycardia, skin and urine color changes, and headache. When available it is the preferred treatment and has the added benefit of low risk if used by pre-hospital personnel [7, 10]. If known threats of chemical weapon attacks exist, a pre-hospital protocol for use of hydroxycobalamin and protocols for sufficient storage of antidote should be in place [11].

18.3.2 Vesicants

Vesicants are chemical agents that cause blistering of skin and mucous membranes. The most commonly used vesicant in war is sulfur mustard (mustard gas).

Sulfur mustard, bis-2-chloroethyl sulfide, smells faintly of mustard when released. Initially mustard gas causes no symptoms, but within 4–12 h causes eye pain, blurred vision and increased lacrimation and potentially temporary blindness, which can last up to 1–2 weeks. Patients may also develop diffuse skin redness and itching followed by edema. Typically, blisters do not develop for several days, but then form in random crops. The skin findings can be very similar to thermal burns, but often are slower healing and are prone to infection. Very high doses of mustard gas can be acutely fatal within an hour [12, 13].

Pulmonary effects of mustard gas can also be severe. Pulmonary injury is the most likely cause of death for patients exposed to mustard gas. Early signs are limited to dry cough and hoarseness. Later, sloughing of tissue and necrosis lead to obstructive symptoms. Patients are at high risk for pulmonary infections as well as ARDS. More frequent than initial symptoms, mustard gas can also lead to chronic obstructive pulmonary dis-

Table 18.1 Cyanide antidotes

Cyanide antidotes	Mechanism of action	Dosing	Side effects
Hydroxycobalamin First-line treatment Safe for pre-hospital use	Binds cyanide to form cyanocobalamin	5 g IV over 15 min Additional doses of up to 10 g may be given if needed	Transient hypertension Bradycardia Headache Skin and urine discoloration
Lilly Cyanide Antidote Kit Not preferred used if hydroxycobalamin unavailable 1. Amyl nitrite 2. Sodium nitrite 3. Sodium thiosulfate	Nitrites form methemoglobin, which preferentially binds cyanide Sodium thiosulfate provides substrate for normal metabolism of cyanide	1. Amyl nitrite 0.3 mL ampoules to be administered by mechanical ventilation or by crushing and inhaling 2. Sodium nitrite 300 mg IV over 5–15 min, additional dose up to 150 mg if needed. For peds 0.33 mL/kg of 10 % solution 3. Sodium thiosulfate 12.5 g IV over 10 min. For peds 1.65 mL/kg of	Reduced oxygen carrying capacity in blood via methemoglobin formation Vasodilation Hypotension
4-DMAP available some countries, not in US	Forms methemoglobin which preferentially binds cyanide	250 mg IV over 1 min	Reduction in oxygen carrying capacity in blood via methemoglobin formation
Dicobalt edetate Due to side effects, not recommended unless other treatments unavailable		300 mg IV over 1 min	Anaphylaxis, hypotension, arrhythmias

Sources: (1) MacLennan L, Moiemen N. Management of cyanide toxicity in patients with burns. Burns. 2015; 41:18–24. (2) Eckstein M. Enhancing public health preparedness for a terrorist attack involving cyanide. J Emerg Med. 2008;35(1):59–65. (3) Rodgers GC, Condurache CT. Antidotes and treatments for chemical warfare/terrorism agents: an evidence based review. Clin Pharm Therapeut. 2010;88(3):318–27

ease as well as chronic bronchiectasis, bronchiolitis obliterans, chronic cough, nasal mucosal abnormalities, and many other long-term respiratory issues [12, 13].

Research concerning treatment of sulfur mustard exposure has not yielded a clear antidote. Studies are limited to animals as no human studies have been conducted to date. Limited animal data have suggested that thiosulfate and *N-acetyl-l*-cysteine may have some benefit, but without verification from human studies, these cannot be routinely recommended at this time [7].

As there are no known antidotes to sulfur mustard, initial management of mustard gas exposure focuses on decontamination. The window for

effective decontamination is very short. Most benefit will be derived from immediate decontamination in the field. For eye exposures, decontamination likely needs to be done within minutes in order to confer any benefit. In order to prevent further spread of the substance, which remains on the skin, patients should be decontaminated on arrival to the hospital, prior to entering any building or hospital structure. Staff should be fully attired in MOPP gear or other approved protective suits as well as a gas mask [12].

The method of decontamination is still an area of uncertainty. Recommendations in the past have included simple soap and water, various oils, and even household bleach, but no studies have been done in humans to evaluate these methods. Limited animal studies have been done showing some benefit of iodine application to exposed areas, but there is not strong enough evidence to recommend one agent over another. Given availability, simple soap and water may be the easiest method for skin decontamination. A simple and thorough saline flush is reasonable for eye decontamination [5, 7].

Following decontamination, management becomes primarily supportive. Eye injuries may be mild or severe. Some studies in rabbits have shown small benefit to topical anti-inflammatory drugs, but there are no comparative studies in humans [7]. Consultation with an ophthalmologist, when available, is recommended.

Treatment of skin injuries is also supportive. Generally, treatment will mirror that of thermal burns with focus on preventing infection. Topical iodine and sodium hypochlorite have been studied in animals with some evidence of benefit, but again no human studies have been done [7]. Recommendations currently are to focus on immediate decontamination to prevent worsening of symptoms, then treat supportively as you would thermal burns.

There is no specific treatment for lung injury in mustard gas exposure. Some animal studies have shown benefit from steroids and from antibiotics, but no human data are available [7, 12]. While in vitro experiments have demonstrated both NAC and doxycycline to result in decreased cellular injury, these data are not robust enough to routinely recommend. Management should focus on aggressive supportive care [14].

Lewisite was a successor to sulfur mustard. It is more volatile and causes almost immediate eye irritation as opposed to the delayed symptoms caused by mustard gas. Lewisite is an organic arsenical compound and has significant vesicant and systemic toxicity [7, 12].

As with mustard gas, decontamination is important. Recommendations for eye and skin decontamination as well as for pulmonary injury are the same as those for mustard gas victims. No specific studies have been done [7]. Treatment for Lewisite exposure is simplified by availability of several antidotes.

During World War II, the British developed an antidote to Lewisite called British anti-Lewisite (BAL) [15]. Fifty-six million tubes of BAL ointment were distributed to US troops during the war [16]. BAL has also been used in civilian medicine to treat multiple heavy metal toxicities. BAL forms a complex with arsenic and was extensively tested in humans during WWII, but these data were not published. Although ointments were distributed during WWII, currently only IM administration of BAL is approved. The commercial preparation is 10 % BAL in peanut oil. Recommended dose is 0.5 mL/25 lb bodyweight up to a maximum of 4.0 mL. This dose can be repeated in 4, 8, and 12 h (see Table 18.2) [16].

BAL does have significant toxicity, resulting in persistently rising systolic and diastolic blood pressures, tachycardia, headaches, nausea, vomiting, anxiety, sweating, and even coma and convulsions at high doses [15]. Newer antidotes to Lewisite are 2,3-dimercapto-1-propanesulfonic acid (DMPS) and meso-dimercaptosuccinnic acid (DMSA), two water-soluble analogs of BAL. DMSA and DMPS are both less toxic than BAL and can be administered orally. There are no routinely recommended dosages for Lewisite exposure as there has been no opportunity to use these drugs in humans exposed to Lewisite. Animals studies show positive results in rabbits exposed to Lewisite who are then treated with DMSA or DMPS up to 90 min post exposure (see Table 18.2) [7, 15].

Treatment of Lewisite should focus on administration of appropriate antidotes. BAL, DMSA, and DMPS have all been shown to benefit patients. DMSA and DMPS have a better safety profile than BAL, but choice of agent will likely depend on availability.

18.3.3 Pulmonary Irritants

Pulmonary irritants are agents that cause lung irritation by penetration into the tissues of the airways. Chlorine and phosgene are the two pulmonary irritants that have been used most frequently in warfare. Both agents act by forming hydrochloric acid on contact with water, causing airway

Table 18.2 Lewisite antidotes

Lewisite antidotes	Mechanism of action	Dosing	Side effects
British anti-Lewisite (BAL) (dimercaprol) [a]contraindicated in renal disease, pregnancy, concurrent use of medicinal iron, and peanut allergy	Chelates arsenic	3–5 mg/kg deep IM injection q4hr for 4 doses, then repeated as needed depending on severity	Usually seen at 5 mg/kg dose: Vomiting, seizures, stupor, coma, headache, anxiety, chest, and throat pain
DMSA (meso-2,3-dimercaptosuccinic acid)	Chelates arsenic	10–30 mg/kg/day in three divided doses (3 days on, 11 days off, for 8 cycles)[a]	Uncommon: GI disturbances, urticaria
DMPS	Chelates arsenic	3–5 mg/kg IV over 5 min q4hr for 24 h, then 400 mg PO q4hr for 1–5 days	Hypotension, allergic reaction, skin rashes

Sources: (1) Agency for toxic substances and disease registry [Internet]. Atlanta: Centers for Disease Control; 2014 [cited 2015 Jun 7]. http://www.atsdr.cdc.gov/mmg/mmg.asp?id=922&tid=190. (2) Alternative Medicine Review. Monograph: meso-2-3-dimercaptosuccinic Acid. [Internet] [place unknown] Thorne Research, Inc; 2001 [cited 2015 Jun 7]. http://www.altmedrev.com/publications/5/3/264.pdf. (3) Ronco C, Bellomo R, Kellum J. Critical Care Nephrology. Elsevier Health Sciences; 2008. (4) Moore DF, O'Callaghan CA, Berlyne G, Ogg CS, Davies HA, House IM, et al. Acute arsenic poisoning: absence of polyneuropathy after treatment with 2,3-dimercaptopropanesulphonate (DMPS). J Neurol Neurosurg Psychiatr. 1994;57:1133–35
[a]*Note:* dosing of DMSA and DMPS based on doses for general heavy metal chelation, not specific to Lewisite exposure

tissue edema and capillary leakage [7]. Chlorine also produces hypochloric acid and an oxygen-free radical on contact with water, all contributing to lung damage [17].

In addition to formation of hydrochloric acid, phosgene also undergoes acylation, a reaction by which phosgene loses carbon and oxygen atoms to nucleophilic components in the tissues, causing direct damage to lung surfactant followed by downstream release of arachadonic acid mediators. Ultimately, this leads to vascular permeability, alveolar leakage, and pulmonary edema [18].

Chlorine is easily obtained and easily dispersed and has a relatively higher water solubility than phosgene. This property results in more immediate noxious effects resulting in victims fleeing the site of exposure and not allowing lower airway effects to occur. However, exposure to large doses may in fact penetrate lower airways [17]. Chlorine may also have effects on the eyes and skin, although these are easily treated with water or saline flushes [7]. Chlorine acts much more rapidly than phosgene, causing symptoms within minutes. If symptomatic, patients usually present with cough, hemoptysis, chest tightness, and dyspnea [14].

Phosgene, in high enough concentrations, smells of musty hay or green corn. Initial exposure to phosgene can cause some mild eye irritation via formation of hydrochloric acid. As with chlorine, simple eye washes and irrigation are effective in treating these symptoms. Phosgene's property of lower water solubility allows victims to have ongoing exposure without immediate upper airway effects. Therefore, the lower airways are more affected than in chlorine gas exposures. After high concentration exposure, immediate symptoms may include throat irritation, cough, headache, nausea, vomiting, and chest tightness. It is important to emphasize that delayed symptoms may not appear for up to 48 h and patients may be symptom free for this period. Later symptoms are secondary to acylation as opposed to hydrochloric acid formation. Delayed symptoms include cough, dyspnea, tachypnea, and respiratory distress caused by pulmonary edema [14, 18].

There are no antidotes to chlorine or phosgene and there is some controversy concerning treatment for lung injury. Management is primarily supportive with positive pressure ventilation and humidified oxygen. Limited animal and human series support this approach, but no controlled studies in humans have been done [7]. Bronchodilators can be given if bronchospasm develops, but otherwise are not routinely recommended [7, 14].

There are some animal studies and case studies supporting the use of nebulized sodium bicarbonate in chlorine inhalation with some improvement in respiratory function. One prospective study in humans exposed to chlorine showed some improvement in FEV1 and quality of life after nebulized sodium bicarbonate, but otherwise no significant difference was found [7, 17]. In animals, N-acetyl-L-cysteine has shown some benefit in decreasing lung pathology after phosgene exposure [14, 18]. Corticosteroids may be of some benefit in both phosgene and chlorine exposure based on success in other inflammatory lung conditions as well as animal studies, but again no human studies exist to confirm this benefit so this cannot be routinely recommended [17, 18].

In summary, care of patients exposed to pulmonary irritants depends on awareness of the likely areas of injury. If a report of chlorine or phosgene attack is given, on-scene providers must decontaminate when possible and use protective gear. In a hospital setting, providers must anticipate need for respiratory support for a large number of patients, initial care likely being limited to humidified oxygen and positive pressure ventilation if indicated.

18.3.4 Nerve Agents

Nerve agents as a group are potent derivatives of organophosphate pesticides. The most notable weaponized forms of organophosphates currently in existence are tabun (GA), sarin (GB), soman (GD), and VX, although there are many others [7]. Nerve agents are colorless, odorless, tasteless, and do not cause skin irritation. They can be dispersed and are harmful as vapor, liquid, or aerosol. Much of the research concerning organophosphates is limited to commercial exposure from pesticides. It is uncertain if these data can

be safely extrapolated to include treatment of nerve agents, but it is currently the best information available [7, 15, 19, 20].

Nerve agents are irreversible inhibitors of cholinesterase enzymes, primarily acetylcholinesterase (AChE). AChE is an enzyme responsible for breaking down acetylcholine (ACh), the neurotransmitter that acts at post-synaptic nicotinic and muscarinic receptors. By inhibiting the breakdown of ACh, nerve agents act to increase activation at these receptors, leading to a cholinergic toxidrome. The relative potency of these agents depends on the time it takes for the bond between the agent and the enzyme to "age," or become an irreversibly inactivated enzyme. While soman ages within minutes, sarin and tabun take hours and VX even days [7, 20].

Symptoms of the cholinergic toxidrome begin immediately. Increased ACh at muscarinic receptors causes miosis, bradycardia, increased airway secretions, vomiting and diarrhea, hypersalivation, and increased urination. ACh at nicotinic receptors causes pupil dilation, tachycardia, bronchodilation, hypertension, sweating, and muscle weakness. At central receptors, increased ACh causes anxiety, confusion, lethargy, coma, and seizures. The overall picture can vary greatly. Significant exposures can cause death within minutes. Mortality is commonly attributed to excessive secretions resulting in pulmonary edema, hypoxia, and ultimately respiratory arrest [15].

Patients are exposed through inhalation or absorption through skin. As with all agents so far discussed, decontamination is extremely important. Emergency personnel should don full protective gear and gas mask. All clothing should be removed from the patient. Simple soap and water, or water alone is likely sufficient to remove residual agent, however this will not break down the agent, so disposal of runoff must be managed so that agent does not reach general water supply or sewer system [7, 15]. There are some formulations for decontamination available through the military that are composed of charcoal or adsorbent resins, but no studies have compared efficacy of these various decontaminants. If they are available, they should be used [15]. Decontamination must occur as soon as possible and prior to patient entering a treatment facility.

Standard antidotes available for treatment of nerve agent exposure are atropine and pralidoxime (2-PAM), with benzodiazepines as needed for seizure activity. Atropine competes with excess acetylcholine by binding and inactivating muscarinic acetylcholine receptors, therefore acting as an antimuscarinic agent [20]. Atropine counters bronchoconstriction and secretions as well as nausea, vomiting, and diarrhea. Atropine also partially counteracts the central respiratory depression caused by nerve agents [15]. Since increased respiratory secretions and respiratory depression are the main cause of death, atropine is the most important initial treatment.

Dosing of atropine will vary according to the severity of exposure. The US military provides Mark 1 kits with autoinjectors of atropine, each containing 2 mg. In minor cases, one injection may suffice, but repeated doses may be needed in more severe cases. Generally, atropine should be initiated intramuscularly or intravenously as soon as possible. Initial dose may range from 2 to 8 mg depending on severity of symptoms. Patients should be re-dosed with atropine every 3–8 min as long as symptoms persist. Atropine dosing in this situation does not have an upper limit. The primary endpoints of atropine therapy are to eliminate respiratory secretions and maintain cardiovascular function (i.e., maintain blood pressure and heart rate) (see Table 18.3) [15, 19, 20].

As evidenced by the Tokyo subway sarin attack in 1995, availability of atropine may become an issue in some facilities given the high doses that might be required and the number of patients that need treatment [2]. In the event that more atropine cannot be obtained, other anticholinergics can be substituted. Glycopyrrolate is one of the alternatives that has been considered and was studied in one small, randomized controlled trial versus atropine, showing no difference in efficacy. Some providers do advocate use of glycopyrrolate in conjunction with atropine to help minimize CNS effects of atropine. From the information we have so far, which is limited, it seems that glycopyrrolate is a reasonable alternative to atropine, especially if atropine supply is limited. Standard dosing for glycopyrrolate in nerve agent or organophosphate pesticide poisoning has not been determined [20].

Another alternative treatment that may be available is scopolamine. It is uncertain if scopolamine would be an effective agent on its own, but some small studies have shown that scopolamine is a useful adjunct to atropine therapy. Scopolamine crosses the blood–brain barrier more readily than atropine and may exert its effect by decreasing CNS symptoms in the acute as well as long-term setting. If atropine is in short supply, it is reasonable to use scopolamine as an adjunct [15, 21].

In the event of severe atropine shortage and large numbers of patients, other alternative treatments may be needed. Most civilian emergency departments have insufficient supply to treat a large number of patients. One study looked at the efficacy of utilizing ophthalmic antimuscarinic agents to treat organophosphate poisoning in rats [22]. In this protocol, four groups of rats were pretreated with saline, atropine, ophthalmic tropicamide, or ophthalmic cyclopentolate solutions. Survival in each of the atropine, tropicamide, and cyclopentolate groups was 90 %, compared to only 10 % in the control group. These preliminary data indicate that parenteral use of ophthalmic solutions may be considered as an alternative to atropine in situations of severe shortages of standard atropine [22].

The other standard therapy for nerve agent or organophosphate exposure is pralidoxime, or other oximes. Oximes act to reactivate acetylcholinesterase by dissociating it from the nerve agent [15]. Reactivation is limited by the aging process of the bond between AChE and nerve agent. Once the bond between nerve agent and acetylcholinesterase is irreversible (i.e., "has aged"), the pralidoxime is no longer effective [15, 20]. Pralidoxime has little to no CNS effect, exerting most of its effects by restoring skeletal muscle function.

In recent years, significant controversy has arisen over the efficacy and safety of oxime use in organophosphate poisoning. Multiple new agents

Table 18.3 Nerve agent antidotes

Nerve agent antidotes	Mechanism of action	Dosing	Side effects
Atropine	Acts at muscarinic receptors by competing with nerve agent	2–8 mg initial dosing IM or IV, re-dosing every 3–8 min until symptoms resolve	Tachycardia, hypertension, high fever, dry mucous membranes, delerium
Pralidoxime	Reactivates acetylcholinesterase	30 mg/kg bolus IV or IM followed by 8 mg/kg/h infusion	Rapid rise in blood pressure (potentially severe), tachycardia, weakness, dizziness, blurred vision

Sources: (1) Munro N, Watson A, Ambrose K, Griffin G. Treating exposure to chemical warfare agents: implications for health care providers and community emergency planning. Environ Health Perspect. 1990;89:205–15. (2) King A, Aaron C. Organophosphate and carbamate poisoning. Emerg Med Clin N Am. 2015;33:133–51. (3) Blain PG. Organophosphorous poisoning. Clin Evid. 2011;05:2102

have been developed showing varying efficacy and varying safety profiles. Patients respond differently depending on the agent of exposure. Overall, the evidence is mixed. There is no evidence good enough to eliminate pralidoxime from the treatment regimen and, as yet, no evidence sufficient to routinely recommend one of the newer oximes over the more traditionally used oximes. Studies are needed to further investigate whether any newer oximes are more broadly active across a spectrum of organophosphates and to further evaluate safety of all of these agents in human subjects. Studies in animals have already begun to focus on both questions [20, 23, 24].

Typical dosing of pralidoxime, according to the World Health Organization (WHO), is 30 mg/kg bolus followed by an 8 mg/kg/h infusion [20]. One small study attempted to evaluate intermittent bolus dosing of pralidoxime, but was not sufficiently powered to recommend this dose over the standard recommended dosing [25]. The WHO also recommends obidoxime as an alternative to pralidoxime. The WHO-recommended dose of obidoxime is a 250 mg bolus followed by 750 mg/24 h. In either case, oxime should be continued until at least 12 h after atropine is no longer required. Continued oxime therapy is warranted for a prolonged period following exposure, even up to 120 h, given that there may be continued reinhibition of AChE at higher concentrations of nerve agent (see Table 18.3) [20, 25].

Nerve agents are among some of the most lethal of the chemical warfare agents. Health care workers should protect themselves fully prior to approaching patients. Primary treatment at present is comprised of immediate decontamination, atropine, an oxime (likely pralidoxime), and supportive care.

18.4 Conclusion

Most health care personnel will never encounter a chemical attack, nevertheless, it is important to be prepared. We must understand the importance of personal protection prior to treatment. If health care workers become patients, our ability to effectively care for patients is only further compromised. Early and close communication between pre-hospital and hospital personnel, when possible, allows early treatment and preparation. Anticipating symptoms and needed treatment, as well as the need for protective gear, is a major step to managing such an event.

Editor's Note: LCDR Jami Hickey, MD is currently serving on Active Duty in the United States Navy. She has served in one combat deployment.

CDR Sean M. Bryant, MD is an Emergency Medicine physician who also works as the Assistant Fellowship Director at the Toxikon Consortium and the Associate Medical Director at the Illinois Poison Center. He serves as a Reservist in the United States Navy.

References

1. Okumura T, Suzuki K, Fukuda A, Kohama A, Takasu N, Ishimatsu S, Hinohara S. The Tokyo subway sarin attack: disaster management, part 1: community emergency response. Acad Emerg Med. 1998;5(6): 613–7.
2. Okumura T, Suzuki K, Fukuda A, Kohama A, Takasu N, Ishimatsu S, Hinohara S. The Tokyo subway sarin attack: disaster management, part 2: hospital response. Acad Emerg Med. 1998;5(6):618–24.
3. Okumura T, Suzuki K, Fukuda A, Kohama A, Takasu N, Ishimatsu S, Hinohara S. The Tokyo subway sarin attack: disaster management, part 3: national and international response. Acad Emerg Med. 1998;5(6): 625–7.
4. Pangi R. Consequence management in the 1995 sarin attacks on the Japanese subway system. BCSIA Discussion Paper 2002-4, ESDP discussion Paper ESDP-2002-01, John F. Kennedy School of Government, Harvard University, 2002.
5. Tuorinsky S. Medical aspects of chemical warfare. Department of the Army. Office of the Surgeon General, Borden Institute (US) Government Printing Office, 2008.
6. Fitzgerald G. Chemical warfare and medical response during World War I. Am J Public Health. 2008;98:611–25.
7. Rodgers GC, Condurache CT. Antidotes and treatments for chemical warfare/terrorism agents: an evidence based review. Clin Pharm Ther. 2010;88(3): 318–27.
8. MacLennan L, Moiemen N. Management of cyanide toxicity in patients with burns. Burns. 2015;41: 18–24.
9. Bebarta V, Pitotti R, Dixon P, Lairet J, Bush A, Tanen D. Hydroxocobalamin vs sodium thiosulfate for the treatment of acute cyanide toxicity in a swine (Sus scrofa) model. Ann Emerg Med. 2012;59(6):532–9.
10. Bebarta V, Tanen D, Lairet J, Dixon P, Valtier S, Bush A. Hydroxocobalamin and sodium thiosulfate versus sodium nitrite and sodium thiosulfate in the treatment of acute cyanide toxicity in a swine (Sus scrofa) model. Ann Emerg Med. 2010;55(4):345–51.
11. Eckstein M. Enhancing public health preparedness for a terrorist attack involving cyanide. J Emerg Med. 2008;35(1):59–65.
12. Baker D. Critical care requirements after mass tox agent release. Crit Care Med. 2005;33(1):S66–74.
13. Ghabili K, Agutter P, Ghanei M, Ansarin K, Shoja M. Mustard gas toxicity: the acute and chronic pathological effects. J Appl Toxicol. 2010;30:627–43.
14. Russell D, Blaine PG, Rice P. Clinical management of casualties exposed to lung damaging agents: a critical review. Emerg Med J. 2006;23:421–4.
15. Munro N, Watson A, Ambrose K, Griffin G. Treating exposure to chemical warfare agents: implications for health care providers and community emergency planning. Environ Health Perspect. 1990;89:205–15.
16. Vilensky J, Redman K. British anti-Lewisite (dimercaprol): an amazing history. Ann Emerg Med. 2003;41(3):378–83.
17. Vajner J, Lung D. Case files of the University of California San Francisco Medical Toxicology Fellowship: acute chlorine gas inhalation and the utility of nebulized sodium bicarbonate. J Med Toxicol. 2013;9:259–65.
18. Grainge C, Rice P. Management of phosgene-induced acute lung injury. Clin Toxicol. 2010;48:497–508.
19. King A, Aaron C. Organophosphate and carbamate poisoning. Emerg Med Clin N Am. 2015;33:133–51.
20. Blain PG. Organophosphorous poisoning. Clin Evid. 2011;05:2102.
21. Koplovitz I, Schulz S. Perspectives on the use of scopolamine as an adjunct treatment to enhance survival following organophosphorus nerve agent poisoning. Mil Med. 2010;175(11):878–82.
22. Bryant SM, Rhee JW, Thompson TM, Lu JJ, Aks SE. Parenteral ophthalmic tropicamide or cyclopentolate protects rats from lethal organophosphate poisoning. Am J Ther. 2009;16(3):231–4.
23. Kassa J, Karasova J, Musilek K, Kuca K, Bajgar J. An evaluation of reactivating and therapeutic efficacy of newly developed oximes (K206, K269) and commonly used oximes (obidoxime, HI-6) in cyclosarin-poisoned rats and mice. Clin Tox. 2009;47:72–6.
24. Wilhelm CM, Snider TH, Babin MC, Jett DA, Platoff Jr GE, Yeung DT. A comprehensive evaluation of the efficacy of leading oxime therapies in guinea pigs exposed to organophosphorus chemical warfare agents or pesticides. Toxicol Appl Pharmacol. 2014; 281:254–65.
25. Tang X, Ruilan W, Xie H, Hu J, Zhao W. Repeated pulse intramuscular injection of pralidoxime chloride in severe acute organophosphorus pesticide poisoning. Am J Emerg Med. 2013;31:946–9.

Providing Surgical Training and Assistance in a Developing Country During Military Assistance

19

Henry Lin

19.1 Introduction

When medical assets are deployed to other nations, there is often an agreement between the host nation and the country placing the asset. The benefits of such a relationship, however, do not have to be limited to political, strategic, or even humanitarian goals. The United States military has placed forces in Djibouti and the United States Navy was tasked with providing the medical support for those forces. The medical asset though can do more than provide this support. Using embedded expertise, the team members can help educate and train host nation physicians, surgeons, anesthesia providers, surgical technicians, and nurses. In addition, they can also promote

H. Lin, M.D. (✉)
General Surgery and Urology, Naval Hospital
Camp LeJeune, Uniformed Services University
of the Health Sciences, 100 Brewster Blvd,
Camp LeJeune, NC 28547, USA
e-mail: StarchMD@gmail.com

and provide resources for preventative care. But despite the altruistic force driving these actions, challenges exist in achieving these goals. This chapter will describe these goals in further details as well as the challenges.

19.2 Why Are We in Djibouti?

Camp Lemonnier is a United States Naval Expeditionary Base situated in the country of Djibouti located in the region of the Horn of Africa as the only US military base in Africa. "The focus is to combat a new generation of terrorist groups across the continent, from Mali to Libya to the Central African Republic." There is a Role II Military Treatment Facility, Expeditionary Medical Facility Djibouti, located there in support of that effort. A surgical team is assigned there for triage and emergency surgical treatment of wounded service members.

Djibouti is generally viewed as a developing country with 40 % of its population below the poverty line and 60 % unemployed. However, there are very small numbers of very wealthy civilians as is not uncommon in poor countries.

© Springer International Publishing Switzerland 2016
C.R.B. Lim (ed.), *Surgery During Natural Disasters, Combat, Terrorist Attacks, and Crisis Situations*, DOI 10.1007/978-3-319-23718-3_19

19.3 What Is the Difference between a MEDCAP (Medical Civilian Action Project) and an Ongoing Relationship in a Memorandum of Understanding between Two Surgical Units of Different Nations?

Generally, a United States military Civilian Action Project is designed to assist an area by using the capabilities and resources of a military force or civilian organization to conduct short-term projects in a particular region. In a MEDCAP, medical doctors and specialists with equipment and supplies usually set up a temporary field clinic to provide limited medical treatment to the local population. MEDCAPs are generally narrow in scope and usually provide targeted assistance, such as inoculations.

Although MEDCAPs have a certain appeal to rendering some medical aid, there has recently been much criticism since the outpouring of generosity can have significant unintended consequences due to the unsustainable nature of these efforts. For example, malignancy resections have, in doctrine, been excluded historically from MEDCAPs since long-term surveillance and adjunctive treatment, like chemoradiation, are not possible in these desperate areas of medical need.

A Memorandum of Understanding, however, generally is an agreement between two entities, frequently between two governments, regarding the conduct of transactions between two nations. A Memorandum of Understanding had been proposed between the government of Djibouti & the government of the United States regarding the conduct of medical exchanges, assistance, and services to promote coordination of care for patients from both nations as well as further training and skills sustainment between medical teams from both nations.

19.4 Why Do We Collaborate with Pelletier General Hospital?

As surgical skills can attrite during the deployment, there have been arrangements made with a local public hospital, Pelletier General Hospital,

to allow for members of the surgical team to operate there a few days per week. (Frequently, forward deployed Role II surgical teams do not perform many operations when not in a "hot spot" or theater of significant hostile military interventions.) This arrangement helps to prevent skill erosion that will inevitably occur if there are no patients for whom to care for. Concurrently, this availability of significant time allows for the training of the local Djiboutian surgeons. In this situation, the Navy surgical team taught the local Djibouti surgical teams the nuances of advanced laparoscopic/minimally invasive surgery.

19.5 How Does the Djiboutian General Surgeon Learn from US Military Surgeons?

Since the Djiboutian general surgeon obtained his surgical training from Tanzania, he had little experience beyond basic laparoscopy, such as a laparoscopic cholecystectomy. Older but very functional equipment was being replaced at EMF Djibouti. After proper approvals, the older but functional laparoscopic equipment were donated to this local public hospital. Equipment without proper instruction, however, has historically been underutilized. The Memorandum of Understanding permitted the United States team to train and mentor the local surgeon and surgery team.

19.6 What Were the Limitations of Teaching? Equipment?

The teaching was not as optimal as it could be. Simulation training, for instance, is the preferred way to start surgical residents on their laparoscopic development. Having a training box, like Fundamentals of Laparoscopic Surgery (FLS), would improve the skill set of the surgical team without putting any patients at risk. Limitations on funds were part of this key problem. The developing nation was so limited in funds that the Djiboutian surgical teams were reusing disposable equipment, like electrosurgical devices, by dipping in "sterilizing solutions" like chlorhexidine gluconate.

Equipment without training is nearly worthless. Until the Naval surgical team re-visited to see if the donated equipment was being used, that equipment initially sat in a storage area. When a follow-on Naval surgical team brought their surgical technicians over to teach the local surgical technicians how to use the equipment, sterilize, and process them, the utilization went up exponentially.

The local Djiboutian surgeon had solid basic general surgery training, so advanced laparoscopy instruction was picked up very quickly. Our surgical team focused on two main goals:

1. Changing the view of the camera to optimize visualization of structures, especially for laparoscopic cholecystectomy.
2. Using endostaplers as well as endoloops for laparoscopic appendectomies.

There were obvious early benefits of bringing laparoscopic surgery to the Djiboutian population in regards to perceived early return to work, return to previous functional status, and a decrease in wound infection rates.

Similar benefits were perceived for laparoscopic appendectomies. But the expensive endostaplers donated from France, another very involved country in the region, quickly ran out and again funding was limited. Demonstration of the laparoscopic approach to appendectomies, however, with an EndoLoop® to ligate the appendiceal stump and mesoappendix, increased the capability of that surgical team with a much less expensive option. The EndoLoop® costs $35 and 3–4 are typically required with this approach while it costs $500 for two sets of laparoscopic staplers that are required for each laparoscopic appendectomy.

19.7 How Did the Djiboutian General Surgeon Teach Our Surgical Team?

Since much of American surgery has progressed to the laparoscopic and endoscopic approach, the experience with open surgery has decreased significantly, especially in the more recently

graduated American surgeons. The Djiboutian surgical team was able to provide additional experience with open common bile duct exploration, open prostatectomies, and complex incarcerated open inguinal herniorrhaphies. A key component was demonstrating how to perform these surgeries with less than optimal equipment, a skill set highly valued in an austere environment.

19.8 Why Did the Collaboration Improve the Process for Both Host Nation and Military Teams?

The local Djiboutian surgical team developed a much better understanding of the new updates in modern surgical technique to help improve their capabilities. The local Djiboutian surgical team was able to refresh the open/traditional approaches to the Naval surgical teams since very frequently, in the far forward setting, advanced equipment was too bulky and cumbersome to mobilize to the field with. Although EMF Djibouti had relatively sophisticated modern equipment, the collaborative surgical practice increased the confidence level of many members of the surgical team. This confidence boost was similar to that gained when previous members of the surgical team had attended the Naval Trauma Training Center at Los Angeles County—University of Southern California prior to other deployments.

19.9 How Did Reuse of Disposable Surgical Equipment by the Djiboutian Surgical Team Give Perspective to How Our Modern Surgical Teams Currently Function?

Our Naval surgical team was obviously dismayed by the Djiboutian team reusing disposable equipment, like the electrosurgical tip and cord, the suction tubing for open cases, the laparoscopic irrigation and suction devices, and the disposable laparoscopic trocars. All of our United States-based training and packaging devices warned us about the potential patient-to-patient transmission of more occult or latent infections, despite utilizing "sterilization" liquids like betadine or chlorhexidine. These concerning infections include hepatitis C and HIV that may not manifest for many years. The Djiboutian surgical team, however, boasted low iatrogenic bacterial and viral infectious rates and felt that their recapture rate was very good since the high indigent population had no other facility to go to in the city of Djibouti, with a population of 600,000. This perception, however, did not find statistical evidence in the first retrospective review of this practice. If these data suggest a low iatrogenic infectious rate in future studies, consideration of this practice for further humanitarian efforts may result in more efficient use of surgical resources.

19.10 How Could Future Collaborative Efforts Be Improved?

There are several factors that interfered with optimal collaboration:

1. There was significant difficulty with funding for surgical equipment.
2. Endoscopy was not readily available.
3. Conflict of interest with other nations' efforts, e.g. Chinese, Egypt.
4. Hospital facilities not conducive to interaction (e.g. clean restrooms, secure areas for surgical team, air conditioning, stable electricity, operating room doors to keep out flies).

Once the stock of initial consumable equipment was utilized, there were problems continuing that type of technique with some of the surgeries. The Endostaplers for the laparoscopic appendectomies were key consumable supplies that created access to care problems. Funding was routed via the Ministry of Health but there were significant difficulties with the final routing of those funds to the purchasing agents. The laparoscopic stapler issue was dealt with substituting for EndoLoop®. The local surgeon then took to requesting supplies be sent directly from donors from France in order for those consumable supplies to reach him. The routing with this method was not completely smooth, however, since intermittently the shipping authorities did not deliver the entire inventory which were purportedly sent.

Additionally, western hospitals routinely donate near-expiring supplies and medications for third world country use, usually in the name of a "Remedy" program. Examples include older model needles or near-expiring meds from crash cart inventory and restocking. Under similar principles, near-expiring medications and consumable materials had historically been donated to the Djiboutian public hospital. But at least two concerns grew over the years. Would an iatrogenic infection or suboptimal outcome be alleged to result from these donations? And what would be the perception in the public eye if reporting occurred that did not balance the desperate needs of the indigent population against the closeness to expiration of these medications and consumable supplies? Hence, these types of fear began to grow and the previously mutually beneficial practices were dropped.

Endoscopic equipment was also attempted to be ordered by the local hospital so that the naval surgical team could help provide the training required to the local team. According to the surgical team at that hospital, the requesting orders appeared to get stuck for many months in the ordering request chain for that nation.

Other nations had ongoing efforts of delivering care to the local population but only on their terms. For example, the Chinese built a new, modern hospital on the western part of the city where many of the affluent officials lived. Unfortunately, there are not many of these officials and their families tended to be were very healthy. Consequently, the hospital remained vastly underutilized, with operations performed on less than 15 patients per week. When our local Djiboutian surgeon attempted to coordinate care with the indigent patients to bring them to this hospital to utilize the underutilized operating rooms, he surprisingly met resistance from the families of the indigent patients. These indigent families could not afford to travel to that nicer Chinese hospital. The culture of the local population was to send significant numbers of the family members to care for their ill family member since less than one nurse per ward of 15 patients would usually be available to provide care per shift.

Frequently there would not be overnight nurses in many of the wards due to limited staffing at Pelletier General Hospital. Even when these families were told that nursing support was much better at the Chinese hospital (comparable ratio to American standards), these families still refused to let their family members travel far, about a 30-min taxi ride that was exceedingly expensive (for an average annual income of $1400), to have care at this Chinese hospital.

Additionally, there was a very elegant Egyptian hospital with capabilities to perform TransUrethral Resection of the Prostate for Benign Prostatic Hypertrophy. But this high end facility staff had not yet been amenable to discussions for payments otherwise by the government of Djibouti. As a result, many elderly Djiboutian men consented to the available open radical prostatectomies to relieve their severe urinary retention from their BPH since they did not have access to a TURP procedure.

There was, however, another NATO (North Atlantic Treaty Organization) country, France, which also had a Role II hospital in Djibouti. But that outstanding and well-staffed facility, Bouffard French Military Hospital, had recently limited its access to care to only cash-paying patients due in part to the financial burdens that that country was facing at home. The United States Naval surgical team also had initiated a Memorandum of Agreement for collaboration with the French Military Hospital. Most of the collaborative work at that hospital was between the French military medical teams and the U.S. Naval surgical teams while caring for the local Djiboutians. There was no collaboration at that facility with the local Djiboutian surgical team. That is, the French MOU did not allow for training of the host nation surgical teams.

Although the staff at Pelletier General Hospital was very hospitable, the physical condition of the facility was not physically conducive to American standards of hospitality. The general surgeon invited the team to his office to use as a changing/locker area but there were no other very clean areas to the hospital. The surgical team would leave their personal gear in the supply closet to the operating rooms since they carried their personnel protective equipment with them, e.g. gowns, gloves, masks, headgear, shoe covers, and scrub brushes.

The toilets were excessively dirty. The staff toilet had water constantly all over the floor and the toilets for the patients were rarely cleaned and frequently had diarrhea from patients. Moreover, they were not usually flushed. Additionally, feral felines roamed the halls, patrolling for rodents.

Air conditioning was frequently not functional outside of the operating room which made travel to the wards for postoperative checks very uncomfortable when the outdoor temperature was frequently 120 °F. Consequently, the ward temperature averaged 90 °F on the cooler days. When the temperature did cool down to 80 °F in the winter, the rains not infrequently caused instability of the electricity, requiring cancellations of elective surgeries.

Even the doors to the operating room were problematic since many of the hinges to these wooden doors were broken and flies frequently entered the room. As a result, the ongoing "joke" was that the surgical teams were not operating fast enough if the flies had time to land in the surgical wound. Initial efforts to donated sophisticated doors were met with worries about the local hospital engineers not having the capabilities to fix the doors should they break in the future. Furthermore, ongoing concerns with the local embassy focused on providing the local facilities with sustainable equipment that the local engineers could maintain. The justification stated was that the generosity of the collaborating nations would not always be present and that developing sustainable independence was a higher priority than potential quick-fixes that relied on current generosity of donor nations and private donors.

19.11 How Was the Local Christian Wound Clinic Affected by U.S. Assistance?

Caritas was a local wound clinic in Djibouti that was run by Catholic volunteers. A few nuns provided this free care to all local Djiboutians and significant efforts were made by American servicepersons, to include those with medical experience. After several months of active participation with improvements in the facility (e.g. constructing shade for the ongoing care in 115 °F weather), there were significant efforts to deter further collaboration. The sources of this deterrence were unclear but varied in etiology. There were claims that Muslims of the mostly Muslim Djibouti did not want this Catholic clinic to receive continued assistance. Additionally, there were concerns about donations of expired medications and dressing supplies, similar to the earlier discussion about perception taken out of context of the local desperateness of the indigent population. Additionally, there developed a focus to decrease funding toward unsustainable charitable efforts and to promote investments in sustainable practices.

Thus, a very robust wound care clinic lost many active volunteers due to concerns about likely misperceptions of potentially second-rate care. This fear, however, resulted in what some medical personnel from several other assisting nations perceived to be understaffing of a desperately needed clinic for long-term complicated wound care.

19.12 How Else Does the Medical Team Provide Assistance?

To increase the probability of providing sustainable assistance, training and language assistance were focused on. Hence, members of EMF Djibouti visited the medical school to provide education on English since that remained the medical language of choice in many of the African countries. Programs were proposed to provide similar training to nursing and laboratory technician students.

19.13 Conclusions

The members of the medical and surgical team at EMF Djibouti did provide many collaborative efforts to assist the development of the hospital at the local public general hospital. The efforts, however, were severely hampered at many points due to worries about potential misperception of "second-rate" care provided to the indigent population. Instead of focusing on the generosity of donors to help desperate patients, there became heightened worries about providing equity of medical care. As a consequence, donations of near-expiring medications and medical consumable supplies stopped and these desperately needed supplies were discarded, contrary to the practice many Remedy organizations at American hospitals that redistribute these supplies to poor countries. Furthermore, the political perception of religious groups interfered with the ability of volunteers to assist medical groups due to the presumed affiliation with certain religions.

Finally, the concern about sustainability led to short-term difficulties with delivering surgical assistance to patients in desperate need. Although the concerns on sustainability are laudable, there were many patients who lost opportunities for good charitable care during the attempts to find sustainable approach. Further thought and plans should be considered to permit charitable care during the attempts for developing sustainable approaches. These lessons from the experience in Djibouti should allow for better short- and long-term planning for both charitable and sustainable aid to developing countries.

Special appreciation goes to Dr. Elias Said Dirie, the local Djiboutian General Surgeon, who provided the critical collaboration in the interest of improving the care for his Djiboutian patients.

Editor's Note: CDR Henry Lin, MD is currently on Active Duty in the United States Navy. He has been deployed five times to the combat zone including this trip to Djibouti. He is fellowship trained via Beth Israel Deaconess Medical Center at Harvard Medical School in Advanced Laparoscopic & Bariatric Surgery.

Use What You've Got: Resource Utilization in a Mass Casualty in Afghanistan

20

Jennifer M. Gurney

Do what you can, with what you have, where you are.
——Theodore Roosevelt

In October 2005, 4 months after completing surgery residency I received Orders from the US Army to deploy with a Forward Surgical Team to Afghanistan. During my surgical residency at Walter Reed Army Medical Center, I was one of many surgical residents who cared for countless combat casualties from the Iraq and Afghanistan wars. Starting in early 2002, almost all wounded service members were evacuated out of theater and were ultimately cared for at Walter Reed Army Medical Center. Despite this experience and training, I had a fair bit of angst about deployment—not just because I was going to a warzone—but essentially because I was a junior surgeon deploying with a small, mobile surgical team to a far-forward position on the battlefield.

20.1 Afghanistan 2005, Uruzgan

Talent wins games, but teamwork and intelligence win championships.
——Michael Jordan

J.M. Gurney, M.D., F.A.C.S. (✉)
Department of Surgery, San Francisco General Hospital, 1001 Potrero Avenue, Ward 3A, San Francisco, CA 94110, USA
e-mail: jennifergurney@hotmail.com

The Forward Surgical Team (FST) to which I was assigned was performing "split operations." While a normal sized FST had 20 members, our group of ten was initially in southern Afghanistan on a small Australian Special Operations Base. Within the first days of arrival into Afghanistan, I quickly learned the value of teamwork and the importance of planning.

As a surgical resident, training emphasized individual skill acquisition, taking care of incredibly sick patients and becoming the best surgeon possible. While teamwork was never taught and rarely emphasized, those individuals who could function well on a team generally had better residency training experiences. As someone who grew up playing sports, I was an okay team player, but during residency I was so very focused on my individual performance and education; I did not foster any teamwork skills. When it came time for me to deploy, I looked around at the nine other individuals with which I would be working and living with for the next 8 months; I honestly believed that as long as they could support *me* and facilitate *me* to get patients to the operating room—then all I had to be was a good surgeon. I learned very quickly that being a good surgeon on an FST was not just getting optimal outcomes in the operating room; I had to be a leader, a planner, and a team player.

Within a few days of arriving in southern Afghanistan we received three patients simultaneously all with penetrating abdominal wounds, all displaying early shock physiology, and all needing expeditious laparotomies. We had one operating room. Each surgical case required myself, the OR tech, the CRNA, the circulator, usually the orthopedic surgeon to assist with bigger cases, and frequently a medic to assist the CRNA. The other five to six personnel were responsible for continuing the triage and resuscitation of other critically injured patients awaiting surgery. Our team's shortcomings that day were blatantly obvious: only one medic knew how to run an I-STAT, our only means of obtaining a very limited amount of laboratory values, three of the medics had never placed IVs in actual trauma patients, only two knew how to run the portable X-ray machine, and our ER nurse had never worked in a trauma center, therefore had no experience in recognizing a decompensating trauma patient.

I was no better. Despite having good training, surgical skills, and judgment, I realized I also had significant shortcomings. I was terrible at communicating with the nurse anesthetist about my expectations of the case timing, resuscitation, and patient physiology. I underestimated the challenge of being able to operate and keep up with the clinical status and triage of the other patients awaiting surgery. I did not recognize the importance of thinking 10 steps ahead when it came to evacuating the patients and preparing for the next potential wave of casualties. Additionally, I certainly did not appreciate the incredible and precious resource of the walking blood bank particularly when our FST's blood supply was only ten units of packed red blood cells. Despite a disorganized approach, these three patients did very well; they were local Afghans, so we were able to see them in follow-up.

From that point on, our team trained. We ensured redundancy in many of the ATLS skills: every team member got good at putting in IVs; everyone could run the I-STAT machine and work the portable X-ray; everyone knew where the essential ATLS equipment was located; and all the medics were trained to be the Trauma Data Recorder. We also emphasized utilitarian communication so that everyone, regardless of rank or experience, was empowered to communicate

his or her concerns or suggestions during our After Action Reviews, which we did after every MassCal Incident (MCI).

To overcome our manpower limitations, our team also reached out to the medical assets on the Forward Operating Base. Every unit has medics and many of them have advanced "Combat Life Saver" skills; some units may even have a Primary Care Physician (PCP) or Physician Assistant (PA). We started involving the medics and Combat Life Savers in our daily operations and refined our Whole Blood Plan to be led by the Australian PCPs and senior medics. The Whole Blood Plan was crucial to our ability to take care of certain patients, but it is labor-intensive to maintain and implement. We therefore organized this vital component so that it did not involve personnel organic to our FST. By doing this, we freed up our team for direct patient care. We also ensured redundancy in the whole blood plan as well our triage system. Our ER Nurse was always the dedicated "triage manager" and he would work with the orthopedic surgeon, the anesthetist, the PCP or myself depending on the situation. And—we practiced and drilled and practiced and rehearsed…good old army training! Chance did indeed favor our preparedness. We were busy, so our plans were frequently implemented, repeatedly discussed, and regularly refined. We *all* got better, and within a few weeks our group of 10 was able to successfully orchestrate and manage many multiple casualty incidents.

20.2 Afghanistan 2006, Kunar

After 3 months at the Australian Forward Operating Base in southern Afghanistan, our team relocated to the Kunar Province in northeast Afghanistan. Close to the Pakistan border, there was heavy fighting and many ongoing combat operations. Our hospital was no longer in a tent, but was in a plywood structure that was approximately 60×25 feet. There was one large open room that we divided into an ATLS/resuscitation area, two-bed operating room, and an ICU consisting of four litters equipped with small portable

Fig. 20.1 Operating area and OR table. ATLS area is just to the right of the operating area

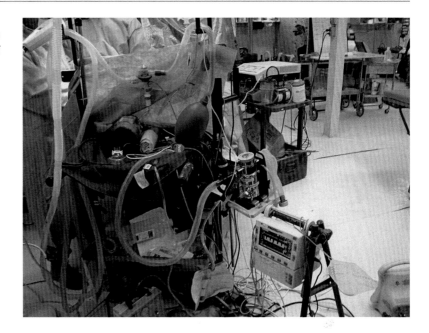

ventilators and IV poles. There was also an area for supplies and a small working/administration area with a desk and a phone (Fig. 20.1).

Our new base, close to the city of Asadabad, was the Forward Operating Base for multiple military elements including the 3rd Marine Regiment, the Army 10th Mountain Division, US Special Operations, and an elite Afghan Army group. A large joint task force operation called Operation Mountain Lion was set to launch on April 11, 2006 involving an estimated 2500 troops; military officials felt it would be the most significant effort to bring stability to the dangerous Korengal Valley (Fig. 20.2). In preparation for this combat operation, our FST received five additional personnel, including an OB-GYN (who, according to Army doctrine, acts in the role of a general surgeon), an OR tech, and a nurse anesthetist. This augmentation enabled our team to run two OR cases simultaneously.

20.3 Planning

> By failing to prepare, you are preparing to fail.
> ——Benjamin Franklin

In anticipation of frequent multiple casualty incidents, we planned, prepared, and rehearsed. See Table 20.1 for a partial overview of our Forward Surgical Team's MASCAL Plan.

My personal preparedness involved: working with the OR techs to ensure they knew what I needed for damage control cases; working with our two outstanding nurse anesthetists with regards to intraoperative management of the trauma patient (minimal crystalloid fluid, blood products, avoiding vasopressors, and communication with me of any changes in the patient's physiology); and working closely with the OB-GYN. During their training and later on in their practices, OB-GYN physicians are not typically exposed to, and do not manage, combat injuries of the magnitude seen during our deployment. However, because of our busy operative tempo, the OB-GYN, who was an exceptional surgeon, became quickly adept at abdominal packing and many damage control surgery techniques in a short period of time.

In terms of overcoming our manpower limitations, we did the same thing on the FOB at Asadabad that we did when we were in the Uruzgan Provence. Since there was a part of a Marine Regiment on the base, there were plenty of Navy Corpsmen (which are the medics of the Marines and Navy) as well as other Army medics. If they were not out on missions, they would be training with us at the FST. We involved the

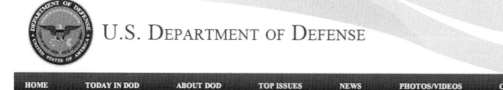

DoD News

NEWS ARTICLE   E-MAIL A COPY | PRINTER FRIENDLY | LATEST NEWS

Operation Mountain Lion Roars Into Korengal Valley

By Sgt. Joe Lindsay, USMC
Special to American Forces Press Service

KORENGAL VALLEY, Afghanistan, May 8, 2006 – Afghan National Army and coalition forces have been taking the war on terrorism to their adversaries in this enemy safe haven in Afghanistan's Kunar province for the past month.

Operation Mountain Lion began April 11 with night helicopter insertions of Afghan and coalition forces at strategic points throughout the valley, followed shortly by troops pushing up on foot through the mouth of the valley.

"We're taking the fight to the terrorists in their own backyard," Army Command Sgt. Maj. James Redmore, of Task Force Spartan, said. "They gave their victims no sanctuary. They'll receive none from us."

An estimated 2,500 Afghan and coalition forces are in the Korengal and surrounding valleys in what military officials are calling the most significant effort yet to bring stability to this war-torn region.

Fig. 20.2 DOD news about Operation Mountain Lion

local Afghan medical providers who had a small clinic on our base about 50 m from the FST. Because of space limitations, our triage area had to be outside; we ensured that the areas were well designated, illuminated, and sheltered. Additionally, we prepositioned three "Trauma Trunks" around the outside of our FST next to the triage areas. Each Trauma Trunk had ATLS supplies for 30 patients; "Trauma Tags" for identification, triage category, injury documentation and vitals; blankets and Sharpie markers.

20.4   April 11, 2006

> In preparing for battle I have always found that plans are useless, but planning is indispensable.
> ——Dwight D. Eisenhower

During the night of Tuesday April 11, 2006 Operation Mountain Lion would commence. That morning there was a different feeling on the base. The FOB was at capacity because none of the units were doing missions but were instead preparing for this huge combat operation. While there were more people at the dining facility for breakfast, it was much quieter. Marines and soldiers were checking their gear, vehicles were being loaded with supplies and there were long lines for the phones to call home. This operation would be ongoing for many weeks and it would be dangerous; the energy on the FOB felt different.

Around 10 AM we heard explosions and the sound of rockets whizzing over our heads. We ran to the bunkers. I remember feeling grateful that the rockets did not land on our FOB; they certainly were close. The retaliation fire from our FOB was impressive, loud and continuous while the Quick Reaction Force (QRF) geared up to race from the base to engage the perpetrators of the attack. As a surgeon, I took care of battlefield injuries every day; however, feeling the reverberation of an M119 Howitzer "charge 8" was a sobering reminder that our unit was amidst a battlefield. The details of the rocket attacks then

Table 20.1 Partial overview of FST MASCAL plan[a]

1. Notification and communication
(a) Recall of personnel to the FST
(b) Communication with base leadership
(c) Activation of our interpreters and the Afghan medical elements if the event involved Afghan civilians
(d) Communication with the CSH and MedEvac to facilitate evacuation to the CSH (the next level of care)
2. Security
(a) Ensuring that patients were disarmed prior to entering the FST
(b) Non-coalition forces were searched for weapons or explosives
(c) Enemy combatants patients were guarded
3. Triage
(a) Triage Officer
• May be fluid depending on the situation
– Requires a "master list"
– Requires excellent communication
(b) Simple Triage scheme (DIME)
• Delayed, immediate, minimal, expectant
(c) Analysis of FST and FOB resources
• Personnel and supply
(d) Ensuring all patients go through one entry point and that all patients get triaged
4. Patient flow
(a) One entry point (through the Triage area) and try to make patient flow in one direction
(b) Direct triage to the operating room is a good option for certain patients
(c) Map demonstrating casualty flow; all personnel understand the "flow of patient traffic"
5. After action review
(a) Performed after all rehearsals and multiple casualty incidents
(b) Involves *all* personnel involved in the event
(c) Review the sequence of events
(d) Each section (Triage, Command, OR, ATLS, Evac, etc.) comments on:
• Three things done well, three things done wrong, three areas of improvement
(e) Chief Surgeon and Command formalize input and changes MASCAL plan if necessary

[a]For a comprehensive review of military triage and mass casualty, please refer to Borden Institute, *Emergency War Surgery*, 4th ed., Fort Sam Houston, TX: 2013, Chapter 3, "Mass Casualty and Triage"

started gradually filtering in: the Taliban had attacked a primary school about a kilometer away. Our team was somewhat used to getting pediatric casualties, for months we had routinely taken care of children who were victims of the war and we were sadly accustomed to children of Afghanistan being among the Taliban's targets (Fig. 20.3).

Once it was confirmed that one of the rockets was a direct hit to the school full of young boys and girls, we immediately activated the MASCALplan. Given the proximity of our FOB to the school, teams quickly assembled to evacuate the casualties both by ground and by helicop-

ter (because of the terrain, 1 km may take 20 min to drive). Our team, the Afghan interpreters, the corpsmen, and medics assembled at the FST. The local Afghan doctors quickly arrived as well. The Afghan Clinic would be used for the minimally wounded and one of the rooms in the clinic would be used for those who were expectant.

Triage by the medics at the scene of the attack was excellent. The first helicopter arrived with four patients, all in need of urgent interventions. Three of the patients were children with penetrating abdominal and extremity wounds, the fourth was the Schoolmaster, and he presented with multiple fragment injuries to his left chest. While

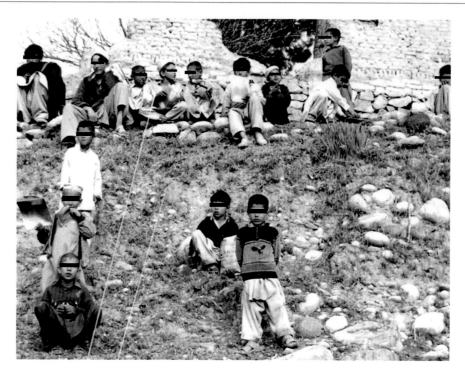

Fig. 20.3 Children in Asadabad, Afghanistan

the children were getting IV access, CXRs, and getting prepared for the OR, I put an IV and a chest tube in the Schoolmaster, who was an older Afghan gentleman. Prior to me doing this the Schoolmaster took my hand; despite being short of breath and in pain from his injuries, he thanked me (in English) for taking care of the children. He then started motioning to the children and spoke to our interpreter in Pashto, the dialect of this region in Afghanistan. He said that wanted me to *only* focus on the children and to not worry about him. The Schoolmaster allowed me to place a chest tube, during which he did not flinch. The chest tube put out 1300 cc of blood immediately. I gave the patient one of our ten, units of blood and activated the Whole Blood Plan for three units, with the stipulation that only people who were *not* leaving that night for Operation Mountain Lion could donate.

The first two cases ran simultaneously. The OR tables were only feet away from each other, making it very easy to communicate with the OB-GYN surgeon who was doing a trauma laparotomy with the orthopedic surgeon as her assis-

tant. Their patient had multiple small bowel injuries and a gastric injury. They resected two segments of small bowel and waited for me to do the gastric repair. My patient had a large amount of hemoperitoneum from a splenic injury and also had small bowel and colon injuries. About ten minutes into these surgeries, our ER Nurse, the designated "Triage Manager", informed me that eight patients had arrived by ground ambulance. The patients were all children, ranging in ages from 6 to 12 years old and were undergoing ATLS protocols in the designated triage areas with more casualties soon arriving. I decided that, given the situation, all surgeries would be "damage control" to expedite each case in order to take care of as many patients as possible. We finished the first two cases rather quickly. I went with our ER nurse to assess the situation as the OB-GYN and orthopedic surgeons placed temporary abdominal closures on each child and they were moved to ICU area of the FST.

When I walked outside the FST to the triage area I was expecting chaos; however, there was no chaos. Eight children had arrived, their litters (tactical Army stretchers) were on the cement slab in the designated Triage Area, and there was at least one medic or corpsman kneeling next to each patient. Six of the eight children were in the immediate area, meaning required immediate care, and two were in the delayed, meaning their care could be delayed. Each child had an IV and a 500 cc bag of crystalloid hanging. A Special Forces medic had intubated a young girl with a severe penetrating brain injury and one of the Marines was carefully bag ventilating her in order not to give her barotrauma. Two of the children had eviscerations and their abdominal contents were covered with moistened ABD dressings. One child had near lower extremity amputation and another had an open lower extremity fracture, both had tourniquets in place. All the other patients with open wounds had dressings on them.

I could not believe my eyes; and to this day, almost 10 years later, reflecting on the manner in which these young Soldiers and Marines cared for these children gives me goose bumps. Our ER nurse took me to each patient, where the medic gave the catalog of patient's injuries and then referred to the Triage Tag (pre-made tags that were in the "Trauma Trunks") to report the vital signs history. Medics were using their manual BP cuffs and portable pulse oximeters to record vital signs every five to ten minutes. Broselow Tapes were being used to determine dosing for pain medications for the younger children. I had our Sonosite to perform FAST (Focused Assessment with Sonography for Trauma) examinations. Our interpreters were in short supply; one moved with us, facilitating communication. Four of the children needed to move inside the FST, two had penetrating chest injuries and two had eviscerations. Of the remaining four patients, they moved into the delayed triage area: two had lower extremity tourniquets, one had a positive FAST exam, and the other was the girl with the penetrating brain injury. I did not think this child was going to survive her injuries, but did not want to move her to the Expectant Area at that time. We brought out one of the portable ventilators from the FST; the Marine, who had been bag-ventilating her, stayed with her, and continued to

record her vitals. The senior OR tech came outside after the first cases finished, to see what to set up for next. Our Admin Officer was already in touch with the Combat Support Hospital (CSH) at Bagram where these patients would be transferred to once they were stabilized. We requested a medical evacuation, anticipating we would need it for ten patients; we also requested additional ventilators (we were only equipped with five), blood products, and interpreters.

As the afternoon proceeded, we continuously operated; the ER nurse did a fantastic job managing the triage, he kept an organized list of the casualties and was in constant communication with us while we continued to operate on the urgent patients. Depending on what was going on in the operating room, one of us would rotate working to re-triage, determining the next operative case (Fig. 20.4) and deciding which patients would move into the FST for closer monitoring, X-rays, or chest tube placement.

The Schoolmaster, who remained in the FST observing the events around him, had over 2 L of blood from his chest tube. He had been transfused two units of PRBCs and one unit of whole blood. He adamantly refused any surgical intervention (which he clearly needed) until "د شام و مانو لوت نش هه," all the children were okay. He would look at me and say in English "the children" and put his right hand over his heart as a sign of gratitude. Despite his significant hemorrhage he remained sitting up on the litter, surprisingly alert and obviously concerned about the injured school children.

I did not help manage the triage for the next hour or so in order to operate on the two children with traumatic eviscerations, and another child with a positive FAST who was decompensating secondary to hemorrhage from small bowel mesentery and liver injuries. When I did return outside to "run the list" with our Triage Manager, the rest of the patients had arrived; 34 in total. Six children were killed at the scene; their parents took the bodies' home. A few of the medics were with the patients in the Immediate Area and ready to present the injuries and vitals while the other medics were circulating, checking, and recording vitals for the other casualties. We no longer had

Fig. 20.4 Completing one of the cases during the MASCAL. This child underwent an exploratory laparotomy as well as a right upper extremity soft tissue debridement. The second operating table was getting set-up for the next case and can be seen in the background

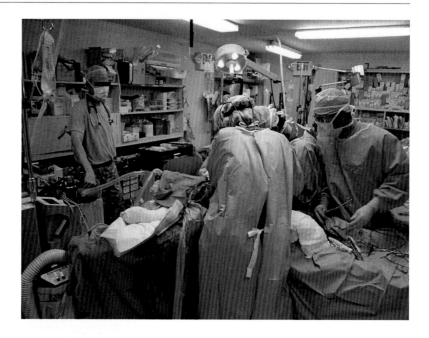

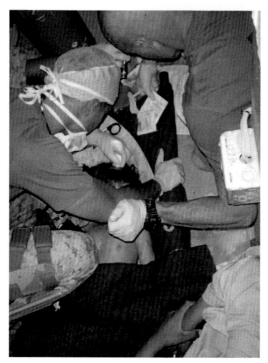

Fig. 20.5 A Navy corpsman and a Marine evaluating a casualty

for them (Figs. 20.5, 20.6, and 20.7). This was actually not part of our MASCAL plan; it was one of the medics' "on the spot" ideas demonstrating the ingenuity, flexibility, and creativity needed for success in this potentially overwhelming situation. Even though these young Soldiers and Marines had not received "medic training," they wanted to, and were capable of, helping. They had already been communicating with the child to which they were assigned and they knew their patient's external signs of trauma and if they were in pain. Fortunately, none of these children had life-threatening injuries, just two required operative debridement of severe soft tissue injuries.

> In spite of everything, I still believe that people are really good at heart.
> ——Anne Frank

The young girl with the penetrating brain injury, who was now hooked up to the ventilator, was not doing well; she had blown both her pupils, the dressing on her head was completely saturated with blood, and she had evidence of Cushing's Reflex (hypertension and bradycardia). When I suggested that we turn off the ventilator and move her to the Afghan clinic where our Expectant Area was designated, the Marine who

enough medics or corpsmen to designate one to each casualty. Instead, casualties had been assigned a "non-medic" Marine or Solider to care

Fig. 20.6 A corpsman and one of the interpreters with a child, note the "D" written on the casualty's forehead indicating that he was in triaged as "Delayed."

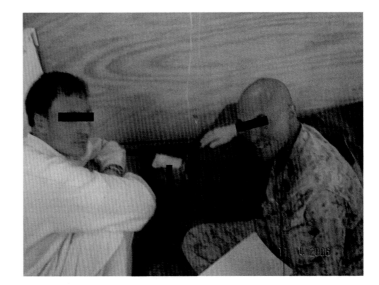

Fig. 20.7 Another child who had been triaged as "Delayed"; he had a wound on his right upper arm bandaged

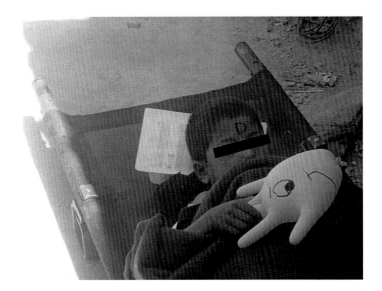

had been by her side since she arrived pleaded with me to not give up on her. One of the hardest things I had to do that day was to tell this Marine that we were not going to be able to save this girl. The young Marine, over 6 feet tall, all muscle, arms covered in tattoos looked at me with tear filled eyes "I understand ma'am."

I later learned that, after moving the child to the Afghan clinic, that Marine along with one of the Afghan physicians, went outside the FOB where the frantic families of the school children had gathered. They found this girl's family and

escorted them onto the base. The Marine brought them to the injured child and stayed with the family and this young girl until she died.

> Anyone who does anything to help a child in his life is a hero to me.
> ——Fred Rogers

This attack on Tuesday, April 11, 2006 by the Taliban regime and the militant enemies of Afghanistan, was the deadliest strike against Afghanistan's education system that the country had experienced since 2001 (Figs. 20.8 and 20.9). Six children were dead at the scene. Our FST

Fig. 20.8 The school that was attacked

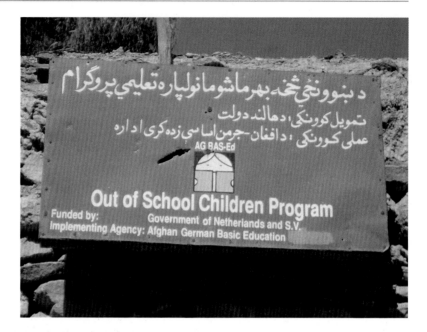

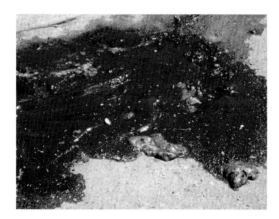

Fig. 20.9 The playground after the attack

along with the great help of the Army medics, Navy corpsmen, and Marines triaged and cared for thirty-four casualties. Those with very minor injuries were triaged, treated, and dispositioned by the medics that were sent to the site of the attack alongside Afghan medical providers. They did not come to the FST to encumber our system; the medics at the scene did not over-triage which would have certainly burdened our system. We were unable to save a young girl with a catastrophic brain injury, but no other children died at the FST that day. We performed eight major operations: six exploratory laparotomies, one

lower extremity amputation, one lower extremity soft tissue debridement, and external fixator. Four patients, the Schoolmaster and three children, had chest tubes placed, one child requiring bilateral chest tubes. Five children underwent operative soft tissue debridement, one for a scalp degloving injury, another for multiple extremity soft tissue injuries and three had concomitant soft tissue debridement while they were also undergoing laparotomy for their abdominal wounds. The rest of the patients underwent local wound care and pain management.

Seven units of PRBCs were transfused: three units to the Schoolmaster; two units to the child with liver, small bowel mesentery, and small bowel injuries who had to wait for over an hour to get to the OR; one unit to the child with a splenic injury; and one to a child with a traumatic evisceration. Three units of whole blood were transfused to the Schoolmaster; two of which he received at the FST and the third while in route to the CSH. The Schoolmaster, the six children with open abdomens and two of the children with chest tubes were flown by CH-47 Chinook helicopter to the CSH at Bagram. At the CSH, the Schoolmaster underwent a thoracotomy and the children all underwent second look laparotomies, restoration of gastrointestinal continuity, and abdominal closure. The rest of the children stayed with us at the FST until they were able to move to the Afghan clinic. We worked with the Afghan care providers on these children and rounded with them until the child's discharge. The ANA (Afghan National Army) reunited the rest of the children with their parents.

Operation Mountain Lion launched as scheduled on the night of April 11, 2006 with helicopter insertions of coalition forces at strategic points throughout the Korengal Valley followed by troops on foot coming through the mouth of the valley. Despite the terrible attack that occurred earlier in the day, unquestionably affecting our entire FOB, these Soldiers and Marines carried out the combat operation as it had been planned. Our FST, and anyone else who had been involved with the MASCAL event, performed an extensive After Action Review (AAR). Much of the discussion involved the emotional impact of caring for the Afghan children who were victims of the despicable terrorist attack. Many spoke about their own children, the events of the day making them miss them more than they already did. Not present at that AAR were many of the Soldiers and Marines who so greatly helped the Afghan children; they instead had to continuing preparing for the operation that would soon ensue.

In the study by Propper et al. >70 % of patients after explosive events require emergent operations [1], our rate was lower. Their study took place at a CSH and the explosive events occurred remote from the hospital; therefore, they only received the patients that were triaged "immediate" or "urgent." In the rocket attack described above, 47 % of those injured required urgent interventions. Of the 34 casualties: eight required major surgery (one amputation, one lower extremity external fixator, and six laparotomies); five children had major soft tissue injuries requiring surgery for either hemorrhage control or debridement (three of which also had parallel abdominal operations); and four patients needed chest tubes. Our rate of operative intervention was likely lower given the proximity of our FOB

to the attack and that only the very minimally injured were not brought to our FST.

> The world breaks everyone, and afterward, some are strong at the broken places.
> ——Ernest Hemingway

The battlefields of the Global War on Terrorism have resulted in unique demands on deployed medical teams. Expected challenges include resource limitations and dangerous environments; an unexpected challenge for our team was such as a high volume of pediatric trauma patients and the overall impact that it had. Forward Surgical Teams, especially when performing "split-operations" will have manpower limitations that can be overcome by involving all medical elements on the Forward Operation Base. As the leaders of the teams, we are lucky if we quickly recognize our strengths and limitations, capitalizing on the former and improving upon all aspects of the latter. There is obviously no substitute for training and preparedness; our FST was undoubtedly successful because of the investment we made in both.

Reflecting on that day in April, 2006 brings up a myriad of emotions, some of which I don't recall having at the time, likely because mission focus took priority. I remember feeling scared, then that fear quickly dissipating, replaced by determination. I remember seeing fear in the eyes of my teammates as we sat in the bunker during the attack and then watching that fear get replaced by courage and commitment. I remember having pride in what we had accomplished as a team and being so impressed by the professionalism, sensitivity, empathy, and skills of the individuals who worked so diligently caring for the casualties. I continue to be proud of how our team and the enitire FOB managed that appalling attack. I witnessed a remarkable display of humanity, amidst the mercilessness of war. As a surgeon I learned the importance of leadership, training, preparedness, and empowering your team. As a person I once again observed the inhumaneness of war but was privileged to witness such compassion, kindness, and humanity amidst the brutality.

Editor's Note: LTC Jennifer Gurney MD is serving on Active Duty in the United States Army. She is currently in fellowship training for Trauma/Critical Care at the University of California at San Francisco and Stanford University. She has been deployed four times to the combat zone and for her work she has received two Bronze Stars and the Navy Commendation Medal amongst several other awards.

Reference

1. Propper BW, Rasmussen TE, Davidson SB, Vandenberg SL, Clouse WD, Burkhardt GE, et al. Surgical response to multiple casualty incidents following single explosive events. Ann Surg. 2009;250(2):311–5.

Index

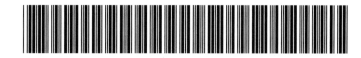